CLINICAL APPLICATIONS
in Surface
Electromyography

Chronic Musculoskeletal Pain

Glenn S. Kasman, MS, PT
Physical Medicine and Rehabilitation
Virginia Mason Medical Center
Seattle, Washington

Jeffrey R. Cram, PhD
Director, Sierra Health Institute
President, Clinical Resources
Nevada City, California

Steven L. Wolf, PhD, PT, FAPTA
Professor
Department of Rehabilitation Medicine
Emory University School of Medicine
Atlanta, Georgia

with
Lisa Barton, MMSc, PT
Area Rehabilitation Manager
Vencor
Lakewood, Washington

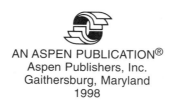

AN ASPEN PUBLICATION®
Aspen Publishers, Inc.
Gaithersburg, Maryland
1998

Library of Congress Cataloging-in-Publication Data

Kasman, Glenn S.
Clinical applications in surface electromyography/
Glenn S. Kasman, Jeffrey R. Cram, Steven Wolf; with Lisa Barton.
p. cm.
Includes bibliographical references and index.
ISBN 0-8342-0752-4 (hardcover)
1. Electromyography. I. Cram, Jeffrey R.
II. Wolf, Steven L.
III. Title.
[DNLM: 1. Musculoskeletal Diseases—therapy.
2. Electromyography. 3. Pain—therapy. WE 500 K19c 1997]
RC77.5.K37 1997
616.7′0645—dc21
DNLM/DLC
for Library of Congress
97–23550
CIP

Orders: (800) 638-8437
Customer Service: (800) 234-1660

About Aspen Publishers • For more than 35 years, Aspen has been a leading professional publisher in a variety of
disciplines. Aspen's vast information resources are available in both print and electronic formats. We are committed to
providing the highest quality information available in the most appropriate format for our customers. Visit Aspen's
Internet site for more information resources, directories, articles, and a searchable version of Aspen's full catalog,
including the most recent publications: **http://www.aspenpub.com**
Aspen Publishers, Inc. • The hallmark of quality in publishing
Member of the worldwide Wolters Kluwer group

The authors have made every effort to ensure the accuracy of the information herein. However, appropriate information sources
should be consulted, especially for new or unfamiliar procedures. It is the responsibility of every practitioner to evaluate the
appropriateness of a particular opinion in the context of actual clinical situations and with due considerations to new develop-
ments. Authors, editors, and the publisher cannot be held responsible for any typographical or other errors found in this book.

Editorial Resources: Jane Colilla

Library of Congress Catalog Card Number: 97-23550
ISBN: 0-8342-0752-4

Printed in the United States of America
1   2   3   4   5

For Little Bear, Carrie, and Gus.

Pay to look skyward
The universe has a price
Ten cents for the moon

—Eric Flaum
1961–1997

Table of Contents

Foreword

Two generations have passed since a young Canadian medical scientist stumbled onto a primitive prototype of an electronic device developed by Canadian and British military medical-engineering teams for improved diagnosis of and prognosis for patients with denervation. That young ex-medical officer was very lucky because he started working as a volunteer in 1949 with the many victims of poliomyelitis at Toronto's Hospital for Sick Children. I was and am that lucky person.

Little did I realize that my expanding research programs in electromyographic diagnosis and kinesiology, along with an increasing international army of independent research centers, would survive. In fact, they blossomed and spread. They grew within the first generation beyond diagnostic and kinesiologic applications to direct therapeutic applications based on my neurophysiologic findings. In the 1950s myoelectric devices had matured and were being prescribed, and by 1970 electromyographic biofeedback was a lusty infant.

I would have been deeply satisfied if those clinical advances had been the culmination of the work in that first generation of progress.

However, the second generation was already being built on the successes of the first. This book is the proud demonstration of how far surface electromyography has advanced. Along with its companion publication, *Introduction to Surface Electromyography*, this book is an instant classic about a vital concern of many clinicians with diverse backgrounds.

Any specialist, therapist, or general health practitioner ignorant of the contents of this book cannot claim to understand fully either surface electromyography or musculoskeletal pain. The subject matter is compulsory reading, and it is absorbing, lucid, and common sensical. How lucky I am to have examined it in manuscript form and thus learned a great deal that I had only guessed about before.

For one who has read many books in neuropsychophysiology (and written a few), I am proud that I was chosen to preview this volume and write this foreword. If this makes me this book's godfather, I am delighted.

J.V. Basmajian
OC, OOnt, MD, FRCPC, FRCPS
(Glasg), FACA, FSBM, FABMR,
FAFRM-RACP (Austral), Hon Dip StLC

Preface

My guess is that 50% of all the therapy done by physicians and therapists worldwide is either useless or harmful to the individual patient. The trouble is I cannot tell you which 50%!

—J.V. Basmajian

Privileged to have received a copy of Dr. Basmajian's autobiography, I randomly opened the book to have a look. The above quotation was the first thing I read, and it has stuck with me ever since. As clinicians, we practice in a time of rapid and radical change. The emergence of managed care in the United States has altered the economic and political stakes of health care delivery. I am challenged daily to try to figure out which components of my practice are part of the good 50%. I have learned to think in terms of value, the concept of which was first thrust on me by my administrators at Virginia Mason Medical Center in Seattle, Washington. Clinical value can be defined as functionally meaningful patient outcomes, plus patient satisfaction, divided by the financial and social costs of providing care.

I believe that surface electromyography (SEMG) can add value to the management of chronic musculoskeletal pain. SEMG offers a window to the movement system that cannot be replicated by any other means. The techniques noninvasively record neuromuscular activity and, within certain limits, allow for quantification and documentation of impairment. When used for patient feedback, the SEMG display provides exquisitely rich cues regarding quality and outcome of motor control strategies, be they consciously planned or automatic. Patients exploit the feedback information to learn more skilled patterns of motor control. When SEMG is combined with other therapies, disability is

reduced and function is enhanced. Both patients and clinicians seem to enjoy the feedback-learning process in SEMG. Sometimes clinical beliefs are confirmed by SEMG data; sometimes they are refuted. On the whole, however, each time an SEMG device is used, a little more knowledge about the movement system is gained.

Chronic musculoskeletal pain is extraordinarily complex. Historically, most material on the use of SEMG in chronic pain has emphasized the psychologic dimension. Feedback training in treatment with SEMG has focused largely on relaxation-based approaches. All along, however, there has been a kinesiologically based school, one that has inherent appeal for physical medicine practitioners and one that seems to be gaining recognition throughout the clinical community prescribing SEMG.

I and my distinguished coauthors have endeavored to respond to clinician requests for a book that brings together aspects of SEMG with regard to chronic musculoskeletal pain. The companion publication to this book is titled *Introduction to Surface Electromyography. Clinical Applications in Surface Electromyography* starts where the companion publication leaves off. We enter deep into the world of SEMG and chronic musculoskeletal pain, discussing sophisticated clinical models and more advanced SEMG techniques. Practitioners trained primarily in psychology will perhaps notice that most words are devoted to kinesiologic issues. This design results not from precedence of one discipline over another but from a plethora of resources relating to relaxation-based methods and fewer resources that integrate SEMG with clinical movement science. Discussion in this book focuses almost exclusively on SEMG. A comprehensive discussion of pathology and treatment is beyond the scope of this book. It is assumed that the reader is experienced with fundamental applications of SEMG and independently trained in other aspects of clinical practice.

Chapters 1 through 7 explore theoretic and practical issues by accenting recurrent principles. The key elements can be applied to any type of musculoskeletal pain presentation, regardless of body region or specific pathology. Chapters 8 through 14 extract evaluation and treatment techniques that are best suited to particular patient problems. The latter chapters are subdivided by body region and share a common organization: review of the pertinent SEMG literature, followed by one or more Application Guides. The Application Guides are practical road maps to evaluation and treatment of frequently encountered syndromes. They are maps in that they show various paths and contain tips on preferred routes. However, clinicians must choose from among the options to determine which will best mesh with their existing practice styles. This approach was inspired by Dr.

Basmajian, who challenges therapists to understand the *why* of intervention methods, instead of just the *how*. Thus rigid protocols have been deliberately avoided. Techniques with demonstrated superior outcomes are detailed, but practitioners are not required to adopt any sort of dogma or fixed intervention sequence. Much clinical research needs to be done to determine optimal methods of delivering value with SEMG. The hope is that readers will be challenged to think through the ideas, discard those that seem to be a poor fit, and incorporate those that resonate. In this process, each operator will realize the greatest clinical potential with SEMG.

I must acknowledge my friend, colleague, and coauthor Jeff Cram for seducing me into this project. In addition, I am honored to have had Steven Wolf's mentoring, which has gone far beyond his written contributions. Kathe Wallace provided early support in innovating clinical ideas. Erik Kramme helped with testing the concepts in educational settings. Rich Bettesworth modeled excellence and made it feasible to find the required time to write. Blair Shular gave valuable commentary. Innumerable others provided inspiration and encouragement; my most grateful appreciation to all.

Glenn S. Kasman

CHAPTER 1

Chronic Musculoskeletal Pain

OVERVIEW AND DEFINITIONS OF PAIN

About one third of the US population between the ages of 25 and 74 years reports musculoskeletal impairments.[1] Musculoskeletal dysfunction and pain are associated with increased health care use, disability, and financial costs.[2,3] Pain is an aspect of experience that signals frank or potential tissue damage. Acute pain tends to be well localized, of sudden onset and relatively short duration, and clinically distinct from chronic pain.[4,5] Acute pain presumably serves a protective role, leading to responses to terminate the noxious stimulus, protect an injured body part, promote healing, and avoid future noxious events.[6] The point at which acute pain becomes chronic pain is arbitrary. However, chronic pain is believed to originate when a time frame beyond that expected for normal healing of the original insult is reached,[5] typically at 3 to 6 months.[7,8] Chronic pain can persist indefinitely in an individual. It does not result in constructive responses and is instead associated with maladaptive biologic and behavioral consequences.[5,9]

Chronic musculoskeletal pain is chronic pain associated with dysfunction of the movement system, owing its genesis to disruption of bone; muscle; fascial, ligamentous, tendinous, synovial, or articular tissue; or to orthopaedic compromise of vascular or nervous system function. Although other factors may coexist, the cause of chronic musculoskeletal pain is related to musculoskeletal dysfunction and not purely a viscerogenic, neurogenic, or psychogenic event. The tissue trauma may occur in a single episode or be related to multiple prior episodes, as well as be perpetuated in a continuous, recurrent, or cumulative manner. Pain is maintained by persistent noxious stimuli from the periphery, dysfunctional central neurophysiologic relationships, and untoward psychologic factors.

PAIN IS A MULTIDIMENSIONAL CONCEPT

It is generally agreed that pain is subjective and idiosyncratic. Pain involves unique perceptual processes, a convergence of sensation and emotion.[10] Clinicians cannot directly discern a subject's experience of pain. Cause, severity, character, and sequelae must be inferred. However, a number of tools have been crafted to measure pain perceptions and behaviors. These can be combined with assessment procedures for musculoskeletal dysfunction, so that treatment can be planned effectively.

Pain is often characterized as extending along sensory and cognitive–affective dimensions.[11] The sensory component is believed to be related directly to nociceptive processes. Nociception is the activation of afferent fibers and subsequent nervous transmission induced by mechanical, chemical, or thermal energy in a potentially injurious range. In the latter part of the nineteenth century, investigators looking at pain focused on sensory processing and postulated that pain was generated by either activation of specific types of sensory end organs or summated intensities and patterns of nerve signals from the periphery.[4] A sensory–physiologic approach has also been the basis for traditional medical models of pain management.[9] These models relate the type and magnitude of peripheral injury to an anticipated pain response. However, the identified physiologic pathology does not always seem to be reflected in observation of patients with pain. The level of apparent disability may be more or less than that which would be predicted by assessing tissue status and expected levels of nociception. For example, athletes are known to continue competing after experiencing severe injuries. On the other hand, profound pain behaviors, functional limitations, and disability can be observed without any evidence of pathology or known physiologic impairment. This does not mean that physiologic changes and impairments are absent. It simply means that they cannot always be detected and that other factors are involved.

With persistent pain, the peripheral response to musculoskeletal injury has been portrayed as a vicious cycle.[12,13] The cycle is triggered by trauma and followed by inflammation (myositis), muscle spasm, restricted movement, metabolite retention, circulatory stasis, muscle guarding, and more pain (Figure 1–1). The various elements feed into each other in a positive closed loop, necessitating some type of clinical intervention to break the cycle. As the degree of chronicity progresses, so does the complexity of dysfunction, and additional elements may be introduced that provoke a downward clinical spiral. These include physiologic agents as well as issues in the psychologic domain.

Pain is inherently unpleasant and will support avoidance behaviors. Arousal, attention, past experiences, beliefs, and emotional set are some of the determinants of the aversiveness attached to sensation. Thus perceptual,[14] personality,[15,16] behavioral,[8] and functional[17,18] considerations have been added to the debate on factors implicated in

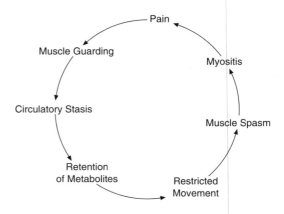

Figure 1–1 Cyclic dysfunction developing in response to musculoskeletal injury. *Source:* Reprinted with permission from HD Saunders, *Evaluation, Treatment, and Prevention of Musculoskeletal Disorders*, p 9, © 1985, The Saunders Group, Inc.

chronic pain. Loeser and Egan[19] provide a framework by stating that nociception usually leads to pain, or recognition of nociceptive stimuli, and pain perception commonly leads to suffering, a negative affective response (Figure 1–2). The degree of suffering is a product of the subject's intrinsic psychologic state as he or she interacts within a social environment. Interpersonal relationships, economic status, life satisfaction, and clinician practice styles contribute to suffering.[20,21] Pain behaviors may then be expressed to communicate suffering to others. The total pain experience flows from a synergistic blending of these factors and varies dynamically across individuals.

MODEL FOR DEVELOPMENT OF CHRONIC MUSCULOSKELETAL PAIN SYNDROME

To establish a context for evaluation and treatment procedures with the use of surface electromyography (SEMG), a model for the development of chronic musculoskeletal pain is presented and discussed next. Although an exhaustive discussion is beyond the scope of this book, salient points for the clinical interventions

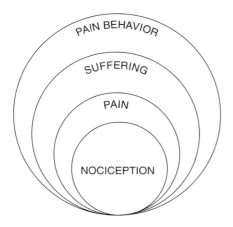

Figure 1–2 Components of the pain experience. *Source:* Reprinted with permission from JD Loeser and KJ Egan, History and Organization of the University of Washington Multidisciplinary Pain Center, in *Managing the Chronic Pain Patient: Theory and Practice at the University of Washington Multidisciplinary Pain Center*, JD Loeser and KJ Egan, eds, p 6, © 1989, Raven Press.

that follow in succeeding chapters have been outlined.

In integrating the concepts in the pain experience with those of soft tissue dysfunction, it is helpful to view development of chronic musculoskeletal pain syndromes along four dimensions. These are depicted in Figure 1–3. The inner circle represents the acute situation, with the potential for trauma, pain, inflammatory responses, and physiologic dysfunction to cycle about one another. Each of the four outer quadrants—histologic dysfunction, psychologic dysfunction, sensorimotor dysfunction, and mechanical dysfunction—represents a set of factors that can lead to the development of a chronic problem in an individual or result from perpetuation of the initial cycle. Each category affects all others. The links are served through metabolic dysregulation; psychophysiologic autonomic effect as well as chronic pain perceptions and behaviors; altered sensorimotor integration; and cumulative mechanical overload. In discussing each category of dysfunction, the order is largely

arbitrary, because it is impossible to define a temporal sequence that would fit all patients.

Histologic Dysfunction

Histologic dysfunction involves responses to soft tissue injury at the microscopic level. The relevant soft tissues are connective tissues and muscle. The former encompass adipose tissue, blood, bone, cartilage, fascia, fibrous joint capsules, synovial tissue, ligaments, and tendons. Histologic dysfunction can occur at varying levels related to the chronicity of the tissue injury and may be implicated in trigger point phenomena.

Connective Tissues

Connective tissues are composed of specific cell types and an extracellular matrix.[22–24] Cells generally include fibroblasts, macrophages, neutrophils, mast cells, other blood cells, and other cells specific to the tissue type that impart unique morphologic properties. The extracellular matrix is made up of a ground substance and fibers. Most of the ground substance is water, which is bound to long-chain carbohydrates or carbohydrate–protein molecules called glycosaminoglycans and proteoglycans. The ground substance forms a viscous medium for the fibers and cells; allows for exchange of cellular nutrients, metabolites, and electrolytes; and contributes to the mechanical properties of the tissue. Collagen, elastin, and reticulin make up the fibrous elements of the matrix. The most common element, collagen, results from formation and hydroxylation (adjoining of hydroxide groups) of polypeptide chains within fibroblasts. Three hydroxylated polypeptide chains are joined in a helix to form one tropocollagen molecule. Tropocollagen molecules are then transported into the extracellular space in which they aggregate with others into collagen fibrils. Groups of fibrils form cross-links to each other to produce collagen fibers. The integrity of the fibers is maintained by intramolecular bonds within tropocollagen molecules and intermolecular bonds between the larger units. Connec-

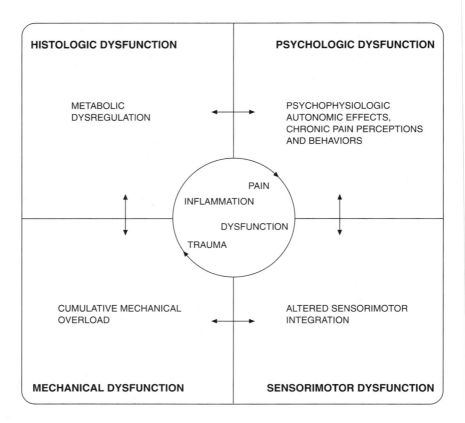

Figure 1–3 Dimensions of dysfunction accompanying chronic musculoskeletal pain syndromes.

tive tissue that is regularly subjected to mechanical stress shows a dense arrangement of fibers. These tissues take the macroscopic forms of aponeuroses and fascial sheets, ligament and tendon bundles, and capsules. When the direction of stress is variable, so is the alignment of fibers. However, tissue stressed in a particular direction develops a highly ordered fiber alignment. Thus in a tendon all fibers are arranged in a direction roughly parallel to the line of tensile stress.

Inflammatory and repair processes occur after injury to connective tissue.[25–27] Cellular damage results in the release of substances, such as histamine, bradykinin, and serotonin, into the extracellular matrix. These mediators initiate a cascade of chemical reactions that alter local blood flow and capillary permeability. Fluid, proteins,

and various other substances move into the extracellular fluid. Edema is produced, coagulation takes place to reduce any blood loss, and a fibrin matrix is formed. The fibrin matrix acts as a chemoattractant for the migration of neutrophils and macrophages to the area. Neutrophils and macrophages protect against bacterial infection, remove cellular debris, and release substances that help attract and differentiate fibroblasts. The fibroblasts proliferate in large numbers as they produce collagen precursors, glycosaminoglycans, and proteoglycans. Capillary ingrowth accompanies the process. The normal extracellular matrix is reconstituted, and a stronger collagenous network is substituted for the provisional fibrin matrix. Usually within a few weeks, the inflammatory cell population subsides, and collagen deposition slows. However, the collagen network continues to remodel for months or longer. The scar must reorganize its fiber volume, cross-linking, and alignment to match those of noninjured tissue in the same structure.

Variations of this basic repair scheme take place in most connective tissue. Disruption of fascial, ligamentous, capsular, meniscal, tendinous, sheath, and bursal tissue can occur because of mechanical trauma. Overload involves stresses that exceed the load limits of the fiber matrix organization. Injury is produced by means of avulsion, in-substance tear, crush, and shear mechanisms.[28] Clinically, these mechanisms result in acute strains and sprains, as well as in chronic adverse tension, impingement, and friction syndromes. Peripheral nerves are also invested with a connective tissue sheath and these structures are vulnerable to adverse mechanical compression and tension syndromes.[29,30]

Movement and loading are necessary for remodeling of new collagen fibers in the matrix.[31] New collagen fibers are deposited in a disorganized manner (Figure 1–4), and until the scar matures with proper fiber alignment, the tissue may be unable to resist high mechanical loads.[27] Mechanical failure can reoccur if the tissue is prematurely subjected to high stress. Repetitive strain injuries are produced in this way. The repair process can also be impeded by immobilization. With immobilization the connective tissue matrix loses glycosaminoglycans and water content, and increased cross-links are formed.[22,31–34] The viscous gel created by the glycosaminoglycans and water provides a lubricated space between collagen fibers that enables the fibers to glide relative to each other. Adequate glide is needed for the normal macroscopic mobility of the connective tissue. The loss of water and glycosaminoglycans reduces the critical distance between collagen fibers. With a lack of normal gliding, abnormal cross-links are formed between randomly oriented new collagen fibrils and older fibers. The result is decreased soft tissue extensibility. Because the collagen fibers of immobilized tissue do not receive a mechanical

stimulus to align in regular directions of tensile loading, they are subject to failure at loads lower than normal.[25,27] Thus immobilization results in tissue weakness and stiffness. Recurrent excessive loading results in microscopic instabilities and chronically immature repair.

Histochemical responses may also complicate connective tissue repair. Lytic enzymes and other factors are released at injury sites, which can have negative consequences. For example, substances liberated from damaged intervertebral discs provoke immunogenic reactions as well as inflammatory responses mediated by a phospholipase, arachadonic acid, leukotrienes, and prostaglandins.[35] Irritative tissue responses follow these chemical triggers, resulting in perineural inflammation, nociceptor activation, and disc degeneration. In addition, protein synthesis plays a role in the rate of tissue repair, along with the degree of vascularity and hence nutrient availability.[36] Nutritionally, iron, ascorbic acid, numerous enzymes, and multiple other substances are required for hydroxylation and tropocollagen formation processes.[26,37] Extreme deficiencies of ascorbic acid lead to wound ruptures in scurvy.[38] Nutritional deficits have also been implicated in carpal tunnel syndrome and some forms of arthritis.[39–41]

Muscle

Like the surrounding connective tissue, muscle can sustain injury and undergo repair. Injury is induced by tensile overload with resulting complete, partial, or microscopic tears, as well as by crush and ischemia.[42] The muscle–tendon junction tends to be most prone to tearing injury, perhaps because of decreased extensibility through this region.[43] Injury and temporary weakness can also be produced by contraction of muscles themselves.[44] Exhaustive, eccentric contractions are most predisposing to exercise injury, although trauma can occur with constant length (isometric) or shortening (concentric) contractions.[45] Eccentric contractions occur when a muscle elongates as it actively generates tension—that is, when the external load exceeds the muscle contractile force. The greater effect

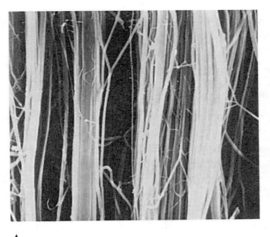
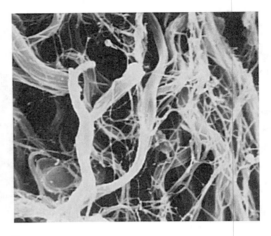

A   B

Figure 1–4 (**A**) Normal ligament. (**B**) Healing scar at 2 weeks. *Source:* Reprinted with permission from T Andriacchi et al, Ligament: Injury and Repair, in *Injury and Repair of Musculoskeletal Soft Tissues*, SLY Woo and JA Buckwalter, eds, p 112, © 1988, American Academy of Orthopaedic Surgeons.

of an eccentric contraction in producing injury has been attributed to high average force levels during this type of contraction, compared with constant length or shortening contraction under maximal loading conditions.[45] With eccentric contractions, individual cross-bridges between actin and myosin filaments may be subjected to greater mechanical stress, and some sarcomeres may be lengthened beyond a tolerable limit.[44]

Muscle regeneration follows a series of steps involving complex biochemical and ultrastructural repair processes.[42–44,46] Muscle tearing or contusion is accompanied by hemorrhage and fiber rupture (Figure 1–5). Trauma is followed by a release of enzymes from damaged fibers, cellular inflammatory responses, and local edema. A vascular-dependent migration of macrophages then acts to remove torn muscle fiber and organelle debris. At the same time, myogenic cells begin to proliferate into myoblasts, which aggregate to form myotubes. These multinucleated fibers synthesize large amounts of protein as they construct and organize contractile filaments, initially at the periphery of the myotube. The T-tubule system, as well as the sarcoplasmic reticulum with its terminal cisterns, is also produced. As the nuclei migrate to the periphery

and myofibrils come to fill the center, the myotube takes on the appearance of a normal muscle fiber. The fiber is then innervated with the creation of a neuromuscular junction and, depending on the type of associated nerve, shows morphologic differentiation of slow or fast twitch characteristics. The extracellular matrix must also be reconstituted, and this may require repair of the basement membrane that lies parallel to the plasma membrane, enveloping the cell in a sheath. The basement membrane isolates cells, transmits and modifies contractile forces, and plays an important role in neural reintegration and composition of the extracellular space. Collagen and muscle-specific proteoglycans contribute to the re-emerging structure of the basement membrane. Proteoglycans in the extracellular matrix interact with water molecules to preserve space with viscous fluid, which is vital to normal muscle micromechanics. The repair process is usually completed in 3 to 4 weeks, but time can vary depending on degree of tissue damage and reoccurrence of trauma.

Regenerated muscle fibers are capable of essentially normal function, but total muscle performance may show lasting deficits in fatigue

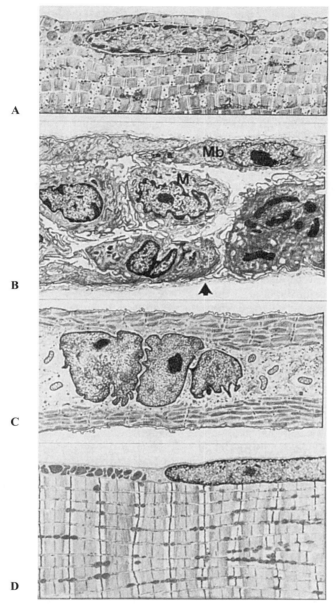

Figure 1–5 Major phases of degeneration and regeneration of a single muscle fiber. (**A**) Early ischemic damage. The mitochondria are swollen and the bundles of contractile filaments are breaking apart throughout the muscle fiber. (**B**) Fragmentation phase. Macrophages (**M**) associated with ingrowing vasculature enter the degenerating muscle fiber and remove bundles of contractile filaments and other cytoplasmic debris. Beneath the basal lamina (**arrow**) spindle-shaped myoblasts (**Mb**) line up in preparation for the formation of new muscle fibers. (**C**) Myotube. Beneath the original basal lamina, myoblasts have fused to form a multinucleated fiber with bundles of newly forming contractile filaments at the periphery. (**D**) Muscle fiber. The mature regenerated muscle fiber is in most respects indistinguishable from a normal muscle fiber. *Source:* Reprinted with permission from A Caplan et al, Skeletal Muscle, in *Injury and Repair of Musculoskeletal Soft Tissues*, SLY Woo and JA Buckwalter, eds, p 248, © 1988, American Academy of Orthopaedic Surgeons.

resistance and contractile tension when a large volume of tissue is damaged.[47,48] In animal muscle graft models, reduced tension is due to a smaller than normal cross-sectional area and fewer than normal muscle fibers.[43,49] Muscle that fails to repair is infiltrated with fibrous connective tissue and fat.[46] Muscle regeneration can be hampered by dense connective tissue formation, denervation, the effects of myotoxic drugs (eg, corticosteroids), and limited microvasculature.[43] For example, disturbances in microcirculation have been identified in the trapezius muscle of patients with posttraumatic chronic neck pain.[50] Damaged muscle that is immobilized after contusion takes longer to regenerate capillaries and to recover tensile strength than nonimmobilized muscle.[51] Inactivity also produces changes in the biochemical milieu of injured muscle tissue and leads to atrophy (particularly of type I fibers), decreased endurance, and reduced strength.[52–55] Muscle immobilized in a shortened position loses sarcomeres, whereas muscle immobilized in a lengthened position gains sarcomeres, with resulting changes in force–length relationships and load to failure.[42,56]

Cumulative Trauma

It is important to recognize that histologic destruction and repair are always occurring. Connective tissue is constantly remodeling and adapting to imposed mechanical loads. Muscle sustains microtrauma, hypertrophy, and atrophy depending on use patterns. Hertling and Kessler[57] maintain that overall tissue status is preserved when an equilibrium exists between tissue repair and breakdown. Function remains within normal limits so long as the rate of breakdown is less than or equal to the feasible rate of repair. When the rate of breakdown exceeds the rate of repair, the tissue is subjected to cumulative breakdown. A heterostasis between the processes of destruction and repair can result from several means (Figure 1–6). Increased breakdown is brought about by recurrent mechanical trauma, which itself is multifactorial. (See discussion later in this chapter.) Repair is hampered by histologic and metabolic issues discussed

earlier. Connective tissue with poor vascularity is especially slow to repair.

Hertling and Kessler[57] emphasize that adaptive tissue changes related to repair must affect joint mechanics when trauma is cumulative or sustained. Increased stiffness of periarticular connective tissue changes the distribution of loads throughout the joint complex. The capsule, ligaments, cartilage surfaces, and subchondral bone become subject to aberrant stresses. Inefficient dissipation of mechanical energy results in further microtrauma, and the cycle continues. Because cartilage lacks nociceptors, early degenerative joint disease may go unnoticed. The person slowly becomes aware of stiffness due to capsular fibrosis, and pain is produced only once low-grade inflammation becomes an accompanying feature. Joint effusion pathologically alters proprioceptive-motor reflexes and causes faulty muscle hyperactivity and inhibition. Myofascial and tenosynovial function is also impaired by histologic adaptations, which change passive mechanical compliance and alter the transmission of force. Impingement syndromes at the subacromial space of the shoulder and the carpal tunnel of the wrist, as well as recurrent tendinitis at the elbow, are examples of cumulative soft tissue microtrauma. Inflammation that occurs in a restricted space around soft tissues causes distention and compression of structures, as it does in a joint capsule. As will be discussed later, efficient muscle recruitment patterns are intimately related to re-establishing suitable mechanics and a homeostasis between histologic breakdown and repair. Clinically, the surface electromyographer assesses muscle function and uses feedback cues to improve patterns of motor control.

Sluka[58] has reviewed evidence for a mechanism by which inflammation is potentiated in musculoskeletal pain syndromes. She argues that peripheral inflammation can be regulated by centrally mediated dorsal root reflexes. Inflammation in muscle and joints sensitizes the afferent responses of small-diameter primary neurons. However, those same afferents also conduct action potentials antidromically follow-

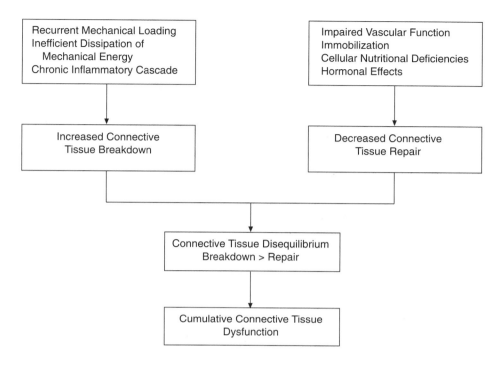

Figure 1–6 Contributory factors to heterostasis between connective tissue breakdown and repair processes, leading to cumulative dysfunction.

ing experimentally induced acute inflammation. The antidromic signals cause neuropeptides such as substance P and calcitonin gene–related peptides to be released from afferent fibers into the joint space, in which they act to further inflammation. This neurogenic edema may be another factor influencing connective tissue heterostasis in chronic states.

Trigger Points

Histologic dysfunction and metabolic distress have been implicated as potential explanations for trigger point phenomena. Trigger points are palpable taut bands that evoke local and referred pain in predictable patterns.[59] Trigger point palpation may also be accompanied by an observable twitch response along the skin which is caused by associated muscle activity. Trigger points have aroused considerable interest in clinicians who use SEMG assessment and feedback techniques as a fundamental construct of myofascial pain syndromes. Aberrant SEMG patterns identified in headache, upper quarter, and lumbar pain syndromes have been associated with trigger points.[60–63] Individual trigger points cannot be visualized with surface recordings, but the implication is that trigger points cause dysfunctional gross muscle behavior that is detectable with surface electrodes.

Travell and Simons[59,64] have reviewed evidence supporting degeneration of filament structure and shortened sarcomeres in the region of trigger points. They have also discussed aberrations in local temperature, tissue oxygenation, and high-energy phosphate levels in relation to trigger point pathophysiology. As a potential mechanism of trigger point formation, a self-perpetuating cycle has been proposed. Elements in the cycle include increased local metabolism, sarcomere shortening, local hypoxia, failure of the sarcoplasmic reticulum calcium pump, and an elevated and sustained calcium concentration in the sarcoplasmic region of the contractile filaments. It is also possible that mechanical disruption of the sarcoplasmic reticulum due to contraction-induced injury could elevate calcium levels in the sarcoplasm,[65] producing involuntary muscle tension.

An alternative line of evidence has emerged from one group, suggesting that trigger points are related to the muscle spindle apparatus.[63,66-68] According to this view, spindle structures are sent into metabolic crisis by sympathetic activity. The investigators have recorded spontaneous electrical discharges from discrete needle electrode placements in trigger points, with relative quiescence at adjacent tissue sites. Intramuscular electromyographic activity recorded from trigger point sites has been increased by deep inspiration or performance of stressful cognitive and emotional tasks. The spontaneous electrical activity recorded from trigger points has been attenuated by an adrenergic antagonist, but not blocked by a pharmacologic antagonist to extrafusal muscle fiber function. These findings provide a potential link between myofascial disorders and sympathetically mediated emotional arousal. The researchers believe that the intrafusal fibers of the spindle complex are tonically innervated by sympathetic efferents. They speculate that there is a resulting distention of the spindle capsule and nociceptor activation. Successful treatment for trigger points therefore may include drugs, physical agents, manual therapies, and exercise, which act peripherally, as well as drugs, relaxation therapy, and psychotherapies, which diminish central sympathetic arousal.

Psychologic Dysfunction

From a psychologic standpoint, patients with chronic pain are a heterogeneous group.[9,69,70] No single measure of psychologic distress or disability can predict treatment outcome across this population.[71] Although many conceptual schemes and patient taxonomies have been proposed for this group,[72] the focus here will be to consider psychologic dysfunction in the pain experience in terms of sensory–perceptual issues, cognition, emotion, behavior, and disability.

Sensory–Perceptual Issues

Awareness of a noxious stimulus comes from the interplay between nociception and various aspects of consciousness. Attributions are made regarding pain intensity, spatial distribution, depth, and quality (eg, sharp or dull), as well as on the basis of whether the perception is well-known or new.[14] An individual's background arousal level plays a major part in determining the outcome of such processing. Arousal is the level of excitation of the individual and refers to both neurophysiologic activity and emotional energy. Traditional SEMG feedback therapy for chronic pain syndromes has focused on facilitating low arousal states.[73,74]

Attention mechanisms also play a prominent role in pain perception. At any given instant in a wakeful state, an individual's sensory systems generate a large amount of information. However, the person actually becomes aware of only a small proportion. Attention is the process by which sensory input is selected for experience, depending on stimulus characteristics and internal factors.[75] Stimuli that are large, intense, novel, repeated, or presented with great contrast tend to be attended to more readily. Internal factors include the set of needs and motivations that the individual has with respect to conscious activity at the moment. For example, a soldier in battle may be highly aroused but not attend to an intense nociceptive event until the fighting has subsided. At the other extreme, some patients with chronic pain attend strongly to relatively weak stimuli, such as superficial palpation during physical examination. Pain perception is heightened when experimental subjects are directed to attend to noxious stimuli and decreased when attention is diverted.[76,77]

Chapman[14] has suggested that some patients with chronic pain become hypervigilant with respect to somatosensory activity. These individuals select nociceptive stimuli for attention, even when the stimuli are of low intensity. Weak or uncertain stimuli are processed with an expectation that they imply harm. Uncertain somatosensory sensations related to passive tightness or active muscle contraction are then amplified and interpreted as noxious. Pain comes to dominate the perceptual field as hypervigilance is reinforced by the responses of caregivers, family members, and workers' compensation and legal systems.

Descending neurophysiologic systems through the brainstem and spinal cord filter transmission of nociceptive signals to higher centers, effectively regulating the contrast of nociceptive signals against background somatosensory activity.[78] If descending inhibitory controls were to become impaired in the presence of persistent noxious stimuli, more nociceptive signals would be transmitted up the neuraxis. A hypothetic ratio of nociceptive signal to background somatosensory noise would be increased, favoring pain perception (Figure 1–7). The normal pattern of background somatosensory activity could also become impaired. Patients who withdraw from activities of daily living and adopt more sedentary lifestyles or restricted movement patterns alter their nonnoxious somesthetic input. A heightened contrast of nociceptive and nonnociceptive signals could therefore result from increased transmission of nociceptive input, decreased background somatosensory activity, or both. For example, patients diagnosed with fibromyalgia display a pattern of hyperresponsiveness to acute, experimentally induced pain.[79] The hyperresponsiveness has been attributed to heightened nociceptive signals from peripheral sensitization, dysregulation of central descending antinociceptive systems, and hypervigilance.

Cognition

Cognition mediates among the sensory–perceptual aspects of pain, emotions, and behaviors. Expectations may be formed that perception of pain will be linked to aversive feelings, or that pain behaviors will produce social rewards or avoidance of unpleasant social contingencies. Those beliefs, appraisals, and expectations held by an individual become intertwined with his or

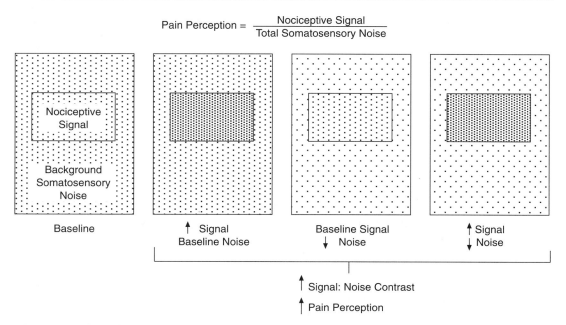

$$\text{Pain Perception} = \frac{\text{Nociceptive Signal}}{\text{Total Somatosensory Noise}}$$

Figure 1–7 Schematic representation of pain perception resulting from signal-to-noise ratio.

her maladaptive coping strategies as the chronic pain cycle is perpetuated.

Common beliefs held by patients with chronic pain involve a mix of cultural and personal convictions about what pain means.[80] Culturally, severe pain is interpreted as a warning that requires medical attention and altered behavior. In turn, there is an expectation that the pain will go away when the medical problem is resolved.[81] These shared beliefs are modified by personal experiences or replaced by other beliefs.[82] Individuals with chronic pain come to believe to varying degrees that

- pain will be a pervasive and enduring part of life
- the cause of their pain is not well defined
- they or others are to blame for their pain
- they have little self-efficacy to deal with the problem
- because of the pain they are disabled[82–87]

The notion that pain will endure can be constructive if it is part of a realistic assessment that enables an individual to adapt and move on with life, or it can be quite unconstructive if it results in hopelessness, helplessness, and passivity.[82,87] Beliefs that the source of the pain problem is biomedical and mysterious and eluding physicians can also intensify dysfunction. Frustration, fear, and poor compliance with therapies may result. Self-blame also may be coupled with poor compliance and depression in patients with chronic pain.[82,88]

Self-efficacy is the belief that one has the ability to manage successfully a specific situation,[89] in this case, to cope with pain. An external locus of control is a set of beliefs that one's life is primarily controlled by external forces. There is little sense of internal choice or accountability. Low self-efficacy and a belief that one's health depends on an external locus of control interact to support pain behaviors.[85] Individuals with low self-efficacy tend to become passive because they believe they cannot effect change and that their pain will endure.[83] As maladaptive coping responses are produced, a sense of failure reinforces low self-efficacy. Patients perceive fur-

ther loss of control and expect others to fix the problem. Thus patients with chronic pain may believe that they are physically disabled and that it is appropriate for others to continue to be solicitous of their needs when they are suffering.[86] Individuals with an external dependency may further conclude that they are entitled to various forms of social compensation.[90]

Coping is the use of cognitive and behavioral strategies to deal with stressful situations.[91] Adaptive cognitive strategies for individuals in managing chronic pain include diverting attention, ignoring pain, praying and hoping, and using positive self-talk and relaxation techniques.[92,93] Maladaptive cognitive strategies include polarizing events into good or bad dichotomous choices, overgeneralizing negative experiences, blaming, maintaining a self-centered perspective, clinging to fallacies related to what is believed to be fair, sustaining an external dependency, and catastrophizing. A propensity to catastrophize is to exaggerate a negative outcome so much that a situation is seen as overwhelming. Catastrophizing has been associated specifically with chronic pain and depression.[93,94] The tendency to catastrophize pain experiences is likely derived from the belief that hurt implies harm, the expectation that suffering will follow pain perception, and the feeling that one's locus of control is external. Protocols have been developed with cognitive restructuring and behavioral techniques to teach patients with chronic musculoskeletal pain improved coping skills.[95]

Emotions

A person's beliefs, attitudes, and expectations help shape the emotions he or she displays with chronic pain. Depression is common,[96] and it is easy to see how decreased social rewards and a perceived loss of control in the pain experience could bring it about.[97] Some investigators have proposed that depression is a consequence of pain and suffering, whereas others have argued that chronic complaints of pain mask an underlying depressive disorder.[94,97–99] Both may be true.[69] The association of depression with chronic pain seems to vary with the anatomic region involved.[99] Neurotransmitter changes involving serotonin, norepinephrine, gamma-aminobutyric acid, and endogenous opioids are potential links between depression and chronic pain.[100,101] Individuals who are depressed may alter the sensory–perceptual component of pain through a hypervigilant somatic focus and in turn foster a negative affect through dysfunctional cognitive assessments.[94]

Besides dysphoria, depression is often accompanied by negative thoughts, sleep disturbances, changes in appetite, loss of libido, fatigue, and decreased physical activity. In depression associated with chronic pain, sleep disturbances and decreased physical energy are particularly common.[69] Poor sleep hygiene, chronic fatigue, and depression are commonly found in patients with fibromyalgia. These patients experience disruptions in restorative non–rapid eye movement stage 4 sleep, which is associated with the emergence of fatigue and tender points.[102] Williams and Kaul[103] note that levels of somatomedin C are decreased in this population. Somatomedin C is secreted mainly during stage 4 sleep, and it affects muscle homeostasis by regulating action of growth hormone. Thus sleep disturbances that accompany chronic pain and depression may be linked to histologic dysfunction in muscle through the endocrine system.

Anxiety, frustration, fear, and anger are also seen in patients with chronic pain.[104,105] Painful experiences are anticipated with anxiety, leading to a focus on pain and expectations of pending aversive experiences.[76] The mysterious nature of the pain creates uncertainty about its meaning, as well as its effects on the individual's future, further contributing to anxiety.[82] Frustration develops as the pain persists, while beliefs that the pain should go away and that care providers should be able to identify a medical cause and cure are maintained. The loss of social rewards provokes more distress. Anger can be directed toward care providers, family members, and employers, as well as toward representatives of insurance companies, workers' compensation, and legal systems when perceived entitlements are denied. Fear is induced by the uncertainty of pain and the suffering that goes with it. Intense pain captivates attention with its aversiveness and drives avoidance behaviors. In a study of fear-avoidance beliefs, Waddell and colleagues conclude that it is the patient's fears and beliefs about pain that dictate behavior, not physical reality.[106]

Pain Behaviors

Pain behaviors are verbal and nonverbal means of communicating the pain experience to others.[8] They are directly observable and play a key role in the interaction between patients and society. Behaviors that are initially adaptive, such as limiting exacerbating physical activity or seeking medical attention, become maladaptive in patients with chronic pain. Pain behaviors include prolific verbal complaints, moaning, frequent sighing, grimacing, furrowing of the brow, protective posturing, gesturing, rubbing affected body parts, limping, frequent and excessive rest periods, and profound guarding responses.[8,83,107,108] Clinical examinations can be punctuated by complaints of pain in nonanatomic or global distributions. Patients may also display dramatic hypersensitivity and withdrawal responses to nonspecific palpation, inconsistent weakness on manual muscle testing with a "ratchety or give-way" quality, provocation with innocuous physical maneuvers, and inconsistencies on formal examination compared with casual functional observation.[107,109] There is no consistent relationship between the degree of pain behavior displayed and the magnitude of apparent tissue damage or nociception.[8] The presence of pain behaviors is predictive of a lowered probability of successful return to work.[110]

Pain behaviors are spontaneously emitted after acute nociception, but according to Fordyce[8] they are operantly reinforced by the responses of significant others. The behaviors increase in frequency when negative experiences are avoided or desirable outcomes are produced. For example, a patient might exhibit exaggerated pain behaviors to a physician if a desired medication or work release is granted after such a display. Interdisciplinary, behaviorally based pain management programs have been developed to counter these effects.[19,107,111] Care providers work to extinguish maladaptive pain behaviors by not reinforcing them and actively encouraging behaviors that characterize normal physical and social function.

Behavioral Effects on Metabolic and Histologic Systems

Excessive use of health care services, abuse of medications, and decreased physical activity are believed to be hallmarks of chronic pain syndromes.[107] These behaviors provide a link to dysfunctional histologic and metabolic responses. Focal restrictions in mobility develop with abnormal posturing and behaviorally limited range of motion. General deconditioning follows withdrawal from physical activities of daily living due to fear-avoidance behaviors. These responses set the stage for maladaptive healing at the histologic level, especially when reinforced with pre-existing conditions such as alcoholism, smoking, and poor nutrition.

Borderline hyperventilation can be associated with faulty postures and psychologic stress states.[112–115] Shallow, rapid respirations may then result in inefficient gas exchange, vasoconstrictive responses, and diffuse metabolic effects.

Associations with the histologic and sensorimotor dimensions are also mediated by the sympathetic nervous system and hypothalamic-pituitary axis. Heightened arousal alters activity in both the limbic system and noradrenergic projections through the brainstem reticular formation.[116–118] Nociceptive input is also routed through the reticular core and into the diencephalon, potentially coupling pain with emotion and inducing dysfunctional peripheral endocrine effects.[118,119] Maladaptive neuroendocrine processing is accepted as a base element of chronic stress states.[120]

Disability

Disability is a restriction in the ability to fulfill socially defined roles expected of an individual.[121,122] Included are roles in vocation, personal care, family care, and recreation. Disability can involve both physical and psychologic elements. In this section, discussion is included on psychologic dysfunction with a view of the disablement process in complex chronic pain syndromes. Here disability is as much or more a function of nonphysical factors than measurable physical impairments.[123–125] Disability is associated with the beliefs that pain implies tissue damage and activity should be avoided.[86] Some patients adopt a sick role, an unwritten agreement between patients and society that relieves individuals of normally expected responsibilities.[70] By acting out a sick role, pain behaviors gain ascendancy over entire dimensions of life experience. The emotional and behavioral displays that accompany the sick role seize the attention of others. They respond with levels of sympathy and solicitousness that operantly reinforce the role.[107] Physicians and therapists may also participate in the process. The idea that chronic pain syndromes might be iatrogenically fostered by well-meaning health care providers is uncomfortable but has been advanced by several clinicians.[20,107,111,125] These clinicians maintain that performance of sophisticated tests with dubious relevance or overprescription of opiate and sedative drugs is not in the patient's best interests. The same is true with an exclusive reliance on passive manual treatments or thermal and electrical therapeutic agents. The patient assumes a dependent role with such modalities. A search for a mysterious medical cause for the patient's suffering is reinforced.

The sick role grows powerful as the patient's time is shifted away from normal vocational, recreational, and household activities (Figure 1–8). In the worst case, the individual becomes profoundly deactivated and "shops" around for care providers who will support disablement. The patient loses the financial and social rewards of work, focuses on compensation claim management, and alters family relationships. Unpleasant responsibilities are often transferred to the spouse or significant other. Underlying conflicts may be suppressed in the name of sym-

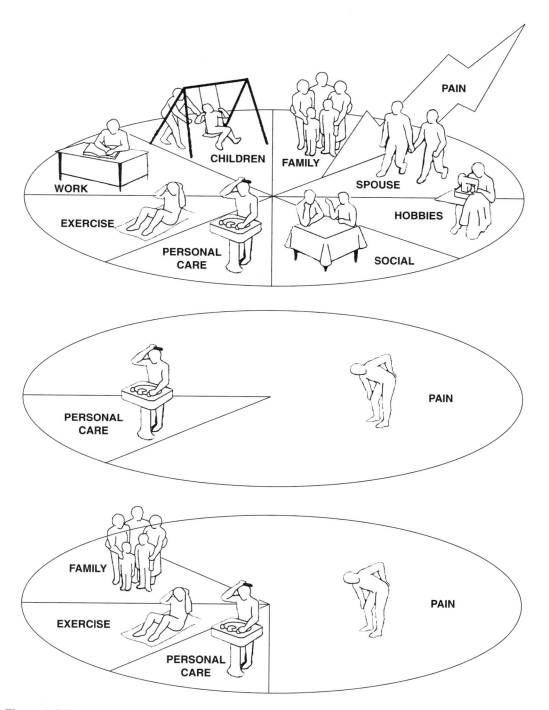

Figure 1–8 Progressive disability and early recovery in patients with chronic pain. *Source:* Reprinted from *Clinical Management.* Sanders, PL. Breaking the Chronic Pain Cycle. 1991: Vol 11, No 4: p 76, with the permission of the APTA.

pathy. Spousal support can be beneficial under certain circumstances, but high levels of perceived solicitousness by spouses are associated with increased pain behavior.[126] If dependency on the spouse increases, patient self-esteem likely declines. Covert resentment between partners may build.

Pain-related vocational disability is positively associated with workers' compensation claims.[127] Disability is greater among workers with low job satisfaction.[123] Nonphysical factors, such as lower educational level and attorney representation, negatively affect return-to-work rates after multidisciplinary work-hardening programs.[110,128] According to operant theory, receipt of financial compensation and avoidance of unpleasant work would likely reinforce disability. However, causal relationships in injury and disability are difficult to determine, and the extent to which compensation actually promotes disability is not clear.[129] Compensation is not itself linked to outcome when patients are treated in a structured, functional rehabilitation program.[130] Individuals who perceive their locus of control as external are more likely to show persistent vocational disability.[131] Gallagher and associates[90] conclude that these persons may benefit by compensation. Workers' compensation may shelter claimants from the full brunt of financial and familial pressures and enable rehabilitation at a lower level of stress. Certainly this is consistent with the social intent of the workers' compensation and legal systems. These researchers also believe, however, that the compensation process may contribute to emotional distress. Pain behaviors may have a negative impact on the responses of clinicians and arbitrators in claims management.

Petersen[110] shares the view that pain behaviors can become counterproductive if clinicians and claims managers perceive them as out of proportion to known injury. In the absence of a well-defined musculoskeletal etiology, pain behaviors may be exhibited in an attempt to legitimize complaints. The patient becomes frustrated if the claims system seems unresponsive. Options may appear limited if the patient has few transfer-

rable job skills. The combination of patient behaviors and attorney actions may alienate a claimant from medical and vocational providers. It is probable that compensation has beneficial effects, but adversarial litigation systems may protract disability.[132]

Sensorimotor Dysfunction

With the normal flow of physical activity, sensory stimuli are processed in the central nervous system (CNS) and motor responses are generated. Changes in sensorimotor function associated with the chronic pain experience will be considered next with a discussion of the afferent limb, followed by implications for motor programming.

Neuroplasticity and Chronic Pain

Many reviews have been published for musculoskeletal clinicians on the anatomic and physiologic bases of pain transmission.[57,58,133–135] Transmission is initiated with peripheral sensory receptors. Nociceptors are free nerve endings that detect noxious stimuli and generate neural codes, which are then conducted to the CNS. Skin, muscle, fascia, and periarticular connective tissue contain nociceptors. The nerve endings are excited by mechanical deformation, thermal energy, or the chemical mediators of inflammatory responses. Action potentials are then conducted along associated small-diameter, thinly myelinated A-delta (group III) fibers and nonmyelinated C (group IV) fibers. Both fiber types are slow conducting, with the C fibers being the slower of the two—as much as two orders of magnitude less than the most rapidly conducting afferent fibers devoted to proprioception. Some nociceptors respond only to robust mechanical stimulation, whereas others respond to multiple stimulus modalities. Polymodal receptors transmit by means of C fibers. A-delta fibers arise from nociceptors with both polymodal and mechanospecific response characteristics. When stimulated, the normally quiescent background activity of nociceptive fibers is replaced by a barrage of impulses.

Nociceptors can habituate to a persistent stimulus or become sensitized in the presence of tissue injury and local inflammation. Polymodal C fiber responses may persist and summate over time, presumably being responsible for the "second" pain that follows A-delta–mediated quick responses. Nociceptive A-delta and C fibers join with nonnociceptive afferent fibers (of the same and different sizes) and efferent fibers in peripheral nerves. Afferent fibers of the nerve pass into the dorsal root as they reach the spinal cord (Figure 1–9). The axons of the nociceptive fibers terminate in specific laminae of the spinal cord dorsal horn. Here they synapse with complex arrays of dorsal horn interneurons and transmission neurons, which give rise to the ascending somatosensory tracts. The fibers of the spinothalamic tracts cross to the contralateral side of the spinal cord and ascend to the thalamus, some directly and others by way of labyrinthian connections through the brainstem reticular formation. Nociresponsive cells are also found in fewer numbers in the dorsal column and medial lemniscal pathways, as well as in other ascending somatosensory pathways. Signals are eventually routed to sensory and association areas of the cerebral cortex. Stimulus information is extracted and processed at all levels of the neuraxis. Antinociceptive systems descend from the diencephalon, periaqueductal gray, nucleus raphe magnus, locus ceruleus, and multiple other reticular nuclei to the spinal cord dorsal horn. These pathways modulate the transmission of nociceptive signals at primary afferent synapses by both presynaptic and postsynaptic mechanisms. Serotonin, norepinephrine, endogenous opioids, and other neuropeptides act as transmitters in the descending inhibitory systems.

There are several possible mechanisms to explain the maintenance of activity in nociresponsive pathways. Chemoreceptive fibers are kept in a sensitized state by the presence of inflammatory mediators, the process of which is facilitated by recurrent cellular damage and circulatory stasis. Sensitized peripheral neurons fire at lower stimulus thresholds and can be facilitated by somatic reflexogenic and sympathetic loops.[12] Mechanical damage to nerve fibers occurs with adverse tension, entrapment, and ischemic syndromes.[29] Trauma results in perineural inflammation, neuropathic pain, and nerve degeneration that is slow to heal.[30] Regenerating sprouts of damaged afferent fibers show spontaneous and aberrant low-threshold discharges, which may be associated with persistent pain.[136,137] Low-level degenerative disease of the spine may produce radiculopathy without axial pain, and the resulting denervation supersensitivity could create pain syndromes that are mistakenly attributed to myofascial or bursal dysfunction.[138]

Damage to peripheral nerves and other structures can result in reflex sympathetic dystrophy (RSD), or causalgia. In its complete expression, RSD is characterized by painful hyperresponsiveness to stimuli, abnormal blood flow, edema, altered sweat gland activity, movement dysfunction, and trophic changes.[137,139,140] The pain can be induced by innocuous touch (allodynia) and is commonly of a burning character. RSD may also be associated with anxiety, depression, and sleep disorders, and it tends to be exacerbated by emotional arousal and movement. As the condition progresses, apparent weakness, spasm, motor reflex changes, soft tissue atrophy, fascial thickening, and contractures may develop from a combination of sympathetic dysfunction and disuse.

The hyperalgesia that accompanies RSD may be a result of sensitization of peripheral nociceptive C fibers by sympathetic activity.[137,139] Alpha-1 receptors, activated by local or circulating norepinephrine, appear to exert a tonic facilitatory effect on C fibers. The activity of C fibers in turn leads to spinal cord activation of wide-dynamic-range neurons, which transmit up the spinal cord. Wide dynamic range neurons respond to both noxious and nonnoxious inputs, and potentially their activation allows for expression of pain by innocuous stimulation of low-threshold mechanoreceptors.

Kramis and associates[141] propose that wide dynamic range neurons are sensitized by central mechanisms, and their subsequent vigorous re-

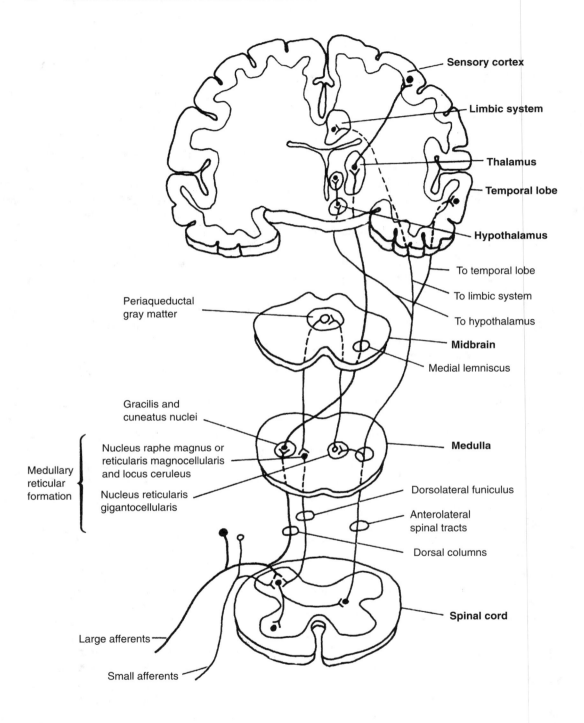

Figure 1–9 Scheme of large- and small-fiber afferent systems and ascending–descending inhibitory loop. *Source:* Reprinted with permission from D Hertling and RM Kessler, *Management of Common Musculoskeletal Disorders*, 2nd ed, p 49, © 1990, JB Lippincott. Illustration by Elizabeth Kessler.

sponses to nonnociceptive input lead to nonnociceptive pain when interpreted by suprasegmental systems. Because wide dynamic spinal neurons receive input from multiple segmental levels, and sympathetic reflexes may be expressed over several segments, the pain and peripheral dysfunction can become relatively diffuse over a region of the body. Sympathetic-maintained pain is therefore subserved by both peripheral and central effects.

Although full-blown cases of RSD are relatively infrequent, sympathetic dysfunction may occur in clinically subtle forms and may contribute to varied chronic pain presentations.[142,143] There is evidence that muscle spindles are activated by sympathetic efferents,[144] which led Kramis and colleagues[141] to link dysfunctional sympathetic responses with aberrant motor activity and myofascial pain syndromes, an issue alluded to earlier with reference to trigger points. The concept of subtle, sympathetic-maintained pain has also been discussed as a basis for intervention with manipulative therapies.[145]

Aside from sympathetic-maintained pain, there is a preponderance of evidence that CNS plasticity contributes to chronic pain states.[141] Coderre and colleagues[136] reviewed clinical and experimental evidence showing that plasticity in the CNS subserves primary and secondary hyperalgesia, phantom limb pain, and chronic referred pain. Primary hyperalgesia refers to increased sensitivity to noxious stimulation at an injured region. Secondary hyperalgesia denotes increased pain sensitivity in a spatial distribution beyond the initially damaged region, including nondermatomal and remote distributions. Hyperalgesia originates with nociceptive input to the CNS but can be maintained by central neurophysiologic mechanisms without ongoing peripheral nociception. After a noxious event, neurons in the spinal cord dorsal horn show reduced firing thresholds, increased spontaneous activity, afterdischarges, expansion of peripheral receptive fields, and increased response to innocuous and noxious stimuli. Sensitization is also observed in somatosensory brainstem and cortical neurons after application of noxious mechanical and inflammatory stimuli.

Coderre and associates[136] also reviewed deafferentiation studies, results of which indicated that a sensitizing central pain "trace" or "memory" can be maintained for many years. After denervation, neurons in the spinal cord dorsal horn and trigeminal nucleus display persistently increased spontaneous activity. Thalamic neurons show increased spontaneous and abnormal bursting activity, as well as receptive field expansion. Peripheral denervation also alters descending inhibitory antinociceptive controls from the nucleus raphe magnus and locus ceruleus.

In addition, Coderre and colleagues[136] reviewed the effects of anesthetic and analgesic pretreatment on postinjury pain. Findings in animal studies show that nociceptive responses to peripheral inflammatory challenge are attenuated by preinjection of a local anesthetic into discrete limbic regions as well as by prior intrathecal injection of an opioid agonist. Postoperative pain in humans is similarly reduced by preoperative treatment with regional anesthetics as well as systemic opiate and nonsteroidal anti-inflammatory drugs. Although the issue has yet to be resolved, Coderre and colleagues attributed the results to a blockade of CNS sensitization, rather than to peripheral effects. They believe that pain-related CNS plasticity is mediated at the cellular and molecular levels by C fiber peptide transmitters, excitatory amino acids, intracellular calcium and second messenger systems, and c-fos gene expression. Figure 1–10 summarizes relationships among nociception, CNS plasticity, and the consequences for sensorimotor function.

Motor Dysfunction

Persistent responses to noxious stimulation are not limited to somatosensory and sympathetic neurons. Spinal motor neurons are also sensitized by tissue injury and inflammation.[146] Flexion reflex thresholds are reduced following superficial and deep noxious activity in animals and humans.[147–149] In animals, flexor excitability is produced in both the stimulated and contralateral limbs and continues after peripheral blockade with a local anesthetic.[150,151] Injection of an

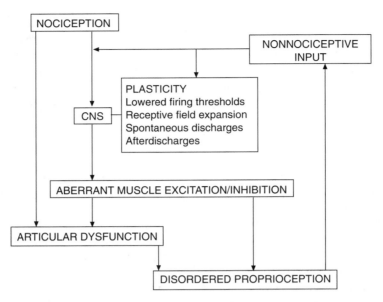

Figure 1–10 Schematic summarizing relationships among nociception, CNS plasticity, and consequences for sensorimotor function.

inflammatory irritant into the deep cervical paraspinal tissues of rats produces increased EMG activity from neck and jaw muscles.[152] Mechanically induced lumbar lesions and irritant injections also result in increased lumbar and hamstring EMG activity in animals.[153]

The extent to which these excitatory reflexes influence patterns of muscle activity in patients with chronic pain is not known, although segmental and suprasegmental facilitatory effects on the motor system have been invoked by a number of clinicians.[154–157] These practitioners have considered muscle spasm as involuntary hypertonicity induced by reflex mechanisms in response to tissue injury. For example, type IV receptors are free nerve endings located in joint capsule, ligament, fat pad, and blood vessel walls.[158] Type IV receptors tend to show high-threshold, nonadapting nociceptive responses. Afferent barrage from these nociceptors results in hypertonicity in the muscles that are functionally related to the involved joint.[159] Hypertonicity may therefore result from articular dysfunction as well as from soft tissue trauma and

perhaps subtle denervation supersensitivity. Ongoing spasm can lead to metabolite accumulation that activates nociceptors in surrounding musculoskeletal tissue and blood vessel walls, exacerbating pain and hypertonicity.[12,159] Pain due to spasm then becomes superimposed on pain from the original insult. Once present, the spasm may continue across different postures and into low-arousal states.[160]

An involuntary neurophysiologic suppression of motor activity, or inhibition, has also been noted in association with pain and joint effusion. Reflex inhibition has been reported after orthopaedic surgery, trauma, and experimentally induced effusion.[161–166] In addition, inhibition has been shown to occur following disruption of normal joint mechanics with a mechanical appliance.[167] Like reflexive hyperactivity, reflex suppression of muscle activity may be brought about by several mechanisms that alter joint function and proprioception. Many clinicians believe that hyperactivity and hypoactivity coexist; that is, where one muscle is overly excited, its antagonist, synergist, or another posturally or functionally related muscle is inhibited.

Basing his ideas on the work of Janda[168–170] and Lewit,[171] Taylor[172] proposes that tonic postural muscles tend to respond to injury with hyperactivity, whereas phasic movers tend to respond with hypoactivity. Taylor agrees with others[173,174] that the concept of resting spasm is insufficient to understand dysfunction in populations with chronic pain. His model goes further to view dysfunctional patterns of muscle activity as postural and movement disorders. At the root of the problem, he sees myofascial pain, trigger point phenomena, and faulty postures as leading to a disruption of normal patterns of muscle reciprocal activity. According to this perspective, a hyperactive postural muscle produces excessive reciprocal inhibition of other muscles through spinal reflexes. A hypoactive phasic muscle disinhibits other muscles. The result is a disturbance of normal patterns of motor control between an agonist and its antagonists or synergists.

Alternative mechanisms of hyperactivity and hypoactivity have been proposed. Edgerton and associates[175] hypothesize that trauma physically disrupts myofascial integrity and leads to decreased muscle force-generating ability. Muscle hypoactivity is thereby produced. The investigators propose that hyperactivity results from excitation of motor neuron pools induced by nociception or from recruitment compensation. Deficits from the hypoactive damaged muscle are detected by proprioceptive systems and relayed to the CNS. To achieve the motor goal, the CNS develops a compensatory motor program that increases the activity of other muscles. Edgerton and colleagues[175] reviewed experimental evidence showing that undamaged synergistic muscles increase their output to compensate for a damaged muscle. They argue that the responses may be maintained over long periods, that the compensating muscles will hypertrophy, and that the process will produce gross motor control changes that are detectable by generation of SEMG ratios among multiple muscles.

Proprioceptive-Motor Integration

Dysfunctional muscle hyperactivity and hypoactivity will inevitably alter proprioceptive responses and guidance of subsequent movement, a point noted by both Taylor[172] and Edgerton and coworkers.[175] Muscle spindles lie parallel to the force generating extrafusal muscle fibers and signal changes in length as well as the rate of length change. When the spindle apparatus is stretched, activity is generated in fast-conducting afferents that synapse in the ventral horn of the spinal cord.[176] The extrafusal fibers of the same muscle become excited, as do synergists, whereas antagonists are inhibited. Spindle responses are biased by the descending control of the gamma motor system, which causes the intrafusal fiber components of the spindle to contract and preload the system.

Golgi tendon organs lie in series at muscle–tendon junctions and signal changes in muscle tension. Afferents from Golgi tendon organs synapse to spinal inhibitory interneurons and act to reduce the tone in the muscle from which they originate, along with synergist inhibition and antagonist excitation. Several types of mechanoreceptors are also located in joint capsules and ligaments, and these cue changes in static joint position, acceleration, and direction of motion.[158] Activation of periarticular mechanoreceptors leads to complex segmental and suprasegmental spinal motor reflexes. Proprioceptive signals are conducted rostral to the brainstem, cerebellum, and cerebral cortex where information is extracted to guide motor execution as well as abstracted with other somatosensory cues and visual information to indicate the results of motor activity.

Functionally, postural control and smooth movement are not possible without these systems. Severe distal lower extremity ligamentous injuries alter local sensory function as well as distal and proximal muscle control.[177,178] The responses of involved somatosensory receptors show adaptation over time, some quickly and others relatively slowly.[158,179,180] Motor control errors may be produced by proprioceptive adaption.[181,182] Clinically, one might envision a patient with chronic neck pain after a motor vehicle accident, with a hyperactive upper trapezius held in a shortened state and abnormal joint posture. Proprioceptive–motor control might become disrupted after the trauma. If proprioceptors were to adapt to the chronic state, the CNS would cease being signaled of the aberrant peripheral event, and it would emerge as a neural status quo. Dysfunctional motor control could be perpetuated with a loss of effective unconscious and conscious proprioception. Indeed, patients with chronically elevated tension do not always seem to be aware of it; pain is their only conscious cue of the dysfunction. Subjects with chronic pain show inferior abilities to discriminate discrete SEMG-based activity levels, compared to control subjects, with a tendency to underestimate tension levels that seems independent of fatigue or attention.[183] In addition, subjects with chronic temporomandibular pain show poor correlation between perceived facial muscle tension and actual SEMG magnitude under conditions of low psychologic stress, compared to healthy control subjects.[184]

Proprioceptive activity may intensify pain because of central plasticity and sensitization of wide dynamic range neurons. Once wide dynamic range neurons are sensitized by previous nociceptive events, they generate hyperexcitable discharges in response to new nociceptive and nonnociceptive input. Proprioceptive signals routed through those wide dynamic range neurons may then induce intense discharges of a type that is normally nociceptive related.[141] Thus an individual in a chronically dysfunctional state could perceive pain during typically innocuous physical activity. Aberrant motor programs might be generated in response, without conscious or normal unconscious feedback and the cycle facilitated by resulting cumulative mechanical trauma.

As will be discussed in some detail in Chapter 3, Schmidt[185] envisions motor response processing in three stages: stimulus identification, motor response selection, and response command programming. In keeping with this perspective, stimuli are misidentified by faulty CNS processing of nociceptive and nonnociceptive inputs. Programming becomes aberrant through somatomotor reflexes that are themselves altered by nociceptive activity, faulty proprioceptive input, and perhaps sympathetic responses. The pattern may become protracted by selection of motor programs that compensate for the impaired action of muscles, hypertrophy of overused muscles and atrophy of underused muscles, and changes in passive stiffness at the histologic level. Dysfunctional motor behaviors are also produced in response to psychologic pressures. The cognitive abstraction of stimulus meaning may be altered by somatic hypervigilance, arousal, beliefs regarding pain avoidance or disability, fear, or depression. Learned guarding and inhibition responses may then result.

With regard to learned inhibition, some patients may become operantly conditioned to avoid activating a muscle that elicits aversive perceptions when contracted. This inhibition is seen as relative hypoactivity on a SEMG display and may be accompanied by compensatory hyperactivity at other sites.

Guarding

Guarding responses are also produced as a learned behavior. With guarding, the subject actively attempts to immobilize a region and prevent anticipated painful movement. Use of muscle tension to restrict a motion segment is often taken as an adaptive response if performed immediately after injury, but maladaptive if maintained for a prolonged period.

Guarding may be conceptualized by using an equilibrium-point spring analogy. Control of a joint by an agonist/antagonist muscle pair is analogous to a pair of complex springs, one on each side of the joint.[185–187] The equilibrium position of the joint is determined by the relative stiffness of each spring-like muscle and its associated connective tissues. The joint will come to rest in the position for which the levels of stiffness of both muscles are balanced (Figure 1–11). To prevent potentially painful movement in one direction, the muscle with an opposite action will be recruited. The joint angle will then change in a way concordant with the

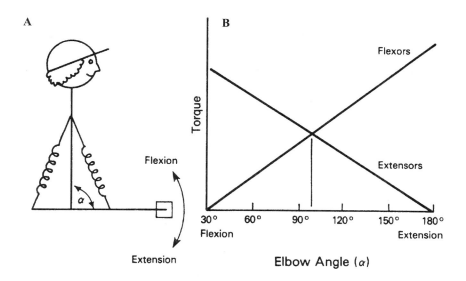

Figure 1–11 The mass-spring, or equilibrium-point, model. (**A**) Muscles seen as springs. (**B**) The length–tension diagrams for flexors and extensors plotted for different elbow angles, with the intersection being the equilibrium point where the tensions in the two muscle groups are equal and opposite. *Source:* Reprinted by permission from RA Schmidt, 1988, *Motor Control and Learning*, 2nd ed (Champaign, IL: Human Kinetics Publishers), 212.

muscle's direction of action until a new equilibrium point is reached. Abnormal posture and stiffness of the joint segment are produced. Compensatory activity from muscles around other joints may be needed to preserve functional use of a limb or to maintain the center of mass within the base of support for upright balance. Thus threatening movement in a particular direction can be prevented by increasing stiffness on one side of the joint and allowing a shift in joint position. The programmed motor response will be seen as hyperactivity of an agonist and its synergists at the involved joint segment and, possibly, as compensatory patterns of hypoactivity or hyperactivity elsewhere. If the individual's goal is to prevent painful movement of the joint in multiple directions, the only effective strategy will be to produce tonic contractions of both agonist and antagonistic musculature. This strategy increases stiffness around the joint in all planes, preventing displacement in any threatened direction while maintaining a fixed equilibrium point in a protective position. Motor programs

that produce diffuse hyperactivity around a joint segment will then be selected.

Muscle Deactivation and Fatigue

Some headache and upper quarter patients appear to manifest problems not because they recruit musculature to extreme levels during a motor task, but because they fail to deactivate muscles periodically. This phenomenon is demonstrated in SEMG tracings as a lack of low-amplitude gaps as well as by decreases in the percentage of total task time spent at low SEMG amplitude levels during continuous functional activities.[188–191] Healthy subjects tend to show gaps, or microrests, on the order of 0.2 second to several seconds, interspersed between bouts of muscle activation. Subjects with pain tend not to show the microrest pattern. Faulty deactivation can also be characterized as a failure to recover to baseline levels during rest periods between repeated discrete experimental movements.[115] Failure to recover intermittently to baseline may produce chronic, low-grade joint stiffness and fatigue. In one study, increased SEMG activity during rest periods was prospectively associated with industrial work injury.[192] Because the aberrant muscle activity patterns were detected before report of symptoms, they could not have been due to reactive guarding. The implication of these study findings is that subjects with musculoskeletal pain continuously recruit low to moderate muscle activity instead of normal activation/deactivation cycling.

It is not known why continual motor activity, rather than rest, is selected and programmed by individuals with musculoskeletal pain. Faulty postures and motor habits are proposed as causes, but the important net results are fatigue and perhaps altered microcirculation.[115] Patients with chronic cervical and lumbar dysfunction can be discriminated from healthy control subjects by fatigue-related SEMG frequency spectral changes.[193–197] High-level isometric contractions induce muscle ischemia by generating intramuscular pressures sufficient to occlude the vascular bed.[198–201] Lower level tonic contractions may also lead to disturbed muscle microcirculation and depleted energy stores.[202] Patients with chronic neck and shoulder pain show impaired abilities to increase microcirculation to the upper trapezius in response to progressively intense isometric contractions.[50] SEMG changes and fatigue are induced at cervical–shoulder girdle musculature within 5 minutes of maintaining 11% of maximum voluntary contractions (MVC), or by 1 hour of 5% MVC.[203–205] Shoulder proprioception is impaired after fatiguing muscle contractions, and this might have further effects on motor control and joint stabilization.[206] In summary, muscle hyperactivity triggers nociception by means of local hypoxemia, contraction-induced injury, fatigue-related metabolic effects, and secondary mechanical strain of connective tissues through motor control imbalances.

Mechanical Dysfunction

In the previous section, the case was made that faulty motor programs are output from the CNS in chronic pain syndromes. Aberrant motor programs include reflexive spasm and inhibition, learned guarding and inhibition, and compensatory patterns of hyperactivity and hypoactivity. Chronically aberrant patterns of muscle activity must logically affect the other components of the movement system. Muscles attach by means of tendons to bones, and in between bones are articulations and periarticular connective tissues.

Effects of Muscle Hyperactivity

As a muscle contracts, a tensile force is generated along the line of attachment of its tendon. Figure 1–12 represents a hypothetic motion segment and muscle contraction. The tensile force is represented as a vector quantity, acting in the direction shown by arrow **A**. Magnitude of force is indicated by the relative length of the line. The muscle force vector can be resolved into several components with a common origin. One component acts perpendicular to the shaft to rotate the moving distal bone about an articular axis that lies perpendicular to the plane of the page. Another component acts parallel to the shaft to produce translation along the plane of the page. Depending on the joint angle, the translatory component will have different effects at the joint. With the joint in a relatively extended position, the translatory component will apply force to the distal bone in a direction toward the other and compress the joint surfaces. If the joint is relatively flexed, the translatory component will apply force to the distal bone in a direction away from the other and separate the joint surfaces. The magnitude of each component vector varies with the magnitude of the muscle force vector. Thus as the muscle contracts with greater intensity, the applied rotary and translatory forces will also increase.

It is obvious from this model that both muscle contraction intensity and joint angle will affect loads at the joint surfaces and periarticular connective tissues. The periarticular connective tissues include the joint capsule, ligaments, articular cartilage, and perhaps a meniscus. Distraction forces that separate the joint surfaces are opposed by the capsule and ligaments.

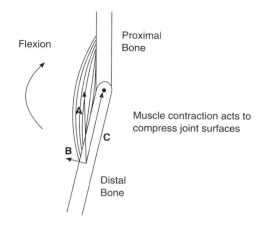

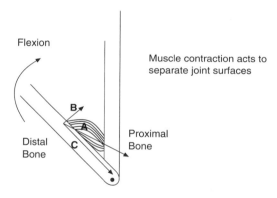

Figure 1–12 Grossly simplified, hypothetic motion segment during flexor contraction. The distance from muscle insertion to joint axis is greater than the distance from muscle origin to joint axis. Muscle contraction causes the distal bone to move on the proximal bone. **Arrow A** represents direction and magnitude of tension developed by the flexor muscle. Component forces that produce rotation and translation of the distal bone are represented by **Arrows B** and **C**, respectively. With a larger angle between the bones, the translatory component (**Arrow C**) acts to compress the joint surfaces. **Bottom**: With a smaller angle between the bones, the translatory component (**Arrow C**) acts to separate the joint surfaces.

Shearing may also be produced at the joint surfaces. Shear force is applied parallel to the surface of the body acted on, generated by an inter-play of muscle forces, joint dynamics, and external loads. A shear force will tend to slide the joint surfaces relative to each other along a line parallel to the joint interface. If the capsular and ligamentous tissues are unable to counteract distraction and shear forces, the joint will be unstable. The joint may sublux (ie, partially dislocate) or fully dislocate. With the hypothetic joint in a flexed position, aberrantly high muscle tension might contribute to ligament and joint capsule damage. If that tissue has already been injured and not fully repaired, the joint segment could incur repeated injury and become chronically unstable in the flexed range.

Norkin and Levangie[207] point out that the action line of most muscles is applied more parallel than perpendicular to the mobile bony lever. They note that the translatory component is usually larger than the rotary component, and most often, the translatory component acts in a compressive direction. The implication is that excessive muscle tension will more often load joints in compression than in distraction. Articular cartilage and meniscal tissue are largely avascular and depend on synovial fluid for nutrient–metabolite exchange.[208] Fluid exchange occurs through periodic compression and unloading of the articular tissue. In a simplified view, compression forces fluid from cartilage and removes metabolites. When the compressive force is lowered, water is imbibed by glycosaminoglycans. Nutrients are carried with the imbibition. Chronically elevated muscle tension might then interfere with joint nutrition by disrupting loading–unloading cycles. In an already traumatized joint, this could contribute to degenerative joint disease and perpetuate articular dysfunction, inflammatory responses, and nociception.

Effects of Muscle Hypoactivity

Muscle hypoactivity has untoward consequences in that it also may disrupt joint mechanics. Primary hypoactivity results from intrinsic contraction injury, externally applied traumatic loads, reflex mechanisms, and learned behaviors. Joints that have an inherently low level of bony stability rely on soft connective tissue and dynamic muscle control to prevent dislocation. The glenohumeral joint, with its shallow cup-and-ball arrangement, is an example. The muscles of the rotator cuff act to maintain joint stability and produce the proper accessory motions at the joint surfaces. Cuff muscles act antagonistically during motions in some planes and synergistically for motions in other planes. Hypoactivity in the cuff muscles due to fatigue and weakness leaves the joint vulnerable to instability and impingement syndromes.[209] Therefore either too little or too much muscle tension will affect joint function.

Arthrokinematics

Arthrokinematics refers to small motions occurring at the joint surfaces that allow for normal gross bony movement. The function of these movements can be understood by comparing a door hinge to a biologic joint.[57] A hinge serves as a joint between the door and its frame. As the door opens and closes, its outer edge inscribes an arc. The door rotates about an axis located at the hinge pin. The movement of the door is pure rotation, and the center of rotation is always located at the hinge pin. Unlike a door, the center of rotation of a biologic joint is not fixed. Figure 1–13 shows a representative biologic joint, the tibial–femoral joint. The gross bony movement is one of rotation, but at the joint surfaces there is a complex rolling–gliding relationship. Of course, the tibial–femoral joint does not have a fixed hinge pin. Hence for bony rotation to occur, there must be a rolling motion at the joint surfaces. If rolling was the only motion to take place, however, the femur would roll off the tibial plateau and the joint would dislocate. The posterior roll that accompanies flexion is instead accompanied by an anterior glide, so that the joint surfaces remain seated. As a consequence, the center of rotation is located at different points throughout the range of motion arc.[210,211]

The instantaneous center of rotation, or centrode, is the point about which one bone rotates relative to another at any given instant. For any joint, the instantaneous centers of rotation can be plotted through a range of motion arc

(Figure 1–14). If the instantaneous centers are connected with a line, a path of the instantaneous centers is generated.[57,210–213] Joint surface velocities are produced in a normal manner, and joint forces are optimally dissipated when the proper centrode path is generated. However, portions of the joint surfaces or periarticular connective tissue will inevitably be subjected to aberrant stress if the centrode path deviates substantially from its standard. That is, joint surfaces will undergo errant compressive loading, and the fibers of the capsule and ligaments will undergo higher than normal tensile stress. Periarticular soft tissues—such as a lax portion of joint capsule, tendinous insertion, or bursa—may also be impinged. Syndromes involving impingement through the subacromial region of the shoulder are examples. Moreover, there is a tendency for different portions of each opposing surface of a joint to contact each other through a range of motion arc. Cartilage sustains fatigue wear from cumulative microscopic damage brought about by repetitive stressing, which can be associated with altered centrodes. With an aberrant centrode path, surface regions will be heavily loaded when they should not be and not sufficiently loaded (normally acting to dissipate force over a larger surface area) when they should be. Portions of joint surfaces that lose periodic compression may not receive adequate nutrition. In other words, some zones of a joint surface will suffer from deficient compression, whereas other parts will sustain excessive loading. A destructive cycle of cartilage fibrillation, impaired lubrication processes, dysfunctional changes in capsular mobility, and altered neuromotor control may then ensue.[57]

The question then arises as to what factors regulate the centrode pattern of a joint. The shapes of the joint surfaces themselves constrain motion at the articulation and therefore help to determine gliding and rolling relationships.[57,210]

Motion at the joint surfaces is also constrained by ligaments and the joint capsule, different parts of which pull taut at different points in the range of motion arc.[210,211] The development of abnormal connective tissue stiffness and abnormal laxity was discussed earlier with respect to

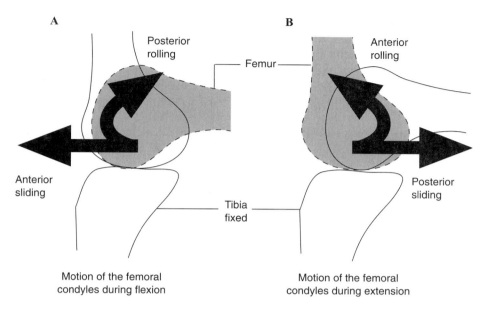

Figure 1–13 Schematic representation of rolling and sliding of femoral condyles on a fixed tibia. (**A**) The femoral condyles roll posteriorly, while simultaneously gliding anteriorly, during flexion. (**B**) The femoral condyles roll anteriorly, while simultaneously gliding posteriorly, during extension. *Source:* Reprinted with permission from CC Norkin and PK Levangie, *Joint Structure and Function*, p 229, © 1983, FA Davis Company.

histologic issues. Hypomobility results from effusion, adaptive shortening of the joint capsule, adhesions formed between the capsule and other connective tissue, and shortening and stiffness of fascial sheets. Connective tissue restraints that are significantly shortened limit the normal arthrokinematic range. Instability of a joint is in part a consequence of elongated or weakened connective tissue restraints, or abnormal joint surfaces. Articular hypomobility and hypermobility both lead to deviation of the centrode path and self-propagating cycles of joint mobility dysfunction.

Combined Muscle Hyperactivity and Hypoactivity

In addition to shape of joint surfaces and connective tissue function, a third factor is implicated in the control of a joint's centrode path. White and Sarhmann[214] believe that a major determinant of the centrode path during active motion is muscle acting in the following way. Sev-

eral muscles contract simultaneously when purposeful movements are produced. For example, upward rotation of the scapula is produced by the combined action of the upper trapezius, middle and lower trapezius, and the lower fibers of the serratus anterior muscles (Figure 1–15). For the scapulothoracic centrode path to be reproduced correctly, each of the three synergists must contract with an appropriate rate of force development. Forces that are too great, too low, or poorly timed cause a deviation of the centrode path. Muscle dominance occurs when the force created by one muscle abnormally exceeds that of its synergists or antagonist. Dominance patterns emerge from long-term combinations of muscle hyperactivity and hypoactivity. The dominant muscle tends to be of decreased passive length and is preferentially recruited during movement. That muscle undergoes hypertrophy over time, whereas the underused muscles atrophy.

White and Sahrmann[214] emphasize that the ability of a muscle to generate tension varies as a

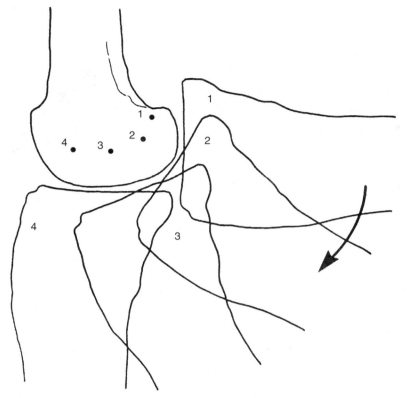

Figure 1–14 Diagram showing four loci of normal instant centers of rotation during flexion and extension of the knee. *Source:* Reprinted with permission from D Hertling and RM Kessler, *Management of Common Musculoskeletal Disorders*, 2nd ed, p 306, © 1990, JB Lippincott. Illustration by Elizabeth Kessler.

function of its length. Peak tension is generated at a length that corresponds to maximal overlap of actin and myosin filaments and, hence, optimal cross-bridging.[211] This is normally near the passive resting length of the muscle. Shortened or lengthened positions are less efficient for cross-bridge formation (Figure 1–16). For muscles that become lengthened by the addition of sarcomeres, the optimal tensile length shifts to a more elongated muscle position.[215] The lengthened muscle is capable of producing greater absolute tension, but is less efficient when tested at normal range and appears weak.[56] Muscles that have shortened also lose efficiency in the functional range; their optimal length has shifted to a shorter position. These muscle length–tension inefficiencies lead to early fa-

tigue and interact with faulty neuromotor control and trophic changes to continue dominance patterns.

Muscle Imbalance

Muscle imbalance involves two or more muscles that participate in concert to execute a specific movement wherein the relative stiffness of participating muscles is inappropriately coordinated. Inefficient patterns of muscle stiffness arise from both passive and active tensile issues. Included are passive myofascial length, active force-generating ability related to length–tension relationships and intrinsic muscle factors, and faulty CNS motor programming. Imbalance may be conceptualized in terms of the relative stiffness developed at each hypothetic phase of

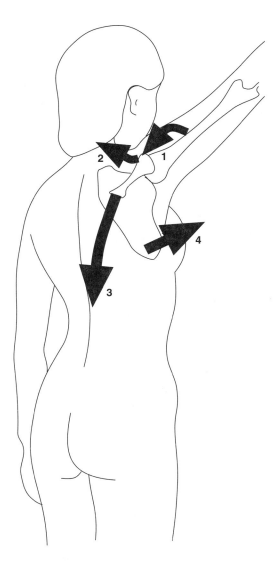

Figure 1–15 Simplified view of muscle forces contributing to upward rotation of the scapula during shoulder flexion. The intrinsic glenohumeral muscles (**1**) produce flexion of the humerus on the glenoid fossa of the scapula. Glenohumeral motion is rhythmically coupled to upward scapular rotation, resulting from the coordinated action of the upper trapezius (**2**), the lower trapezius (**3**), and the lower fibers of the serratus anterior (**4**). *Source:* Reprinted with permission from IA Kapandji, Vol 1: Upper Limbs, *The Physiology of the Joints*, 5th ed, p 65, © 1982, Churchill Livingstone.

movement. Tension generation is aberrant in both time and amplitude domains. Each muscle generates too much or too little force at particular portions of the range of motion arc. The result is that muscles co-contract when they should not, fail to fire in a synchronous manner when they should, or otherwise function disproportionately out of phase. At any given point in the movement arc, the equilibrium position of the involved joint surfaces and the instantaneous center of rotation are altered from the ideal. Thus the inefficient coupling of forces from the participating muscles causes a deviation of the ideal centrode path of the involved joint. Pathologic consequences are produced for articular and myofascial structures (Figure 1–17).

Patterns of imbalance occur at a single joint between an agonist and its antagonists and synergists, but the effects may be transmitted across motion segments that function in a kinetic chain. Muscles act as phasic prime movers of body parts, tonic postural stabilizers, and phasic stabilizers. If the goal movement requires harmonized control of adjacent joint segments and one of those segments functions in an imbalanced way, other segments must compensate in some way to achieve the movement goal. Imbalances involving muscles that act over two joints and in multiple planes are even more complex. Motion segments that function in a closed kinetic chain, in which the distal segment is fixed against an extrinsic surface, must further transmit and dissipate aberrant reaction forces from that surface. Muscle imbalances therefore have broad impact on, and are widely affected by, other elements of the movement system. Imbalanced muscle action has been associated with a diverse range of musculoskeletal disorders, such as patellofemoral dysfunction, degenerative lumbar disease, shoulder impingement syndrome, cervical muscle dysfunction, trigger points, and headache.[61,154,209,216] By monitoring muscle recruitment levels in real time, SEMG offers a means of observing aspects of muscle imbalance. The electromyographer can exploit this detection as a window into chronic musculoskeletal dysfunction, and it seems likely that the area of muscle

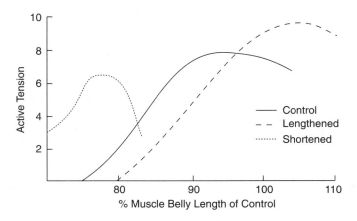

Figure 1–16 Schematic of active length–tension curves for adult animal muscles immobilized in shortened and lengthened positions versus control subjects. For each of the muscle groups, peak tension is developed at a particular length range and is lower in shortened or elongated positions. Loss or addition of sarcomeres induced by immobilization in shortened or lengthened positions, respectively, alters the peak tension–length relationship relative to control preparations. *Source:* Adapted with permission from PE Williams and G Goldspink, Changes in Sarcomere Length and Physiological Properties in Immobilized Muscle, *Journal of Anatomy*, Vol 127, © 1978, Cambridge University Press.

imbalance will emerge as a major focus for clinical users of SEMG.

Behavioral–Mechanical Interactions

Many clinicians consider inefficient postural and ergonomic habits as primary factors in the precipitation and perpetuation of chronic pain. Considerable educational and material resources are devoted to correcting perceived problems. In general, repeated or sustained use of faulty body mechanics places undue strain on joint structures, resulting in greater spinal intradiscal pressures; higher compressive loads across joint surfaces; and increased tensile strain on ligaments, joint capsules, tendons, and perhaps blood vessels.[13,57,217,218] Motor unit activity may be increased to compensate for inefficient joint alignment. Muscles can also be predisposed to a faulty length–tension relationship if the posture results in a chronically shortened or lengthened position. Fatigue and overuse syndromes follow.

Middaugh and associates[115] describe relationships among faulty posture, motor habits, muscle overuse, adaptive shortening, poor ergonomics, and inefficient respiratory patterns as contributory factors for cumulative trauma disorders. They note that forward head posture is associated with increased suboccipital SEMG activity. Dynamic upper extremity work performed with a forward head posture is accompanied by increased upper trapezius SEMG activity, a finding consistent with the work of others.[219,220] As the head is displaced anteriorly, the posterior musculature increases tension to counteract the greater flexion moment. Adaptive shortening of passive myofascial elements occurs as the posture is maintained over long periods. Aberrant joint relationships are produced through the craniomandibular region, and normal cervical muscular force couples are disturbed.[115,221] Figure 1–18 shows SEMG activity during head rotation recorded from the cervical paraspinal and sternomastoid muscles of an individual in erect versus forward head posture. Note the increase in cervical paraspinal activity and the decrease in sternomastoid activity that occur with adoption of the forward head posture. Faulty postures predispose individuals to inefficient motion control.

The individuals at greatest risk for inefficient motion control may be those who combine

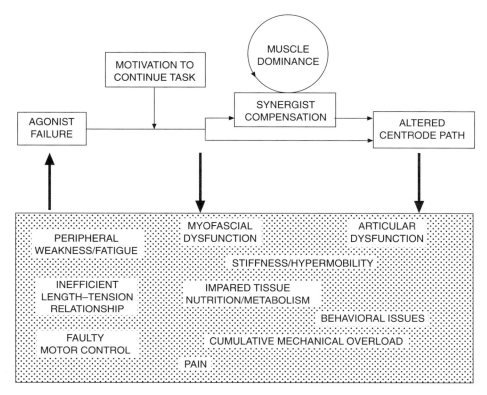

Figure 1–17 Schematic representation of relationship of muscle imbalance to chronic musculoskeletal dysfunction.

faulty postures and body mechanics with poor activity pacing. These persons tend to sustain performance of high-intensity tasks with insufficient rest periods or task rotation. Tissue is loaded in a particular direction over many task repetitions or for long static periods. When the pattern is sustained as a routine part of a subject's daily activities, it is considered to be a high risk factor for musculoskeletal injury.[218,222] Poor pacing may result from externally applied job demands or internal cognition related to job efficacy and time management. The situation is made all the worse if emotional stressors trigger increased tonic muscle contractions during task performance. Job stressors and satisfaction levels are known to be associated with cumulative trauma disorders.[223] Thus mechanical and psychodynamic factors interact in the maintenance of workplace musculoskeletal dysfunction.

CLINICAL INTERVENTION NOTES

The state of nature is complex with respect to chronic musculoskeletal dysfunction and pain. Patients with pain over a particular body region may be affected along histologic, psychologic, sensorimotor, and mechanical dimensions in different ways. Factor combinations are represented in Figure 1–19. With low back pain, for example, one patient might have histologic degenerative disease along the vertebral column, mechanical impairments, modest neuromuscular dysfunction, and little psychologic dysfunction. For another patient, affective disturbance and disability beliefs could be primary limiting factors. Various interactions are possible, and patients who show serious dysfunction along all dimensions require an interdisciplinary approach.

A

Forward Head
Cervical Rotation

Retracted Head
Cervical Rotation

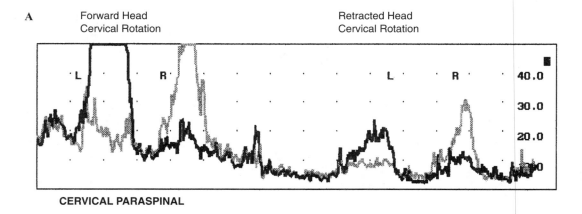

CERVICAL PARASPINAL

B

Forward Head
Cervical Rotation

Retracted Head
Cervical Rotation

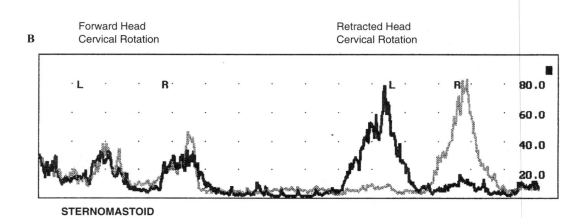

STERNOMASTOID

Figure 1–18 SEMG activity of (**A**) left (black) and right (gray) cervical paraspinals and (**B**) left (black) and right (gray) sternomastoid muscles during head rotation left (**L**) and right (**R**) in forward head versus retracted head postures. Peak activity of cervical paraspinals is increased, whereas that of sternomastoids is reduced, in forward head posture compared with retracted head posture.

Numerous clinicians have discussed the merits of interdisciplinary programs with patients who are severely disabled and have chronic pain.[19,107,110,224,225] These programs involve a team of care providers and incorporate a range of medical, manual, psychologic, physical, occupational, and vocational therapies. Various provider skills are brought into play to meet the unique combination of factors contributing to each patient's presentation. Less intensive work "conditioning" programs have also become popular, and patients with focal problems may do well with single-discipline or simpler multidisciplinary care. In any event, a broad array of evaluation and treatment tools is called for. Saunders[13] has candidly challenged clinicians to go beyond discipline-specific biases and deal with the whole patient (Table 1–1). Jette[226] has argued that the primary need now is to understand how different physiologic (and psychologic) impairments are linked to improvements in functional outcomes. This understanding is necessary to provide quality care and

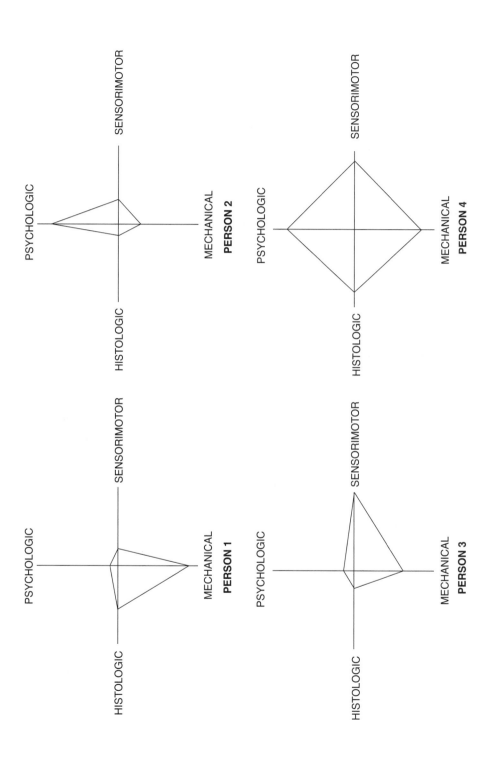

Figure 1–19 Relative contributions of histologic, psychologic, sensorimotor, and mechanical factors to chronic musculoskeletal dysfunction and pain in four persons. Each factor is represented as contributing in proportion to the graphed distance to the origin along its axis. The four factors are modeled as variably interacting across patient cases, even though all persons may share a similar original pathologic mechanism.

Table 1–1 Health Care Practitioners Tend To Stereotype Persons with Chronic Back Pain into Groups That Correspond with Their Conceptual Models and Methods of Treatment. It May Be More Productive To View Chronic Disorders as Multifactorial and Plan Multidisciplinary Intervention.

My Treatment Is	Therefore 90% of My Patients Have
Manipulation	Fixations and Subluxations
Disc Surgery	Disc Disease
Exercise	Weakness, Stiffness
Muscle Relaxants	Muscle Spasm
Antidepressants	Depression
Rhizotomy	Facet Disease
Pain Medication	Pain
Anti-Inflammation Medication	Inflammation
Nothing	Hysteria or Malingering

Source: Reprinted with permission from HD Saunders, *Evaluation, Treatment, and Prevention of Musculoskeletal Disorders*, p 9, © 1985, The Saunders Group, Inc.

patient satisfaction with contained costs. Clinicians must identify ways to stratify patient variables, so that the right treatment is provided at the right time in the right patient.

SEMG is a useful assessment tool for chronic musculoskeletal pain syndromes that involve aberrant patterns of motor activity. The methods described in this book help delineate contributory neuromuscular relationships, but they can only be an adjunct to the evaluation process. SEMG recordings in and of themselves resolve little in the way of psychologic and musculoskeletal questions. The recordings do not measure pain, stress, anxiety, coping, joint position, soft tissue extensibility, or strength. Nevertheless, the information derived from the

SEMG signal is unique in muscle evaluation. The SEMG system also possesses peculiar benefits in treatment. SEMG feedback is used to augment motor learning. In this way, aberrant patterns of muscle hypoactivity and hyperactivity can be modified.

Healthy physical function requires flexibility, strength, endurance, and an appropriate rate of force development. Also involved are modulation of reflex activity, integrated control of joint chains incorporating the body axis with the extremities, and perceptual–cognitive factors related to motor planning and pain. As will be discussed, SEMG may be integrated with other methods in the practitioner's armamentarium to address each of these issues.

REFERENCES

1. Cunningham LS, Kelsy JL. Epidemiology of musculoskeletal impairments and associated disability. *Am J Public Health.* 1984;74:574–579.

2. Frymoyer JW, Cats-Baril WL. An overview of the incidence and costs of low back pain. *Orthop Clin North Am.* 1991;22:263–271.

3. Murt H, Parsons PE, Harlan WR, et al. Disability, utilization, and costs associated with musculoskeletal conditions. *Natl Med Care Util Expend Surv C.* 1986; 5(Sept):1–64.

4. Bonica JJ. Introduction. In: Bonica JJ, ed. *Pain.* New York: Raven Press; 1980;1–9.

5. Sternbach RA. *Pain Patients: Traits and Treatment.* New York: Academic Press; 1974.

6. Wall PD. On the relation of injury to pain. *Pain.* 1979;6:253–264.

7. Bigos S, Bowyer O, Braen G, et al. *Acute Low Back Problems in Adults.* Rockville, MD: Agency for Health Care Policy and Research, Public Health Service, US Dept of Health and Human Services; 1994. Clinical Practice Guideline No. 14, AHCPR publication 95-0642.

8. Fordyce WE. *Behavioral Methods for Chronic Pain and Illness.* St. Louis, MO: CV Mosby; 1976.

9. Turk DC, Rudy TE. Towards a comprehensive assessment of chronic pain patients. *Behav Res Ther.* 1987;25:237–249.

10. Merskey H. Pain terms: a list with definitions and notes on usage. International Association for the Study of Pain, Subcommittee on Taxonomy Report. *Pain.* 1979;6:249–252.

11. Melzack R. Psychologic aspects of pain. In: Bonica JJ, ed. *Pain.* New York: Raven Press; 1980;111–142.

12. Livingston WK. *Pain Mechanisms.* New York: MacMillan Publishing USA; 1943.

13. Saunders HD, Saunders R. *Evaluation, Treatment, and Prevention of Musculoskeletal Disorders.* 3rd ed. Chaska, MN: Educational Opportunities (a Saunders Company); 1993.

14. Chapman CR. Pain and perception: comparison of sensory decision theory and evoked potential methods. In: Bonica JJ, ed. *Pain.* New York: Raven Press; 1980.

15. Deardoff WW, Chino AF, Scott DW. Characteristics of chronic pain patients: factor analysis of the MMPI-2. *Pain.* 1993;54:153–158.

16. Pietri-Taleb F, Riihimaki H, Viikari-Juntura E, Lindstrom K. Longitudinal study on the role of personality characteristics and psychological distress in neck trouble among working men. *Pain.* 1994;58:261–267.

17. Delitto A. Are measures of function and disability important in low back care? *Phys Ther.* 1994;74:452–462.

18. Deyo RA. Measuring the functional status of patients with low back pain. *Arch Phys Med Rehabil.* 1988; 69:1044–1053.

19. Loeser JD, Egan KJ. History and organization of the University of Washington Multidisciplinary Pain Center. In: Loeser JD, Egan KJ, eds. *Managing the Chronic Pain Patient: Theory and Practice at the University of Washington Multidisciplinary Pain Center.* New York: Raven Press; 1989;3–20.

20. Loeser JD. What is chronic pain? *Theor Med.* 1991;12:213–225.

21. Volnin EP, Lai D, McKinney S, Loeser JD. When pain becomes disabling: a regional analysis. *Pain.* 1988; 33:33–39.

22. Donatelli R, Owens-Burkhart H. Effects of immobilization on the extensibility of periarticular connective tissue. *J Orthop Sports Phys Ther.* 1981;3:67–72.

23. Nimin ME, Marcel E. The molecular organization of collagen and its role in determining the biophysical properties of the connective tissues. *Biorheology.* 1980;17:51–82.

24. Williams PL, Bannister LH, Berry MM, et al, eds. *Gray's Anatomy.* 38th ed. New York: Churchill Livingstone; 1995.

25. Andriacchi T, Sabiston P, DeHaven K, et al. Ligament: injury and repair. In: Woo SLY, Buckwalter JA, eds. *Injury and Repair of Musculoskeletal Soft Tissues.* Park Ridge, IL: American Academy of Orthopaedic Surgeons; 1988;103–128.

26. Davidson JM: Wound repair. In: Gallin JI, Goldstein IM, Snyderman R, eds. *Inflammation: Basic Principles and Clinical Correlates.* New York: Raven Press; 1992;809–819.

27. Gelberman R, Goldberg V, An KN, Banes A. Tendon. In: Woo SLY, Buckwalter JA, eds. *Injury and Repair of Musculoskeletal Soft Tissues.* Park Ridge, IL: American Academy of Orthopaedic Surgeons; 1988;5–40.

28. Woo SLY, Buckwalter JA, eds. *Injury and Repair of Musculoskeletal Soft Tissues.* Park Ridge, IL: American Academy of Orthopaedic Surgeons; 1988.

29. Butler DS. *Mobilisation of the Nervous System.* Melbourne, Australia: Churchill Livingstone; 1991.

30. Lundborg G, Rydevik B, Manthorpe M, Varon S, Lewis J. Peripheral nerve: the physiology of injury and repair. In: Woo SLY, Buckwalter JA, eds. *Injury and Repair of Musculoskeletal Soft Tissues.* Park Ridge, IL: American Academy of Orthopaedic Surgeons; 1988;297–352.

31. Akeson WH, Amiel D, Woo S. Immobility effects of synovial joints: the pathomechanics of joint contracture. *Biorheology.* 1980;17:95–110.

32. Akeson WH, Amiel D, Mechanic GL, Woo S, Harwood FL, Hamer ML. Collagen crosslinking alterations in joint contractures: changes in reducible crosslinks in periarticular connective tissue collagen after nine weeks of immobilization. *Connect Tissue Res.* 1977;5:5–19.

33. Woo SLY, Gomez MA, Woo YK, Akeson WH. The relationship of immobilization and exercise on tissue remodeling. *Biorheology.* 1982;19:397–408.

34. Woo S, Matthews JV, Akeson WH, Amiel D, Convery R. Connective tissue response to immobility: correlative study of biomechanical measurements of normal and immobilized rabbit knees. *Arthritis Rheum.* 1975;18:257–264.

35. Saal JS. The role of inflammation in lumbar pain. *Spine.* 1995;20:1821–1827.

36. Banes AJ, Enterline D, Bevin AG, et al. Effects of trauma and partial devascularization on protein synthesis in the avian flexor profundus tendon. *J Trauma.* 1981;21:505–512.

37. Frank C, Woo S, Andriacchi T, et al. Normal ligament: structure, function, and composition. In: Woo SLY, Buckwalter JA, eds. *Injury and Repair of Musculoskeletal Soft Tissues.* Park Ridge, IL: American Academy of Orthopaedic Surgeons; 1988;45–101.

38. Hunt AH. The role of vitamin C in wound healing. *Br J Surg.* 1941;28:436–439.

39. Fuhr JE, Farrow A, Nelson S. Vitamin B6 levels in patients with carpal tunnel syndrome. *Arch Surg.* 1989:124:1329–1330.

40. Kieldsen-Kragh J, Haugen M, Borchgrevink CF, et al. Controlled trial of fasting and one-year vegetarian diet in rheumatoid arthritis. *Lancet.* 1991;338:899–902.

41. Russell TI. Magnesium requirements in patients with chronic inflammatory disease receiving intravenous nutrition. *J Am Coll Nutr.* 1985;4:553–558.

42. Garret W, Tidball J. Myotendinous junction: structure, function, and failure. In: Woo SLY, Buckwalter JA, eds. *Injury and Repair of Musculoskeletal Soft Tissues.* Park Ridge, IL: American Academy of Orthopaedic Surgeons; 1988;171–207.

43. Caplan A, Carlson B, Faulkner J, Fischman D, Garrett W. Skeletal muscle. In: Woo SLY, Buckwalter JA, eds. *Injury and Repair of Musculoskeletal Soft Tissues.* Park Ridge, IL: American Academy of Orthopaedic Surgeons; 1988;209–291.

44. Faulkner JA, Brooks SV, Opiteck JA. Injury to skeletal muscle fibers during contractions: conditions of occurrence and prevention. *Phys Ther.* 1993;73:911–921.

45. McCully KK, Faulkner JA. Injury to skeletal muscle fibers of mice following lengthening contraction. *J Appl Physiol.* 1985;59:119–126.

46. Carlson BM, Faulkner JA. The regeneration of skeletal muscle fibers following injury: a review. *Med Sci Sports Exerc.* 1983;15:187–198.

47. Faulkner JA, Cote C. Functional deficits in skeletal muscle grafts. *Fed Proc.* 1986;45:1466–1499.

48. Faulkner JA, Niemeyer JH, Maxwell LC, et al. Contractile properties of transplanted extensor digitorum longus muscles of cats. *Am J Physiol.* 1980;238:C120–C126.

49. Thomas D, Kleuber K, Bourke D, et al. The size of myofibers in mature grafts of the mouse extensor digitorum longus muscle. *Muscle Nerve.* 1984;7:226–231.

50. Larsson SE, Alund M, Cai H, Oberg PA. Chronic pain after soft tissue injury of the cervical spine: trapezius muscle blood flow and electromyography at static loads and fatigue. *Pain.* 1994;57:173–180.

51. Jarvinen M. Healing of a crush injury in rat striated muscle. *Acta Pathol Microbiol Scand.* 1976;142:47–56.

52. Davies CTM, Sargeant AJ. Effects of exercise therapy on total and component tissue leg volumes of patients undergoing rehabilitation from lower limb injury. *Ann Hum Biol.* 1975;2:327–334.

53. Eriksson E. Rehabilitation of muscle function after sport injury: major problems in sports medicine. *Int J Sports Med.* 1981;2:1–11.

54. Haggmark T, Jansson E, Eriksson E. Fiber type area and metabolic potential of the thigh muscle in man after knee injury and immobilization. *Int J Sports Med.* 1981;2:12.

55. Stanish WD, Valiant GA, Bonen A, Belcastro AN. The effects of immobilization and electrical stimulation on muscle glycogen and myofibrillar ATPase. *Can J Appl Sport Sci.* 1982;7:267–271.

56. Gossman MR, Sahrman SA, Rose SJ. Review of length associated changes in muscle: experimental evidence and clinical implications. *Phys Ther.* 1982;62:1799–1808.

57. Hertling D, Kessler RM. *Management of Common Musculoskeletal Disorders.* 2nd ed. Philadelphia: JB Lippincott Co; 1990.

58. Sluka KA. Pain mechanisms involved in musculoskeletal disorders. *J Orthop Sports Phys Ther.* 1996; 24:240–254.

59. Travell JG, Simons DG. *Myofascial Pain and Dysfunction: The Trigger Point Manual.* Vol 1. Baltimore: Williams &Wilkins; 1983.

60. Donaldson CCS, Romney D, Donaldson M, Skubick D. Randomized study of the application of single motor unit biofeedback training to chronic low back pain. *J Occup Rehab.* 1994; 4:31–44.

61. Donaldson CCS, Skubick DL, Clasby RG, Cram J. The evaluation of trigger point activity using dynamic EMG techniques. *Am J Pain Manage.* 1994;4:118–122.

62. Headley BJ. Evaluation and treatment of myofascial pain syndrome using biofeedback. In: Cram JR, ed. *Clinical EMG for Surface Recordings.* Vol 2. Nevada City, CA: Clinical Resources; 1990;235–254.

63. Hubbard DR, Berkoff GM. Myofascial trigger points show spontaneous needle EMG activity. *Spine.* 1993;18:1803–1807.

64. Simons DG. *Myofascial Pain Syndrome Due to Trigger Points.* Cleveland, OH: Gebauer Co; 1987. International Rehabilitation Medicine Association Monograph Series No. 1.

65. Armstrong RB. Initial events in exercise-induced muscular injury. *Med Sci Sports Exerc.* 1990;22:429–437.

66. Hubbard DR. Psychophysiology of muscle tension and tension myalgia. In: *Proceedings of the Association for Applied Psychophysiology and Biofeedback (AAPB) 27th Annual Meeting, Albuquerque, New Mexico, March 1996.* Wheat Ridge, CO: AAPB; 1996;18.

67. Lewis C, Gervitz R, Hubbard D, Berkoff G. Needle trigger point and surface frontal EMG measurements of psychophysiological responses in tension-type headache patients. *Biofeedback Self Regul.* 1994; 19:274–275.

68. McNulty W, Gervitz R, Berkoff G, Hubbard D. Needle electromyographic evaluation of trigger point responses to a psychophysiological stressor. *Psychophysiology.* 1994;31:313–316.

69. Magni G, Moreschi C, Rigatti-Luchini S, Merskey H. Prospective study on the relationship between depressive symptoms and chronic musculoskeletal pain. *Pain*. 1994;56:289–297.

70. Waddell G, Pilowsky I, Bond M. Clinical assessment and interpretation of abnormal illness behavior in low back pain. *Pain*. 1989;39:41–53.

71. Hazard RG, Bendix A, Fenwick JW. Disability exaggeration as a predictor of functional restoration outcomes for patients with chronic low back pain. *Spine*. 1991;16:1063–1067.

72. Jamison RN, Rudy TE, Penzien DB, Mosley TH Jr. Cognitive-behavioral classifications of chronic pain: replication and extension of empirically derived patient profiles. *Pain*. 1994;57:277–292.

73. Basmajian JV, ed. *Biofeedback: Principles and Practice for Clinicians*. 3rd ed. Baltimore: Williams & Wilkins; 1989.

74. Schwartz MS, ed. *Biofeedback: A Practitioner's Guide*. 2nd ed. New York: Guilford Press; 1995.

75. Morgan CT, King RA, Robinson NM. *Introduction to Psychology*. 6th ed. New York: McGraw-Hill; 1979.

76. Arntz A, Dreessen L, De Jong P. The influence of anxiety on pain: attention and attributional mediators. *Pain*. 1994; 56:307–314.

77. Turk DC, Meichenbaum D, Genest M. *Pain and Behavioral Medicine*. New York: Guilford Press; 1983.

78. Le Bars D, Dickenson AH, Besson JM. Diffuse noxious inhibitory controls (DNIC), II: lack of effect on non-convergent neurones, supraspinal involvement and theoretical implications. *Pain*. 1979;6:305–327.

79. Lautenbacher S, Rollman GB, McCain GA. Multimethod assessment of experimental and clinical pain in patients with fibromyalgia. *Pain*. 1994;59:45–53.

80. Bates MS, Edwards WT, Anderson KO. Ethnocultural influences on variation in chronic pain perception. *Pain*. 1993;52:101–112.

81. DeGood DE, Shutty MS Jr. Assessment of pain beliefs, coping, and self-efficacy. In: Turk DC, Melzack R, eds. *Handbook of Pain Assessment*. New York: Guilford Press; 1992;199–240.

82. Williams DA, Robinson ME, Geisser ME. Pain beliefs: assessment and utility. *Pain*. 1994;59:71–78.

83. Buckelew SP, Parker JC, Keefe FJ, et al. Self-efficacy and pain behavior among subjects with fibromyalgia. *Pain*. 1994;59:377–384.

84. Feuerstein M, Beattie P. Biobehavioral factors affecting pain and disability in low back pain: mechanisms and assessment. *Phys Ther*. 1995;75:267–280.

85. Headley BJ. Self-efficacy and chronic pain. *Clin Manage*. 1990;10:47–51.

86. Jensen MP, Turner JA, Romano JM, Lawler BK. Relationship of pain-specific beliefs to chronic pain adjustment. *Pain*. 1994;57:301–309.

87. Morley S, Wilkinson L. The pain beliefs and perceptions inventory: a British replication. *Pain*. 1995; 61:427–433.

88. Williams DA, Thorn BE. An empirical assessment of pain beliefs. *Pain*. 1989;36:351–358.

89. Bandura, A. Self-efficacy: toward a unifying theory of behavioral change. *Psychol Rev*. 1977;84:191–215.

90. Gallagher RM, Williams RA, Skelly J, et al. Workers' compensation and return to work in low back pain. *Pain*. 1995;61:299–307.

91. Lazarus RS, Folkman S. *Stress, Appraisal, and Coping*. New York: Springer Publishing Co; 1984.

92. Jensen MP, Turner JA, Romano JM, Strom SE. The chronic pain coping inventory: development and preliminary validation. *Pain*. 1995;60:203–216.

93. Morley S, Pallin V. Scaling the affective domain of pain: a study of the dimensionality of verbal descriptors. *Pain*. 1995;62:39–49.

94. Geisser ME, Robinson ME, Keefe FJ, Weiner ML. Catastrophizing, depression and the sensory, affective and evaluative aspects of chronic pain. *Pain*. 1994;59:79–83.

95. Keefe FJ, Kashikar-Zuck S, Opiteck J, Hage E, Dalrymple L, Blumenthal JA. Pain in arthritis and musculoskeletal disorders: the role of coping skills training and exercise interventions. *J Orthop Sports Phys Ther*. 1996;24:279–290.

96. Romano JM, Turner JA. Chronic pain and depression: does the evidence support a relationship? *Psychol Bull*. 1985;97:18–34.

97. Turk DC, Okifuji A, Scharff L. Chronic pain and depression: role of perceived impact and perceived control in different age cohorts. *Pain*. 1995;61:93–101.

98. Leino P, Magni G. Depressive and distress symptoms as predictors of low back pain, neck-shoulder pain, and other musculoskeletal morbidity: a 10 year follow-up of metal industry employees. *Pain*. 1993;53:89–94.

99. Von Korff M, Le Resche L, Dworkin SF. First onset of common pain symptoms: a prospective study of depression as a risk factor. *Pain*. 1993;55:251–258.

100. Fields HL. *Pain*. New York: McGraw-Hill; 1987.

101. Magni G. On the relationship between chronic pain and depression when there is no organic lesion. *Pain*. 1987; 31:1–21.

102. Boissevain MD, McCain GA. Toward an integrated understanding of fibromyalgia syndrome, I: medical and pathophysiological aspects. *Pain*. 1991;44:227–238.

103. Williams FH, Kaul MP. Fibromyalgia and myofascial pain. In: Lemoke D, Pattison J, Marshall L, Crowley D, eds. *Primary Care of Women*. Stanford, CT: Lange Publishers; 1995;348–359.

104. Wade JB, Price DD, Hamer RM, Schwartz SM, Hart RP. An emotional component analysis of chronic pain. *Pain*. 1990;40:303–310.

105. McCrakken LM, Zayfert C, Gross RT. The Pain Anxiety Symptoms Scale: development and validation of a scale to measure fear of pain. *Pain*. 1992;50:67–73.

106. Waddell G, Newton M, Henderson I, Somerville D, Main CJ. A fear-avoidance beliefs questionnaire (FABQ) and the role of fear-avoidance beliefs in chronic low back pain and disability. *Pain*. 1993;52:157–168.

107. Fey SG, Williamson-Kirkland TE. Chronic pain: psychology and rehabilitation. In: Caplan B, ed. *Rehabilitation Psychology Desk Reference*. Rockville, MD: Aspen Publishers; 1987;101–129.

108. Keefe FJ, Williams DA. Assessment of pain behaviors. In: Turk DC, Melzack R, eds. *Handbook of Pain Assessment*. New York: Guilford Press; 1992;275–294.

109. Waddell G, McCulloch JA, Kummel EG, et al. Nonorganic physical signs in low back pain. *Spine*. 1980;5:117–125.

110. Petersen M. Nonphysical factors that affect work hardening success: a retrospective study. *J Orthop Sports Phys Ther*. 1995;22(6):238–246.

111. Fey SG, Fordyce WE. Behavioral rehabilitation of the chronic pain patient. In: Pan EL, Backer TE, Vash CJ, eds. *Annual Review of Rehabilitation*. Vol 3. New York: Springer Publishing Co; 1983;32–63.

112. Fried R. *The Hyperventilation Syndrome*. Baltimore: Johns Hopkins University Press; 1987.

113. Harris V, Katlick E, Lick J, Habberfield T. Paced respiration as a technique for modification of autonomic responses to stress. *Psychophysiology*. 1976;13:386–391.

114. Janis I, Defares P, Grossman P. Hypervigilant reactions to threat. In: Selye H, ed. *Selye's Guide to Stress Research*. Vol 3. New York: Scientific and Academic Editions; 1983.

115. Middaugh SJ, Kee WG, Nicholson JA. Muscle overuse and posture as factors in the development and maintenance of chronic musculoskeletal pain. In: Grzesiak RC, Ciccone DS, eds. *Psychological Vulnerability to Chronic Pain*. New York: Springer Publishing Co; 1994;55–89.

116. Henry JP. Neuroendocrine patterns of emotional response. In: Plutchik R, Kellerman H, eds. *Emotion: Theory, Research and Practice*. Vol 3. Orlando, FL: Academic Press; 1986;37–60.

117. Panksepp J. The anatomy of emotions. In: Plutchik R, Kellerman H, eds. *Emotion: Theory, Research and Practice*. Vol 3. Orlando, FL: Academic Press; 1986;91–124.

118. Panksepp J, Sacks DS, Crepeau LJ, Abbott BB. The psycho- and neuro-biology of fear systems in the brain. In: Denny MR, ed. *Fear, Avoidance and Phobias: A Fundamental Analysis*. Hillsdale, NJ: Lawrence Erlbaum Associates; 1991;7–59.

119. Chapman CR. Mechanisms of pain: a basis for its emotional aspects. In: *Integrating Pain Management in the Rehabilitation Process: The Fourth Annual Northwest Regional Conference for Occupational Therapy and Physical Therapy*. Seattle, WA: University of Washington; 1993;2.1–2.13.

120. Selye H. *The Stress of Life*. New York: McGraw-Hill; 1978.

121. Jette AM. Physical disablement concepts for physical therapy research and practice. *Phys Ther*. 1994; 74:380–386.

122. Nagi S. Disability concepts revisited: Implications for prevention. In: Pope A, Tarlov A, eds. *Disability in America: Toward a National Agenda for Prevention*. Washington, DC: National Academy Press; 1991;309–327.

123. Bigos SJ, Battie MC, Spengler DM, et al. A prospective study on work perceptions and psychosocial factors affecting report of back injury. *Spine*. 1991;16:1–6.

124. Lancourt J, Kettelhut M. Predicting return to work for lower back pain patients receiving workers' compensation. *Spine*. 1992;17:629–638.

125. Waddell G. A new clinical model for the treatment of low-back pain. *Spine*. 1987;12:632–644.

126. Paulsen JS, Altmaier EM. The effects of perceived versus enacted social support on the discriminative cue function of spouses for pain behaviors. *Pain*. 1995;60:103–110.

127. Greenough CG, Fraser RD. The effects of compensation on recovery from low back injury. *Spine*. 1989;14:947–955.

128. Haddad G. Analysis of 2932 workers' compensation back injury cases. *Spine*. 1987;12:765–769.

129. Dworkin RH. Compensation in chronic pain patients: cause or consequence? *Pain*. 1991;43:387–388.

130. Ambrosius FM, Kremer AM, Herkner PB, Dekraker M, Bartz S. Outcome comparison of workers' compensation and noncompensation low back pain in a highly structured functional restoration program. *J Orthop Sports Phys Ther*. 1995; 21:7–12.

131. Gallagher RM, Raugh V, Haugh L, et al. Determinants of return to work in low back pain. *Pain*. 1989;39:55–68.

132. Carron H, DeGood DE, Tait R. A comparison of low back pain patients in the United States and New Zealand: psychosocial and economic factors affecting severity of disability. *Pain*. 1985;21:77–89.

133. Hanegan JL. Principles of nociception. In: Gersh MR, ed. *Electrotherapy in Rehabilitation*. Philadelphia: FA Davis; 1992;26–48.

134. Porterfield JA, DeRosa C. *Mechanical Neck Pain: Perspectives in Functional Anatomy*. Philadelphia: WB Saunders Co; 1995.

135. Wolf SL. Neurophysiologic mechanisms in pain modulation: relevance to TENS. In: Mannheimer JS, Lampe GN, eds. *Clinical Transcutaneous Electrical Nerve Stimulation*. Philadelphia: FA Davis; 1984;41–56.

136. Coderre TJ, Katz J, Vaccarino AL, Melzack R. Contribution of central neuroplasticity to pathological pain: review of clinical and experimental evidence. *Pain*. 1993;52:259–285.

137. Schwartzman RJ. Reflex sympathetic dystrophy. *Curr Opinion Neurol Neurosurg*. 1993;6:531–536.

138. Gunn CC. "Prespondylosis" and some pain syndromes following denervation supersensitivity. *Spine*. 1980;5:21–28.

139. Dotson R. Causalgia-reflex sympathetic dystrophy maintained pain: myth and reality. *Muscle Nerve*. 1993;16:1049–1055.

140. Van Houdenhove B, Vasquez G, Onghena P, et al. Etiopathogenesis of reflex sympathetic dystrophy: a review and biopsychosocial hypothesis. *Clin J Pain*. 1992;3:300–306.

141. Kramis RC, Roberts WJ, Gillette RG. Non-nociceptive aspects of persistent musculoskeletal pain. *J Orthop Sports Phys Ther*. 1996;24:255–267.

142. Perelman RB, Adler D, Humphreys M. Reflex sympathetic dystrophy: electronic thermography as an aid in diagnosis. *Ortho Rev*. 1987;16:561–566.

143. Roberts WJ. A hypothesis on the physiological basis for causalgia and related pains. *Pain*. 1986;24:297–311.

144. Selkowitz DM. The sympathetic nervous system in neuromotor function and dysfunction and pain: a brief review and discussion. *Funct Neurol*. 1992;7:89–95.

145. Korr IM. The spinal cord as organizer of disease processes, III: hyperactivity of sympathetic innervation as a common factor in disease. *J Am Osteopath Assoc*. 1979;79:232–249.

146. Woolf CJ. Evidence for a central component of postinjury pain hypersensitivity. *Nature*. 1983;306:686–688.

147. Dahl JB, Erichsen CJ, Fugslang-fredriksen A, Kehlet H. Pain sensation and nociceptive reflex excitability in surgical patients and human volunteers. *Br J Anaesth*. 1992;69:117–121.

148. Woolf CJ. Long term alterations in the excitability of the flexion reflex produced by peripheral tissue injury in the chronic decerebrate rat. *Pain*. 1984;18:325–343.

149. Woolf CJ, Wall PD. Relative effectiveness of C primary afferent fibers of different origins in evoking a prolonged facilitation of the flexion reflex in the rat. *J Neurosci*. 1986;6:1433–1442.

150. Wall PD, Woolf CJ. Muscle but not cutaneous C-afferent input produces prolonged increases in the excitability of the flexion reflex in the rat. *J Physiol (Lond)*. 1984;356:443–458.

151. Woolf CJ, McMahon SB. Injury-induced plasticity of the flexor reflex in chronic decerebrate rats. *Neuroscience*. 1985;16:395–404.

152. Hu JW, Yu X-M, Vernon H, Sessle BJ. Excitatory effects on neck and jaw muscle activity of inflammatory irritant applied to cervical paraspinal tissues. *Pain*. 1993;55:243–250.

153. Pedersen HS, Blunck CFJ, Gardner E. The anatomy of lumbosacral rami and meningeal branches of spinal nerves (sinu-vertebral nerves) with an experimental study. *J Bone Joint Surg Am*. 1956;38A:377–388.

154. Grieve GP. *Common Vertebral Joint Problems*. Edinburgh, Scotland: Churchill Livingstone; 1991.

155. Korr IM. Proprioceptors and somatic dysfunction. *J Am Osteopath Assoc*. 1975;74:638–650.

156. Kraus H. Muscle spasm. In: Kraus H, ed. *Diagnosis and Treatment of Muscle Pain*. Chicago: Quintessence Publishing Co; 1988;11–20.

157. Patterson MM. A model mechanism for spinal segmental facilitation. *J Am Osteopath Assoc*. 1976;76:121–131.

158. Wyke BD. Articular neurology—a review. *Physiotherapy*. 1972;3:94–99.

159. Wyke BD. The neurological basis of thoracic spinal pain. *Rheum Phys Med*. 1970;10:356–372.

160. Fischer AA, Chang CH. Electromyographic evidence of paraspinal muscle spasm during sleep in patients with low back pain. *Clin J Pain*. 1985;1:147–154.

161. Blockey NJ. An observation concerning the flexor muscles during recovery of function after dislocation of the elbow. *J Bone Joint Surg Am*. 1954;36-A:S33–S40.

162. de Andrade JR, Grant C, Dixon A. Joint distension and reflex muscle inhibition in the knee. *J Bone Joint Surg Am*. 1965;47-A:313–322.

163. Shakespeare DT, Stokes M, Sherman KP, Young A. Reflex inhibition of the quadriceps after meniscectomy: lack of association with pain. *Clin Physiol*. 1985;5:137–144.

164. Spencer JD, Hayes KC, Alexander J. Knee joint effusion and quadriceps reflex inhibition in man. *Arch Phys Med Rehabil*. 1984;65:171–177.

165. Stokes M, Young A. The contribution of reflex inhibition to arthrogenous muscle weakness. *Clin Sci*. 1984;67:7–14.

166. Swearingen RL, Dehne E. A study of pathological muscle function following injury to a joint. *J Bone Joint Surg Am.* 1964;46-A:1364–1369.

167. Kleinberg IJ, Greenfield BE, Wyke B. Contribution to the reflex control of mastication from mechanoreceptors in the temporomandibular joint capsule. *Dent Pract.* 1970;21:73–74.

168. Janda V. Muscles and cervicogenic pain syndromes. In: Grant R, ed. *Physical Therapy of the Cervical and Thoracic Spine.* New York: Churchill Livingstone; 1988;153–166.

169. Janda V. On the concept of postural muscles and posture in man. *Aust J Physiother.* 1983;29:83.

170. Janda V. Muscles, central nervous motor regulation and back problems. In: Korr IM, ed. *The Neurobiologic Mechanisms in Manipulative Therapy.* New York: Plenum Publishing; 1978;124–141.

171. Lewit K. *Manipulative Therapy in Rehabilitation of the Locomotor System.* London, England: Butterworths; 1985.

172. Taylor W. Dynamic EMG biofeedback in assessment and treatment using a neuromuscular re-education model: In: Cram JR, ed. *Clinical EMG for Surface Recordings.* Vol 2. Nevada City, CA: Clinical Resources; 1990;175–196.

173. Dolce JJ, Racynski JM. Neuromuscular activity and electromyography in painful backs: psychological and biomechanical models in assessment and treatment. *Psychol Bull.* 1985;97(3):502–520.

174. Nouwen A, Bush C. The relationship between paraspinal EMG and chronic low back pain. *Pain.* 1984;20:109–123.

175. Edgerton VR, Wolf SL, Levendowski DJ, Roy R. Theoretical basis for patterning EMG amplitudes to assess muscle dysfunction. *Med Sci Sports Exerc.* 1996;28:744–751.

176. Hagbarth KE. Microneurography and applications to issues of motor control: fifth annual Stuart Reiner Memorial Lecture. *Muscle Nerve.* 1993;16:693–705.

177. Bullock-Saxton JE. Local sensation changes and altered hip muscle control function following severe ankle sprain. *Phys Ther.* 1994;74:17–31.

178. Gauffin H, Pettersson Y, Tenger Y, Tropp H. Function testing in patients with old ruptures of the anterior cruciate ligament. *Int J Sports Med.* 1990;11:73–77.

179. Hutton RS, Atwater SW. Acute and chronic adaptations of muscle proprioceptors in responses to increased use. *Sports Med.* 1992;14:406–421.

180. Guyton AC. *Human Physiology and Mechanisms of Disease.* 3rd ed. Philadelphia: WB Saunders Co; 1982.

181. Hutton RS, Kaiya K, Suzuki S, Watanabe S. Post-contraction errors in human force production are reduced by muscle stretch. *J Physiol.* 1987;393:247–259.

182. Thompson S, Gregory JE, Proske U. Errors in force estimation can be explained by tendon organ desensitization. *Exp Brain Res.* 1990;79:365–372.

183. Flor H, Schugens MM, Birbaumer N. Discrimination of muscle tension in chronic pain patients and healthy controls. *Biofeedback Self Regul.* 1992;17:165–177.

184. Glaros AG. Awareness of physiological responding under stress and nonstress conditions in temporomandibular disorders. *Biofeedback Self Regul.* 1996; 21:261–272.

185. Schmidt RA. *Motor Control and Learning.* 2nd ed. Champaign, IL: Human Kinetics; 1988.

186. Feldman AG. Once more on the equilibrium point hypothesis (model) for motor control. *J Mot Behav.* 1986;18:17–54.

187. Latash ML. *Control of Human Movement.* Champaign, IL: Human Kinetics; 1993.

188. Milerad E, Ericson MO, Nisell R, Kilbom A. An electromyographic study of dental work. *Ergonomics.* 1991;34(7):953–962.

189. Winkel J, Westgaard RH. Occupational and individual risk factors for shoulder-neck complaints, Part II: the scientific basis (literature review) for the guide. *Int J Indust Ergo.* 1992;10:85–104.

190. Veiersted KB, Westgaard RH, Andersen P. Electromyographic evaluation of muscular work pattern as a predictor of trapezius myalgia. *Scand J Work Environ Health.* 1993;19:284–290.

191. Veiersted KB, Westgaard RH, Andersen P. Pattern of muscle activity during stereotyped work and its relation to muscle pain. *Int Arch Occup Environ Health.* 1990;62:3–41.

192. Veiersted KB. Sustained muscle tension as a risk factor for trapezius myalgia. In: Nielsen R, Jorgensen K, eds. *Advances in Industrial Ergonomics and Safety.* London, England: Taylor & Francis; 1993;15–19.

193. Gogia P, Sabbahi M. Median frequency of the myoelectric signal in cervical paraspinal muscles. *Arch Phys Med Rehabil.* 1990;71:408–414.

194. Klein AB, Snyder-Mackler L, Roy SH, De Luca CJ. Comparison of spinal mobility and isometric trunk extensor forces with electromyographic spectral analysis in identifying low back pain. *Phys Ther.* 1991;71:445–454.

195. Roy SH, De Luca CJ, Casavant DA. Lumbar muscle fatigue and chronic lower back pain. *Spine.* 1989; 14:992–1001.

196. Roy SH, De Luca CJ, Emley M, Bijs RJC. Spectral electromyographic assessment of back muscles in patients with low back pain undergoing rehabilitation. *Spine.* 1995;20:38–48.

197. Roy SH, De Luca CJ, Snyder-Mackler L, Emley MS, Crenshaw RL, Lyons JP. Fatigue, recovery, and low

back pain in elite varsity rowers. *Med Sci Sports Exerc.* 1990;22:463–469.

198. Ashton H. The effect of increased tissue pressure on blood flow. *Clin Orthop.* 1975;113:15–26.

199. Barcroft H, Millen JLE. The blood flow through muscle during sustained isometric contraction. *J Physiol.* 1939;97:17–31.

200. Hill AV. The pressure developed in muscle during contraction. *J Physiol.* 1948;107:518–526.

201. Reneman RS, Slaaf DW, Lindbloom L, Tangelder G, Arfors KE. Muscle blood flow disturbances produced by simultaneously elevated venous and total muscle pressure. *Microvasc Res.* 1980;20:307–318.

202. Hagberg M, Kvarnstrom S. Muscular endurance and electromyographic fatigue in myofascial shoulder pain. *Arch Phys Med Rehabil.* 1984;65:522–525.

203. Chaffin DB. Localized muscle fatigue-definition and measurement. *J Occup Med.* 1973;15:346–354.

204. Hagberg M. Electromyographic signs of shoulder fatigue in two elevated arm positions. *Am J Phys Med.* 1981;60:11–21.

205. Jorgenson K, Falletin N, Krogh-Lund C, Jensen B. Electromyography and fatigue during prolonged low-level static contractions. *Eur J Appl Physiol.* 1988; 57:316–321.

206. Voight ML, Hardin JA, Blackburn TA, Tippett S, Canner GC. The effects of muscle fatigue on the relationship of arm dominance to shoulder proprioception. *J Orthop Sports Phys Ther.* 1996;23:348–352.

207. Norkin CC, Levangie PK. *Joint Structure and Function: A Comprehensive Analysis.* Philadelphia: FA Davis; 1983.

208. Mow V, Resoenwasser M. Articular cartilage: biomechanics. In: Woo SLY, Buckwalter JA, eds. *Injury and Repair of Musculoskeletal Soft Tissues.* Park Ridge, IL: American Academy of Orthopaedic Surgeons; 1988; 427–463.

209. Kamkar A, Irrgang JJ, Whitney SL. Nonoperative management of secondary impingement syndrome. *J Orthop Sports Phys Ther.* 1993;17:212–224.

210. Kapandji IA. *The Physiology of the Joints, Volume One, Upper Limbs.* 5th ed. New York: Churchill Livingstone; 1982.

211. Nordin M, Frankel VH. *Basic Biomechanics of the Musculoskeletal System.* 2nd ed. Philadelphia: Lea & Febiger; 1989.

212. Frankel VH, Burstein AH, Brooks DB. Biomechanics of internal derangement of the knee. *J Bone Joint Surg Am.* 1971;53-A:945–963.

213. Gertzbein SD. Centrode patterns and segmental insta-bility in degenerative disc disease. *Spine.* 1985; 10:257–267.

214. White S, Sahrmann S. A movement system balance approach to management of musculoskeletal pain syndromes. In: Grant R, ed. *Clinics in Physical Therapy: Physical Therapy of the Cervical and Thoracic Spine.* 2nd ed. New York: Churchill Livingstone; 1994.

215. Williams PE, Goldspink G. Changes in sarcomere length and physiological properties in immobilized muscle. *J Anat.* 1978;127:459–468.

216. Shelton GL, Thigpen LK. Rehabilitation of patellofemoral dysfunction: a review of literature. *J Orthop Sports Phys Ther.* 1991;14:243–249.

217. Chaffin DB, Andersson GBJ. *Occupational Biomechanics.* 2nd ed. New York: John Wiley & Sons; 1991.

218. Linton SJ. Risk factors for neck and back pain in a working population in Sweden. *Work Stress.* 1990; 4:41–49.

219. Enwemeka C, Bonet I, Jayant A, et al. Postural correction in persons with neck pain, II: integrated electromyography of the upper trapezius in three simulated neck positions. *J Orthop Sports Phys Ther.* 1986; 8:240–242.

220. Schuldt K, Ekholm J, Harms-Ringdahl K, Nemeth G, Arborelius UP. Effects of changes in sitting work posture on static neck and shoulder muscle activity. *Ergonomics.* 1986;29:1525–1537.

221. Kraus S. Cervical spine influences on the craniomandibular region. In: Kraus S, ed. *TMJ Disorders: Management of the Craniomandibular Complex.* New York: Churchill Livingstone; 1988;367–404.

222. Ohlsson K, Attewell R, Skerfing S. Self-reported symptoms in the neck and upper limbs of female assembly workers: impact of length of employment, work pace, and selection. *Scand J Work Environ Health.* 1989;15:75–80.

223. Smith MJ, Cohen BGF, Stammerjohn JR, Happ A. An investigation of health complaints and job stress in video display operations. *Hum Factors.* 1981;23:387–400.

224. Hazard RG. Spine update functional restoration. *Spine.* 1995;20:2345–2348.

225. Hazard RG, Fenwick JW, Kalisch SM, et al. Functional restoration with behavioral support: a one-year prospective study of patients with chronic low back pain. *Spine.* 1989;14:157–161.

226. Jette, AM. Outcomes research: shifting the dominant research paradigm in physical therapy. *Phys Ther.* 1995;75:965–970.

CHAPTER 2

SEMG Assessment

This chapter will focus on an assessment scheme that can be applied to any case in which faulty patterns of muscle activity are suspected. Evaluation will be framed with a staged algorithm for patient classification. In addition, a series of surface electromyography (SEMG) profiles will be elaborated to characterize aberrant activity. These profiles are presented as a menu of choices for evaluation. In Chapter 5, a menu of SEMG feedback treatment techniques will be presented, and in Chapter 7, the two series will be linked together conceptually. Menu items that are most applicable to specific clinical problems will be extracted and set into practical sequences in Chapters 8–14. The same principles, however, apply no matter what the clinical problem or involved body area. Rather than a strict protocol approach, recurrent themes in evaluation and treatment will be emphasized.

In the discussion that follows, various screening procedures are proposed, but considerations other than those relating to setup of SEMG are largely omitted. This focus should not be taken to imply that SEMG stands alone as an evaluation or treatment modality. It does not. SEMG monitors muscle activity, activity that is used as a vehicle for emotional expression or posture and movement control (Figure 2–1). A rational interpretation of SEMG findings is not possible without an appreciation of potential psychologic and movement system deficiencies. Aberrant patterns of muscle activity are but one of many dimensions that contribute to chronic pain presentations. Therefore, SEMG should be inte-

grated into a comprehensive approach to patient management.

All patients should be assessed with a thorough intake and examination, if not by the SEMG practitioner, then by a close associate with whom information can be shared. Consider, for example, a patient with persistent neck pain and trapezius hyperactivity after a motor vehicle accident. Assume that this patient presents with a forward head posture, displays apparent anxiety regarding pain and perceived injury, and shows patterns of soft tissue tightness and intervertebral joint dysfunction on examination. The hyperactivity seen on the SEMG display could be attributed to psychologic issues, active tension, passive mechanical problems, or some combination thereof. Case management would proceed in different directions, depending on the particular causal agents. Sorting the factors would not be possible without a thorough evaluation.

The objectives of evaluation with SEMG are threefold:

1. To clarify aberrant patterns of muscle activity.
2. To define related physiologic and psychologic impairments.
3. To recognize how objectives 1 and 2 are linked together in preparation for treatment.

Treatment resources can then be selected to address the base musculoskeletal, neurophysiologic, or psychosocial dysfunction in a cost-ef-

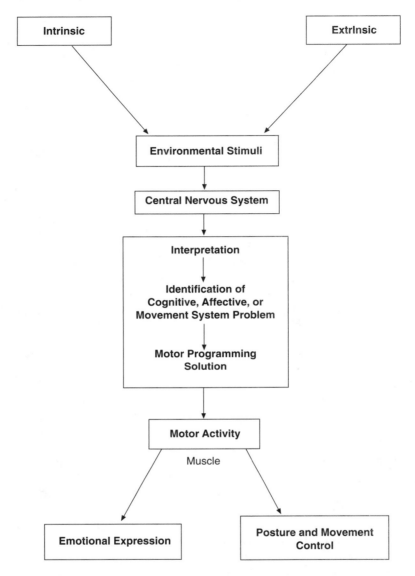

Figure 2–1 Schematic representation of the relationship of SEMG monitoring to environmental stimuli and functional motor activity.

fective manner that respects the needs of the total person.

Delitto and colleagues have proposed a three-level assessment scheme—aspects of which have been chosen as the model of this chapter—for therapists classifying patients with acute low back problems.[1]

LEVEL 1 ASSESSMENT

In the first level of assessment, Delitto and associates[1] propose that patients be screened for occult medical problems and psychologic dysfunction. Practitioners determine whether the patient is an appropriate candidate for therapeutic intervention and whether referral or additional consultation is indicated. The remaining two assessment levels stage the patient with respect to severity of problem and provide syndrome categorization for treatment. In this discussion, it is proposed that a level 1 assessment similar to that of Delitto and coworkers[1] be used with interdisciplinary SEMG interventions for chronic musculoskeletal pain, incorporated into a trilevel assessment model (Figure 2–2).

For the present purpose, level 1 assessment provides answers to the following questions:

1. Is evaluation with SEMG appropriate?
2. Is additional referral or consultation indicated?

3. Assuming evaluation with SEMG is indicated, should assessment proceed along psychophysiologic lines, kinesiologic lines, or both?

There should be some rational suggestion of inappropriate muscle activity before conducting a SEMG evaluation. In other words, not every patient with chronic pain requires intervention with SEMG. In Chapter 1, the case was made that chronic musculoskeletal pain is complex and multifactorial. If there is a low index of suspicion for neuromuscular involvement, then care resources are better directed elsewhere. Level 1 assessment is made on the basis of referral criteria, history and intake, physical ex-

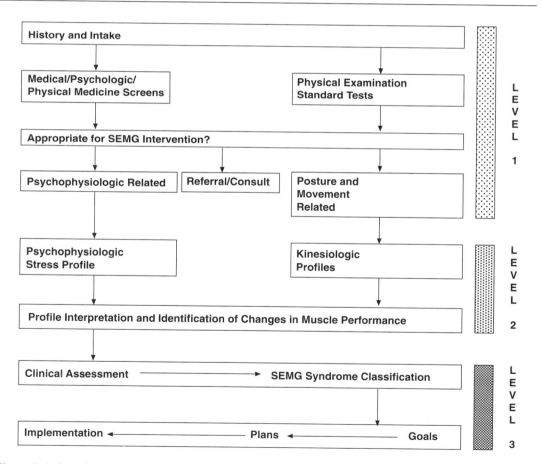

Figure 2–2 Overview of patient evaluation algorithm.

amination, and pencil and paper screening questionnaires.

SEMG evaluation is indicated if all of the following conditions exist:

1. There are clearly identifiable functional limitations and disability.
2. Neuromuscular impairments are suspected as contributory factors.
3. Serious medical or psychologic pathology is unlikely or is otherwise being addressed by an attending care provider.
4. Information regarding muscle activity is likely to contribute new insight into the case and have an impact on care planning.

Exhibits 2–1 and 2–2 summarize intake and examination considerations for any patient with chronic musculoskeletal pain. Of course, all interactions should be maintained within the boundaries of the operator's professional and legal scope of practice.

Screening for Neuromuscular Involvement

Suspicion of neuromuscular involvement is raised by a number of considerations (Exhibit 2–3). One factor is the patient's perception of chronic, pain-related muscle tension. Perception of tension may be described as a feeling of soft tissue tightness, pressure, or spasm, which acts as an antecedent to or accompanies the presenting symptoms. Another relevant complaint is abnormal posturing before or during symptom exacerbation. Included are anomalous head and trunk positions, jaw clenching, elevated shoulders, and protective limb guarding.

Evidence for an active tension problem also comes from the physical examination. A lesion in the contractile muscle–tendon–bony insertion unit is implied when active movement in a particular direction is restricted and painful, while passive movement in the same direction is full and painless and passive movement in the opposite direction is painful at end range.[2] The contractile lesion is confirmed by manual muscle testing, palpation, and other physical examination maneuvers. There may also be palpatory

Exhibit 2–1 Possible Intake Considerations for Patients with Complex Chronic Musculoskeletal Pain

- chief and secondary complaints
- location/distribution/pain drawing
- symptom character
- onset and course
- intensity: maximum/minimum/average; verbal "0–10/10" or rating instrument
- episodic/constant
- frequency/duration
- exacerbating/alleviating factors
- temporal patterns: day, week, month
- associated neurologic symptoms
- medical, systemic complaints
- previous consults/tests
- previous treatments
- medications
- past medical history
- family medical history
- exercise routines
- functional limitations
- response to activities of daily living
- work: work disability, work station, physical requirements, behavioral demands, interpersonal relationships
- recreational activities
- sleep: latency, awakenings, physical positions
- appetite/weight changes/energy levels
- dietary issues
- caffeine/alcohol/smoke/other
- major stressors
- family of origin psychosocial history
- present family dynamics/interpersonal stressors
- present family/friend support systems
- open claim/litigation
- feelings of depression, anxiety, fear, anger
- patient goals

findings of increased muscle tone, local tenderness, or trigger points.

Other clues are generated by observations of faulty kinematics. Kinematics refers to the pattern of displacement of body parts without regard for the forces that produce them. A clinician may notice a winging scapula during eccentric return from shoulder flexion, de-

Exhibit 2–2 Examination Considerations for Patients with Complex Chronic Musculoskeletal Pain

Presentation

- general appearance
- gait
- transfers/casual activity
- pain behaviors—verbal, nonverbal
- cooperation/apprehension

Psychologic Examination

- mental status examination
- affect
- thought—insight, judgment, memory, problem solving, content, impulsivity/planning, sequencing
- language and communication
- personality type
- somatic focus
- disability conviction
- psychometric testing

Physical Examination

- observation—height:weight, soft tissue bulk, swelling, skin
- structural examination—posture, alignment
- active range of motion—quantity, quality
- passive range of motion—quantity, quality, end feel
- accessory joint play, segmental mobility
- muscle length
- muscle accessory play/myofascial extensibility
- palpation—tenderness, texture, temperature, trigger points
- manual muscle tests; isokinetic and functional tests for strength, power, endurance
- neurologic examination—dermatomes, myotomes, reflexes, dural stretch
- special tests for ligamentous stability
- functional capacities simulations

Exhibit 2–3 Screening for Neuromuscular Involvement in Patients with Chronic Musculoskeletal Pain

- patient perception of chronic soft tissue tension, tightness, pressure, or spasm
- abnormal posturing before or during symptom exacerbation
- faulty kinematics
- guarding responses during active or passive range of motion, or functional activity
- replication of complaints with trigger point palpation
- palpable hypertonicity
- altered muscle length or fascial extensibility associated with strength/power deficits

evaluation is indicated by patterns of altered muscle length, or fascial extensibility, that are associated with weakness on manual muscle testing or deficits in the ability to sustain power during functional movements.

The reader is reminded that in this discussion persistent problems are being emphasized, which tend to be refractory to other conservative therapies. It is not being suggested that SEMG evaluation be instituted when simple exercise will do. Formal evaluation with SEMG is indicated for patients with hypertonicity, weakness, or muscle length–strength imbalances who have not responded to acute management. There also may be times when the clinician finds physical examination results that are suggestive of muscle dysfunction but are too subtle or too complex to meaningfully assemble. The SEMG record then acts as an extension of the practitioner's eyes and hands.

In addition, the clinician must discriminate between passive tightness and active tone when using palpatory findings. A shortened muscle will feel firm when it is palpated in a stretched position; that is, when all the passive slack has been removed. This is a different situation from firmness caused by active muscle contraction. The two conditions will impart to the practitioner a different kinesthetic feel in static positions and during passive range of motion testing. Thus clinicians who use palpatory findings to justify use of SEMG should be versed in basic physical ex-

creased lumbar intervertebral recruitment during trunk flexion, or inability to hold the pelvis level during unilateral stance. In each case, the related muscles could then be isolated and tested for length, strength, and neural integrity. SEMG

Exhibit 2–4 "Red Flags" Indicating Need for Consultation with Physician in Patients Presenting for Musculoskeletal Evaluation

- trauma
- failure of conservative therapy
- gross joint instability
- severe, unremitting spasm
- significant medical history of any type
- pain unrelated to movement, unremitting night pain
- fever, malaise, unusual fatigue, unexplained weight loss
- abdominal or groin pain
- menstrual irregularities, unusual genital discharge
- sexual dysfunction
- blood in stool or urine
- polyarthralgias, stiffness, dermatologic lesions
- cardiorespiratory distress or related pain
- receiving prescription medications
- over-the-counter or recreational drug abuse
- chronic headache
- visual disturbance, dizziness, balance dysfunction
- cognitive dysfunction
- urinary or bowel incontinence or retention
- radiating pain, parasthesia, numbness, abnormal reflex activity
- new or progressive weakness
- inability to reproduce/affect symptoms on physical examination
- inconsistencies on physical examination, copious pain behaviors
- vocational limitations
- positive medical screening questionnaire

amination methods. SEMG evaluation is not recommended just because muscles feel hard to the touch, nor is SEMG intervention advocated solely because there is apparent psychologic distress with pain. Before SEMG is initiated, there should be evidence of a coupling of reactive muscle tension with untoward affect and cognition.

Screening Need for Additional Consultation

The patient's responses to past medical history and current symptoms can be used to screen for the need for additional medical consultation. Exhibit 2–4 lists manifestations or "red flags" that indicate potentially serious underlying medical problems in patients presenting for musculoskeletal evaluation.[1,3–9] Positive findings on questioning or examination call for immediate review with a physician.

Exhibit 2–5 lists screening criteria for psychologic consultation. Apparent life stressors or psychologic distress can be probed with standardized evaluation instruments. A number of these tests have been used with chronic pain populations and are easy to administer.[10] If indicated, screening can be followed by consultation with a trained mental health practitioner. Formal evaluation and psychometric testing can clarify the best direction for treatment, which may or may not include SEMG feedback tracking.

Exhibit 2–6 lists screening criteria for physical dysfunction and disability. These can also be quantified with standardized questionnaires.[11–15] Functional screening instruments use patient self-report to assess the impact of perceived pain on activities of daily living and life roles. Chronic restrictions in the ability to perform specific physical tasks indicate referral to a therapist or physician trained in assessment of the musculoskeletal system and function. Physical medicine practitioners can help to create an integrated treatment plan to restore physical capacities for home, work, and recreation. Multidisciplinary team relationships are recommended, with referral criteria delineated for each member.

Psychophysiologic versus Kinesiologic Assessment with SEMG

The final step of the level 1 assessment is to decide whether the patient's suspected muscular involvement is due to psychophysiologic arousal versus kinesiologic dysfunction. Psychophysiologic arousal is the level of excitation in related cognitive, affective, and physiologic systems. For example, anxiety may be linked with tachycardia, hypertension, increased muscle tension, and a host of other changes associated with increased sympathetic nervous sys-

Exhibit 2–5 "Red Flags" Indicating Need for Consultation with Mental Health Practitioner Trained in Chronic Pain Management in Patients Presenting for Musculoskeletal Evaluation

---

- chronic sleep disturbance
- substance abuse
- major life stressors
- apparently poor coping
- family/work discord
- markedly depressed or aroused affect
- chronic alteration of appetite or energy levels
- inexplicable inconsistencies on physical examination during distraction, simulated loading
- copious pain behaviors in excess of those expected on basis of identifiable impairments
- nonanatomic pain, numbness, weakness
- abnormalities identified on cognitive/perceptual/affective screening questionnaires

---

Exhibit 2–6 "Red Flags" Indicating Need for Consultation with Physical Medicine Practitioner in Patients Presenting for Musculoskeletal Evaluation

---

- pain related to movement
- range of motion impairment
- restricted physical activities of daily living
- abnormalities identified on functional assessment screening questionnaire

---

tem tone.[16] The concern during SEMG evaluation is for elevations in muscle tension that are due to emotional stressors. Kinesiologic dysfunction is a direct abnormality of the movement system related to neuromuscular, myofascial, and biomechanical elements. Additional screening procedures can be used to determine which types of assessments are appropriate for an individual.

An obvious clue of psychophysiologic dysfunction is the patient's self-report of active muscle tension and symptom exacerbation linked to emotional arousal. Patients may describe a sense of spasm that is triggered in emotionally charged situations and followed by pain, most commonly about the head, neck, or shoulder girdle. Clinicians may observe an increase in guarding behavior, pressured speech, or pain complaint while discussing psychologic stressors with the patient. Subjects should be carefully questioned to identify when their symptoms become better or worse. If pain is regularly increased in a manner preceding, during, or following a particular social context, further exploration of psychosocial issues is warranted. The same is true if symptoms vary across the week, such as during the workweek compared with the weekend. The line of questioning should be funneled to separate potentially exacerbating physical factors from psychologic issues. A patient with exacerbation of symptoms at work might be questioned regarding time pressures, perceptions of self-efficacy, and relationships with co-workers. Physical work demands and ergonomic conditions would also be assessed. Any referral from a psychologic practitioner or positive finding on psychophysiologic screen should be followed with a psychophysiologic stress profile. Referral with confirmed musculoskeletal pathology, symptoms associated with specific physical tasks, or a positive finding on physical examination should be followed by kinesiological SEMG profiles. Exacerbating and alleviating situations are then reproduced as closely as possible during SEMG recording.

LEVEL 2 ASSESSMENT

During the level 2 assessment, specific factors that exacerbate or ameliorate aberrant patterns of muscle activity are identified. The results guide syndrome classification during the level 3 assessment, as well as development of a treatment plan. The level 2 assessment consists of options for detailed psychophysiologic stress profiling or kinesiologic profiling (or both). Level 2 assessment is summarized in Figure 2–3.

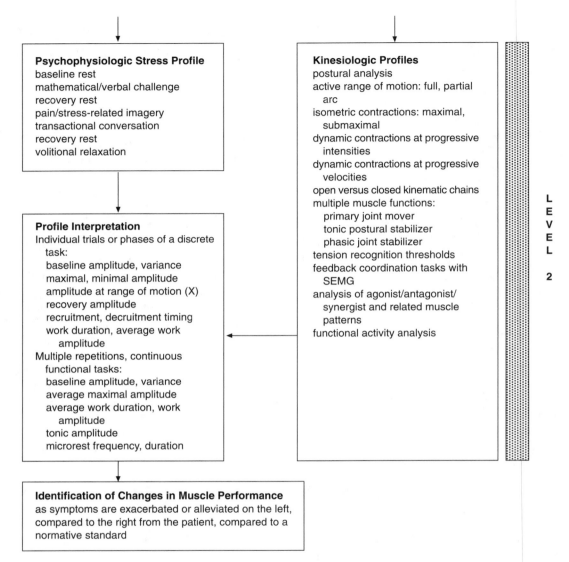

Figure 2–3 Summary representation of level 2 assessment.

Psychophysiologic Stress Profile

The psychophysiologic stress profile is recommended when arousal responses are thought to be contributory to the patient's complaints. SEMG electrodes can be placed according to a variety of schemes. The activity of muscles underlying the area of complaint should be monitored. Recordings may also be considered for muscles that are tense on palpation or in which trigger points or focal tender points are identified. Muscles in the involved body region that are shortened or for which there seems to be decreased myofascial extensibility may also be included. Alternatively, the static postural SEMG scanning procedure (see Chapters 5 and 6 of the companion book, *Introduction to Surface Electromyography*)[17] can be used to identify problem areas. If the number of potential recording sites exceeds the number of available SEMG channels, then priorities must be set or nonspecific placements must be used. Nonspecific placements are achieved by placing one of each of the active electrodes of a channel at the left and right side of the forehead, as well as at left and right temporalis, masseter, and upper trapezius muscles or forearm, respectively. One of the active electrodes of a single channel might also be located at the cervical paraspinal area, with its match placed over the center of the upper trapezius on the same side or perhaps at the cervical paraspinal region paired with the center of the forehead. (These generalized placements, along with specific placements, are detailed in Chapter 14 of the companion book.[17])

Specific placements are preferred when equipment allows. An elevated SEMG amplitude that is found with a nonspecific recording could be produced by one muscle, a few particular muscles, or a very diffuse arousal pattern. Clinically, it is most useful to relate abnormal profiles to individual muscles. This specificity contributes to precise documentation of evaluation results and facilitates efficient planning of treatment. If the problem lies in a muscle that can be reasonably isolated with surface electrodes, feedback training techniques can be used to facilitate focal proprioceptive awareness. Specific stretching exercises or postural correction may also be prescribed. Treatment is therefore matched to the peculiar needs of the patient, as opposed to using a "shotgun" approach and hoping for the best. If multiple muscles are found to be involved, a broad-based program is justified.

Psychophysiologic stress profiling is a common procedure, with different formats employed by clinical and research practitioners. The fundamental steps, however, are classic components of biofeedback evaluation,[18,19] and the following sequence is advocated in this book. Any type of display available with the practitioner's equipment is acceptable, based on operator preference. The suggested time frames are minimums; longer periods are preferred by some operators. See the box "Clinical Procedure— Psychophysiologic Stress Profile."

When used as a screening tool, interpretation of the psychophysiologic stress profile is relatively straightforward. The patient's baseline av-

erage may be compared with an expected range if standardized SEMG baseline values are available for the operator's equipment and recording setup. This might be characterized as a number of standard deviations above or below a control sample mean. During the stress challenge periods (steps 3 and 5), any subject's SEMG amplitude might increase. The increase, however, is expected to be a modest percentage of the baseline average. A complete recovery to baseline should occur within 1 to 2 minutes of the recovery period. Positive findings include an appreciable increase in SEMG amplitude during challenge periods and a prolonged failure to recover during rest periods. If the evaluation is computer assisted, the mean amplitude during each challenge period may be characterized as the number of standard deviations above or below the baseline mean for that subject. If recovery to baseline appears delayed after a stressor period, the rest period may be lengthened and the challenge repeated. Evidence that shows changes in SEMG activity that are time locked to specific challenge and rest periods is most meaningful.

The final period, step 7, is used to assess what relaxation skills the patient brings into training. If the patient successfully lowers his or her SEMG activity, and it is discovered that the subject has experience with a particular type of relaxation skill, the therapist will probably capitalize on that method during feedback training. Even if the patient is unable to lower SEMG activity, his or her remarks may provide clues as to what type of relaxation technique may be most suitable. For example, one patient may say, "I concentrated on my breathing and felt my muscles let go." Another might reply, "I visualized myself sitting by a peaceful pond on a beautiful summer's day." Still another might say, "I counted backward from 10 to 1 and then concentrated on stopping my self-talk." Relaxation training for these patients might be initiated with techniques that focus on kinesthetic sensations, imagery, or sequential intellectual processing, respectively. A sample psychophysiologic profile with positive findings is provided in Figure 2–4.

Clinical Procedure—Psychophysiologic Stress Profile

1. Prepare the subject by instructing him or her to sit comfortably, but symmetrically, in an upright chair. Explain the rationale for psychophysiologic monitoring and what the patient should expect to feel during the procedure. After consent has been obtained, attach the sensors. Prepare the equipment, with the display turned away from the patient.

2. Record baseline activity levels for 2 to 3 minutes. During this period, instruct the patient to sit quietly and try not to think about anything in particular. If the patient appears anxious regarding the procedure or electronic recording apparatus, answer any questions and provide reassurance. Assuming the results are stable, proceed to the first challenge period.

3. Ask the subject to perform difficult verbal and mathematical tasks for 2 to 3 minutes. Possibilities include counting backward from 1,000 by subtracting sevens, repeating three- to four-digit sequences in reverse order, saying the alphabet backward, spelling three- or four-letter words in reverse, or associating each letter of the alphabet with a word that begins with the same letter (eg, "A is for apple, B is for boy, C is for cat," etc). Have the patient perform the tasks aloud. Periodically coach the patient to think faster and speak louder. It is not necessary to check whether the answers are correct, as long as the patient is appropriately challenged. The selected tasks should be challenging but not so difficult that the patient becomes overwhelmed and gives up.

4. Instruct the patient to sit quietly for a 2- to 3-minute recovery period. Ask him or her to let go mentally of the previous exercises. Explain that you were simply monitoring physiologic responses to the challenging tasks and that the answers were not important.

5. Ask the patient to visualize a stressful situation for 3 to 5 minutes. Begin by instructing the patient to think of stressful circumstances related to the injury or symptoms or, more generally, a repetitive life stressor or "the most stressful thing that happened to you this week." Guide the patient to visualize explicitly the relevant environment. Include, for example, the color of the walls in the room, the furniture in the room, and the faces of any involved persons. Also guide imagery related to any sounds, smells, and kinesthetic sensations associated with the event. After about 2 minutes, ask the patient if he or she feels successful in constructing meaningful imagery. Then ask permission to discuss the patient's thoughts and feelings about the intended stressor. If it is within your scope of practice, conduct a brief transactional conversation to determine the subject's experiences.

6. Instruct the patient to let go mentally of the stressful image for a 2- to 3-minute recovery period. Again, ask the patient to sit comfortably without doing or thinking about anything in particular.

7. Ask the patient to use any technique desired to relax for 3 to 5 minutes, so long as he or she maintains a stable posture. At the end of the period, ask the subject what he or she did to try to relax.

The effects of mental arithmetic on forehead frontal SEMG activity are reliable across sessions in normal subjects.[20] However, the modulating effects of anxiety on SEMG responses vary in patient groups.[20-25] Anxiety is not universally associated with increased muscle activity. The psychophysiologic profile is designed to reveal an arousal muscle–tension relationship in individuals prone to such a response, when suitable test stimuli are provided.[26] Sandrini and coworkers[27] observed that algometric and frontal muscle SEMG measures were more impaired among patients with episodic tension-type headache than among control subjects or patients with

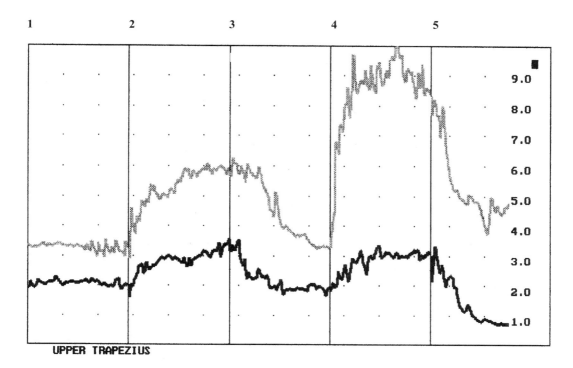

Figure 2–4 Psychophysiologic stress profile from a patient with right cervical paraspinal and suprascapular pain 4 months after motor vehicle accident. SEMG activity is shown from left (gray) and right (black) upper trapezius muscles during five consecutive recording periods. (**1**) Baseline, (**2**) Backward counting and reverse digit sequencing, (**3**) Recovery, no task, (**4**) Guided stressful imagery related to driving, (**5**) Recovery followed by volitional relaxation. Note increased right side baseline activity (**1**), increased right side activity during challenge (**2**, **4**), and increased duration of elevated activity (delayed baseline recovery) on right side during recovery (**3**,**5**).

migraine when all were subjected to mental arithmetic stressors. Flor and associates[28] used mental stressors to find increased lumbar paraspinal SEMG activity as well as a delayed return to baseline, in patients with chronic low back pain. The lumbar muscle responses were not observed in healthy control subjects, nor in patients with chronic pain problems at regions other than the low back. Further, aberrant muscle activity in patients with low back pain was not generalized to the frontalis; the effects were specific to the lumbar recording site. In subsequent work by Flor and colleagues,[29] patients with chronic low back or temporomandibular pain showed topographically related SEMG hyperreactivity associated with stressful imagery. Healthy control subjects did not demonstrate this type of SEMG hyperreactivity, nor a change in skin conductance levels. They did, however, experience a significant increase in heart rate.

Multiple measures of autonomic arousal provide a more robust assessment of psychophysiologic effects. Thus arousal responses should be routinely investigated with physiologic modalities in addition to SEMG. These modalities include recordings of skin temperature, electrodermographic activity, heart rate, photoplethysmographic activity, and respiratory patterns.[30–34]

A few other cautions should be kept in mind when the psychophysiologic stress profile is conducted. The operator must observe the patient as well as the SEMG display during the procedure. Shifts in posture or fidgeting may bring about spurious changes in SEMG scores. The test is intended to provoke SEMG changes coupled with cognitions and emotion, not with movement.

This procedure rarely provokes frank emotional upset. If a subject becomes overtly distressed or serious psychologic issues are suspected, appropriate counseling must be provided. Steps should be taken for timely consultation with a licensed mental health practitioner, if not already in progress. (Additional discussion pertaining to stress-profiling methods, reliability, and interpretation of results, can be found in Chapter 7 of the companion publication.[17])

Kinesiologic Profiles

The kinesiologic profiles are a series of procedures designed to characterize muscle function under different movement circumstances. Inherently, they have nothing to do with SEMG. The profiles are used to gain specificity in the evaluation; that is, to identify the conditions under which motor control is faulty and when it is not. Target muscles are selected for monitoring on the basis of symptom location, musculoskeletal impairments identified on physical examination, and the practitioner's working hypothesis of the underlying abnormality. The lumbar paraspinal muscles would be an obvious recording choice for a patient who has low back pain. Additional recording channels also could be of interest. For example, the abdominal, hamstring, or gluteal muscles might be selected if tightness, weakness, or trigger points were identified at those locations on physical examination. SEMG would then be used to assess how those muscles work together during purposeful movements.

Activity of the target muscles is monitored during assumption of various postures, volitional contractions, and functional activities. The list of kinesiologic procedures should be thought of as a catalog of options. It is not necessary to perform all procedures. For any particular patient, the clinician may scan the roster (see Figure 2–3), select the techniques that are relevant for the case at hand, and leave the others. Tasks are selected on the basis of the involved body region and what types of movements make the symptoms better or worse. Activities that match the elements of the physical examination

that reproduce, exacerbate, or alleviate symptoms are specifically included.

Oftentimes, multiple muscles that are spatially adjacent or partially covered by other layers of muscles are selected for recording. Powerful contractions may be called for during profiling. Hence, volume conduction of SEMG activity may be a major concern. Without the ability to isolate the activity of a particular muscle or muscle group, the assessment will be meaningless. The kinesiologic profiles therefore require meticulous attention to recording technique. Electrode placements must be exacting and almost always applied with a close bipolar arrangement parallel to muscle fiber direction. Miniature electrodes may be required for smaller muscles. A frequency bandpass filter with a low cutoff in the range of 20 to 25 Hz is generally recommended. (Additional considerations for isolated recording technique and instrumentation are described in Chapters 3 and 4 of the companion book.[17]) See the box "Clinical Procedure—Preliminary Instructions for Kinesiologic Profiles."

The preliminary recording period is used to ensure a stable signal with minimal noise, as well as to gauge baseline levels of muscle activity for comparisons that follow. During the profiles, a minimum of five to six repetitions should be performed for discrete test tasks. The initial two repetitions may be discarded, and key parameters can be averaged over the remaining trials. A prolonged postural hold time or many repetitions of a task may be required to replicate real-life conditions and reproduce symptoms.

**Interpretation of the Kinesiologic Profiles—
General Principles**

Interpretation of the kinesiologic profiles is made on the basis of several variables (see Figure 2–3). Individual repetitions of a discrete task (one of relatively short duration that has easily definable starting and ending points, such as a trial of shoulder flexion active range of motion) can be inspected. The effects of multiple repetitions of a discrete movement or a continuous functional task can also be examined.

Clinical Procedure—Preliminary Instructions for Kinesiologic Profiles

1. Begin by explaining to the patient the rationale for monitoring with SEMG and what he or she should expect to feel during the procedures.
2. After consent has been obtained, apply the electrodes over the target muscle(s).
3. Select a visual display that combines a continuous digital readout with moving line tracings as the ideal for evaluation. Bar graphs are adequate for most procedures if line tracings are not available. Use a raw visual or audio display to discriminate subtle movement artifacts. Select a full wave rectified display, with the signals overlaid, to ease timing and amplitude comparisons.
4. Document the average SEMG amplitude during a 30- to 60-second baseline period in quiet sitting or standing position, along with some indication of signal stability. This can be a qualitative statement based on visual observation of the signal, or better, a statistical measure of variance if the SEMG device is computer assisted.

For single trials, baseline amplitude and variance are noted, as are maximal amplitude, minimal amplitude (if evaluating relaxation ability), and recovery amplitude on movement cessation (Figure 2–5). Desirable baseline, maximal, and minimal amplitude levels will vary with the specific task and recording setup. (Additional guidelines are provided where relevant in the remaining sections of this book, as well as in the companion book, *Introduction to Surface Electromyography*.[17])

For general purposes with current commercial equipment, satisfactory baseline recovery is operationally defined (with a smoothing time constant of 0.1 second or less) as a return to a SEMG amplitude within two standard deviations of the original baseline mean, within 3 seconds of movement cessation, and maintenance within that amplitude range for at least 30 seconds or until the next movement is initiated. Recovery may be characterized by the latency to achieve this amplitude criterion. More simply, the amplitude percentage of baseline observed 1 to 3 seconds after movement termination can be identified. Any amplitude deflection that is stereotypically reproduced at a particular point in the range of motion arc is also documented. In addition, the recruitment rise from baseline and the decruitment fall back to baseline are observed. These timing features may be qualitatively assessed as smooth and well timed, or

quantified in various ways with computer processing, for example, as the time from baseline to peak or with average slope calculations. Finally, if the task is associated with a discrete recruitment rise from a stable baseline and a discrete decruitment fall to the same baseline, the work duration and average work amplitude may be of interest. Duration can be quantified as the time between onset (the point at which the amplitude rises to a value 2 standard deviations above the baseline mean) and recovery (amplitude recovery within 2 standard deviations of the baseline mean). Any procedure that generates positive findings may be repeated with the subject in a non–weight-bearing position to assess whether the aberrant pattern is replicated when mechanical load is minimized.

The same variables can be averaged for assessment across multiple repetitions of task performance. In addition, the tonic amplitude and the presence, duration, and relative frequency of low amplitude gaps or microrests may be examined. Employment tasks (for example, repeated trials of an assembly line task or a continuous keyboard typing assignment) are most often studied with these latter measures. Both the tonic amplitude and presence of microrests can be determined by visual inspection of a rectified moving line tracing with a smoothing time constant of 0.1 second or less, SEMG sampling at 100 Hz or faster, and a frequency bandwidth fil-

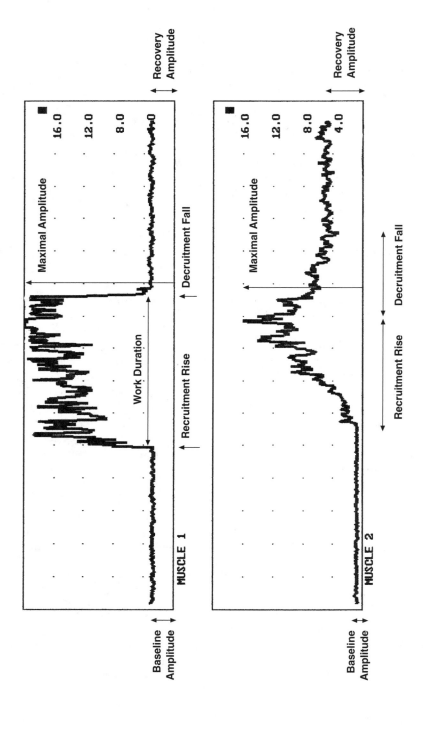

Figure 2–5 SEMG tracings of two muscle contractions, illustrating common assessment parameters.

ter low cutoff of 25 Hz or less. The tonic amplitude appears as the amplitude from which a muscle is phasically activated during repeated trials of a discrete movement (Figure 2–6). Essentially, the tonic amplitude can be thought of as the average intertrial amplitude, a "running baseline." The tonic amplitude represents the approximate minimal level of muscle activity during the work period.

A similar but more sophisticated concept is the static level, the SEMG amplitude above which there is a 0.9 probability of finding individual microvolt samples during the recording period.[35–38] In other words, only a small percentage of the total task time is spent below the static level. A high static level may imply that a muscle has insufficient opportunity for rest. When calibrated to force recordings and represented as a percentage of maximal volitional isometric contraction (%MVIC), higher static muscle load has been associated retrospectively and prospectively with upper quadrant musculoskeletal complaints.[39–41] SEMG amplitude and frequency spectral changes and other physiologic indexes of fatigue have been reported with 5% to 10% MVIC sustained for 1 hour,[42,43] and 2% to 5% MVIC has been recommended as acceptable static level limits.[38,44] As most clinicians currently do not have the means to calculate static levels as discussed above, and the static level will vary with the individual subject, specific task, electrode configuration, sampling rate, frequency bandwidth filter low cutoff, and smoothing time constant or integration time, the tonic amplitude proposed here serves as a practical compromise. With a satisfactory, low noise commercial recording setup, an acceptable tonic amplitude is operationally defined as less than a 5% to 10% MVIC amplitude range for tasks that are functionally performed for about 1 hour or longer. This definition, as well as that for satisfactory baseline recovery described previously, appears physiologically and clinically reasonable but has not been subjected to the formal scrutiny that other SEMG parameters have received.

The tonic amplitude is noted initially and every 2 to 3 minutes of task performance thereafter until symptoms are reproduced or exacerbated.

Values for the tonic amplitude are monitored over time to assess whether a significant rise is produced and associated with a change in symptoms. Left and right sides are compared if the functional task involves symmetric movements and the patient has involvement unilaterally. A representative screen sweep at indicated time intervals or, even better, the entire session should be saved to enable retrospective analysis. Many commercial devices save only maximal, minimal, average, and standard deviation statistics. Because of uncontrolled differences in subject movement across trials, potential influences of fatigue on the SEMG amplitude, and inherent variability, these statistics will not be of any help with this type of analysis. The clinician may therefore wish to estimate the tonic amplitude level visually at each assessment epoch or, if feasible, print hard copies of representative screen sweeps without interrupting the patient.

A microrest is a short pause in muscle activity (approximately 0.2–20 seconds). Short microrests are seen as low amplitude gaps in the SEMG tracing during uninterrupted performance of a continuous task.[40,41] Short pauses are naturally produced with transient muscle relaxation during a task routine. Longer pauses can be consciously planned or relatively automatic during respites in a work process.[45] A lack of both long and short pauses has been associated with musculoskeletal problems in work settings.

The microrest frequency is found by setting a visible threshold marker at a microvolt value of about 5% MVIC (Figure 2–7). A threshold value of two standard deviations above the initial baseline might be used if reliable maximal contractions are unattainable. If the patient's postural baseline range exceeds 5% MVIC, the assessment should be deferred. With suitable precautions for patient safety, task performance is maintained until the patient reports reproduction or exacerbation of symptoms. A tracing of the entire session is ideally saved for off-line analysis. Otherwise, a 30- to 60-second representative display sweep is frozen and quickly analyzed (or a hard copy is printed) without patient interruption at the start and every 2 to 3 minutes of task performance. Each threshold crossing is counted as one

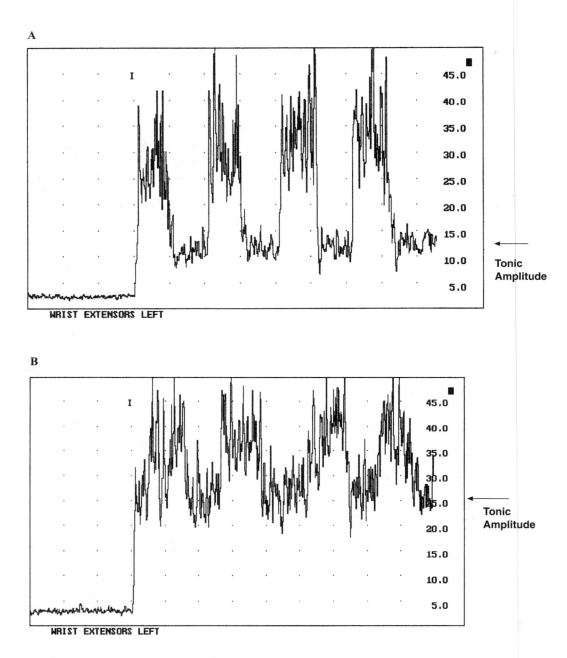

Figure 2–6 SEMG tracings of wrist extensor activity during four repletions of an industrial task. (**I**) denotes initiation of the trials from complete rest. (**A**) Activity in a healthy subject. (**B**) Activity in a worker with chronic lateral epicondylitis. Note the higher tonic amplitude in **B** compared with **A**. The tonic amplitude in **A** is less than 5% of the subject's maximal volitional isometric contraction amplitude (not shown), whereas that of **B** exceeds 22% of that person's maximum. On the basis of these tracings, it is presumed that the total work of the wrist extensors shown in **B** is greater (despite that peak activity of the two subjects is within 10% of respective maximal values), with inadequate opportunities for muscle rest when the pattern is repeated over a work shift.

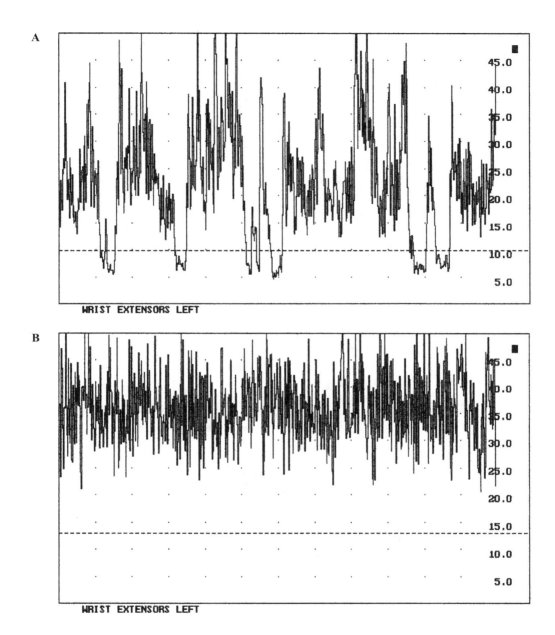

Figure 2–7 SEMG tracings of wrist extensor activity during a computer keyboard task performed by two persons. Subjects were required to scan a form, perform simple mental mathematical computations, and enter data onto a new computer spreadsheet. Dashed lines represent 5% of maximal volitional isometric contraction amplitude for each subject. (**A**) Activity from a healthy subject. (**B**) Activity from a worker with chronic wrist pain and diagnosis of carpal tunnel syndrome. Both subjects spontaneously paused keyboarding at irregular intervals to scan the form or perform mental calculations. The pauses are apparent in **A**, corresponding to the low amplitude gaps. No low amplitude periods are seen in **B**, indicating a lack of interspersed microrests, which might contribute to overuse syndromes if repeated over the work day.

microrest. The typical microrest duration for each epoch is also assessed, either visually estimated or calculated by a computer.

Values for the relative microrest frequency and duration are monitored over time to assess whether significant changes are produced and associated with reproduction or exacerbation of symptoms. Left and right sides are compared if the functional task involves symmetric movements and the patient has involvement unilaterally. This method of microrest assessment is again a practical, operational compromise for clinicians. Assessment of microrests is best accomplished with SEMG devices with high temporal resolution and sophisticated processing. Microrest counts can vary because of the same variables that affect determination of a tonic amplitude. It is impossible to state an absolute microrest frequency that should be produced in all circumstances.

A patient who manifests cumulative work injury may show a decreased microrest frequency and duration or an increased tonic amplitude (or both) as the problematic task is continued. Also, the average SEMG amplitude and variance may increase. Recruitment and decruitment timing may become less discrete across repetitions, and recovery to baseline with task cessation may become delayed across task bouts.

Other options become available with advanced software and hardware. Included are amplitude probability distributions (Figure 2–8) and frequency spectral analyses (Figure 2–9), both of which are regarded as specialized procedures. (See Chapters 3 and 8 in the companion book.[17]) Conventional interpretation is made on the basis of factors in the amplitude (usually root mean square or integral average methods) and time domains. For a given phase of movement, the activity of a particular muscle may show insufficient or excessive magnitude, delayed or premature recruitment, as well as insufficient or excessive duration.[46]

Normalized Comparisons with SEMG

As described above, amplitude and timing comparisons are made across different movement phases for the same muscle. The activity of one muscle also is compared with that of its contralateral homologue. During unilateral movements of the extremities, as well as during side-bending and rotation movements of the spine, similar levels of left-right coactivation are often considered aberrant. Motor activity is expected to be simultaneously symmetric for bilateral simultaneous symmetric movements (eg, bilateral symmetric shoulder flexion). Reciprocally symmetric SEMG patterns are expected for reciprocally symmetric movements (eg, left shoulder flexion followed by right shoulder flexion through an equivalent range of motion excursion).

Asymmetry is most often quantified as percent difference in peak activity produced during a task. Several methods of calculation are possible. Assume peak activity for some test averages 20 microvolts on the left and 40 microvolts on the right. The left side score can simply be divided by the right side score and multiplied by 100, such as $20/40 \times 100 = 50\%$. If the scores were reversed, the equation would yield $40/20 \times 100 = 200\%$. A simple way to deal with the discrepancy is to subtract whichever score is lower from whichever score is higher (or the absolute value of the difference between the scores) and then divide by the higher score and multiply the quotient by 100. For the previous example, the equation would yield $[(40 - 20)/40] \times 100 = 50\%$, regardless of whether the left or the right side happens to be greater. Calculated in this way, asymmetry exceeding a range of 20% to 35% has been reported experimentally to be of significance from upper trapezius, thoracic, and lumbar paraspinal recording sites.[47,48]

Further comparisons can be made among the activity of agonists, antagonists, and synergists. Because of potential differences in recording setup, impedance, muscle cross-sectional area, and numerous other factors, SEMG values are typically normalized for comparisons between different muscles.[39,46,49–55] (See Chapter 3 of the companion book.[17]) A relatively straightforward normalization method for clinicians is to convert raw SEMG scores to a percent MVIC score. First, a standardized isometric position is identi-

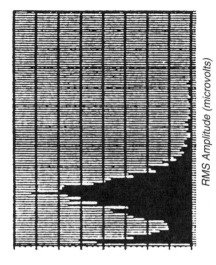

B

No. of ½-second intervals spent at given
EMG level during 10-minute task

RMS Amplitude (microvolts)

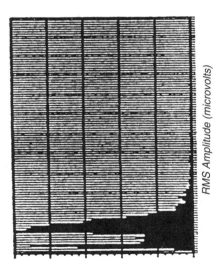

A

No. of ½-second intervals spent at given
EMG level during 10-minute task

RMS Amplitude (microvolts)

Figure 2–8 Sample amplitude probability distributions. SEMG activity was averaged over 0.5 second epochs for a total of 10 minutes of a typing task from left (**A**) and right (**B**) upper trapezii of a subject with right side neck pain. The plots represent the relative proportion (Y axis) that each average EMG value (X axis) was observed. (**A**) Amplitude probability distribution from nonpainful left side. (**B**) Amplitude probability distribution from painful right side. Lower amplitude values are seen less frequently, and higher amplitude values more frequently, on the right side compared with the left side. On the whole, there appears to be fewer opportunities for muscle rest on the right. Courtesy of Dr. Will Taylor, Blue Hills, Maine.

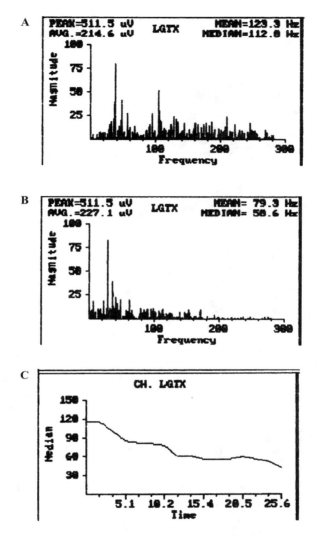

Figure 2–9 An illustration of the compression of the SEMG frequency spectrum associated with muscle fatigue. Frequency analyses were derived from signals recorded from the wrist extensor group at (**A**) the start and (**B**) near the end of a high intensity isometric contraction. The progressive shift in median frequency versus contraction time is illustrated in (**C**). Increased frequency shifts or delayed return to initial frequencies after designated rest periods can be indicative of impaired resistance to fatigue.

fied (eg, the manual muscle test position[56,57] for the desired muscle). Maximal isometric resistance is applied for a defined period, such as 6 seconds. SEMG activity is then averaged over the middle 2 seconds and averaged again over 3 trials. This mean becomes the normalization reference value for the muscle. Next, the movement task of clinical interest is performed, and an average or peak score is obtained—also averaged across three trials. The clinical task mean is divided by the MVIC mean and multiplied by 100 to complete the calculation.

Consider as an example comparison of function in quadriceps and hamstring muscles. The clinical objective is to assess the degree of co-contraction during a squat maneuver in a patient undergoing rehabilitation after a ligament injury. The normalization procedure is illustrated in Table 2–1. Maximal effort contractions are performed for quadriceps and then hamstring muscles. Data are subsequently collected for both quadriceps and hamstring muscles during the same squat maneuver. SEMG scores obtained during the squats are converted to %MVIC scores for the quadriceps and the hamstrings, respectively. Once expressed as %MVIC, SEMG activity can be compared across recording sites, across patients, or to a published standard. A ratio of the %MVIC of one muscle to the %MVIC of another may be constructed as a measure of the relative recruitment of the two during a particular task. Each muscle's MVIC reference value may be different over time, and the full procedure should be repeated on follow-up testing.

This normalization method is only appropriate if the patient can reliably produce a maximal effort contraction. If he or she is unwilling to do so, another method must be found. Normalizing as %MVIC is also inappropriate when a motor control fault is suspected of biasing the maximal contractions.[58] There may be times when the patient is motivated to provide maximal voluntary effort but neurophysiologic inhibition limits recruitment. A true motor problem could be masked if muscle activity is aberrant for the normalizing reference contraction and the clinical test contraction in the same way. Numerous other approaches to normalization can be found.

Activity during a dynamic task of interest could be expressed as a percentage of the activity displayed in any other controlled static posture. For a clinical stair-stepping task, the normalization reference value could be obtained from the quadriceps while the patient isometrically holds 60 degrees of squat, with a scale under each foot to ensure a constant level of weight bearing. The patient's average quadriceps score during the stepping task would be divided by his or her average score during the 60-degree squat, and the resulting quotient would be multiplied by 100. Hence activity during stair stepping would be expressed as the percentage of 60-degree isometric squat score. Activity for the quadriceps could then be compared with that of another muscle or the quadriceps in another subject. Upper trapezius activity during typing could be normalized to a reference value obtained while maintaining 90 degrees of shoulder

Table 2–1 Sample Normalization to Percentage of Maximal Volitional Isometric Contraction (MVIC)

Muscles	Maximal Effort Test Position	Maximal Effort SEMG Scores, Trials 1–3	Average Maximal Effort EMG	Squat Peak SEMG Scores, Trials 1–3	Average Squat Peak EMG	MVIC
Quadriceps	Seated isometric knee extension	94 μV 100 μV 106 μV	100 μV	22 μV 18 μV 20 μV	20 μV	20%
Hamstrings	Prone isometric knee flexion	55 μV 45 μV 50 μV	50 μV	5 μV 4 μV 6 μV	5 μV	10%

Normalized quadriceps:hamstrings ratio = 2:1

Note: SEMG scores are hypothetic microvolt amplitudes. %MVIC = (average squat/average maximum) × 100.

abduction. The patient's average typing amplitude would be divided by his or her average abduction hold amplitude, with the resulting quotient multiplied by 100. Muscle activity during typing would then be expressed as a percentage of isometric abduction activity. Lumbar musculature could be addressed by positioning a patient prone with pelvic support and lower extremity straps and no chest support. A reference value would be derived while isometrically maintaining a horizontal trunk position (monitoring with an inclinometer) against gravity. A lumbar activity score during a functional lifting task would then be divided by the prone isometric reference score, with the resulting quotient multiplied by 100.

The examples are identical to the procedure for normalization to MVIC, simply with a lower intensity contraction. The important point is that individual site differences need to be accounted for before comparing one muscle in one person with anything other than itself. Effects due to variations in electrode placement, adipose tissue, and muscle geometry hopefully are neutralized by the normalization process. A measure of relative recruitment intensity is generated, which can be applied to other recording sites and persons. It should be obvious, though, that these and like procedures are not suitable for all patients. The contractions can be difficult to standardize, and the alternatives tend to be complex for the typical clinician to perform.

Experimental results are sometimes reported by using normalization to submaximal contraction levels, standardized with a dynamometer. Here, a MVIC is generated and force is measured. Typically 30% or 50% of that force level is then calculated. Force feedback is provided to the patient, who isometrically maintains the target force level for a set time. SEMG activity is measured during this interval, and the average amplitude becomes the normalization reference value for SEMG data collection during a subsequent, purposeful movement. An unencumbered MVIC is again required with this method but the process can yield greater end reliability. Clinicians can implement this method by using a hand-held dynamometer designed to complement manual muscle strength testing, or a dynamometer associated with isokinetic apparatus, set to an isometric mode.

Simpler variations on this theme can be performed with an exercise weight system. The maximum load that can be moved through a set range of motion arc by using the target muscle in one repetition—or perhaps 10 repetitions—is identified. Alternatively, the patient's body weight is measured. Some percentage of body weight, the one-repetition maximal lift, or the 10-repetition maximal lift, is calculated. The patient then isometrically holds this load at a recorded joint angle in a position that can be easily replicated, and the reference SEMG value is determined. The SEMG average value obtained during a clinical test is divided by the reference value, with the quotient multiplied by 100 to complete the normalization process. Although this method does not require an expensive dynamometer, exercise equipment, extra time, and additional skill are needed.

Another set of techniques relates to creating an ensemble average of SEMG amplitude obtained over multiple trials of a movement task. The movement task must have definable starting and ending points and, often, specific phases in each cycle. SEMG activity is continuously recorded throughout the cycle, and by matching the start/end/phase points over each trial, an average SEMG pattern is generated from the ensemble of trials. Gait, bicycling, and repeated shoulder abduction movements are studied in this way. The mean SEMG amplitude during an ensemble phase of clinical interest is expressed as a percentage of the ensemble peak, as a percentage of the ensemble average of a different phase, or as a percentage of the ensemble average value for the entire movement. Sophisticated computerized kinematic measurement systems must be synchronized to SEMG recordings to apply this technique with precision.

SEMG quantification and normalization are difficult areas for clinicians. The methods can be confusing, and the procedures are always imperfect and take up valuable time. Nevertheless, interpretation of SEMG literature is compromised without at least a superficial awareness of the issues. Meaningful clinical comparisons are often made within subjects (eg, from involved to uninvolved side or pretreatment versus posttreatment) and tied to other objective measures and changes in functional performance. Clinicians may reasonably be expected to calculate percentages of asymmetry, MVIC, or a standardized submaximal reference contraction. If this is not feasible, most clinicians will either have to refrain from cross-site and cross-subjects recording comparisons or reconcile the use of nonnormalized data. Practitioners may decide that nonnormalized data are valid and reliable for some particular evaluation process. The problem is that nonnormalized comparisons can be less reliable in many circumstances, and operators may fall prey to faulty clinical judgments. If the range of variation is very large in healthy populations, it becomes difficult to distinguish correctly between healthy persons and those with musculoskeletal abnormalities. By avoiding cross-site and cross-subject comparisons, the clinician eliminates the need for such calculations. SEMG activity from each site is separately compared across movements. The majority of kinesiologic profiles are developed in this way. Computation of asymmetry and MVIC percentages allows for full interpretation with the other profiles.

Procedures for Profiles

The 11 kinesiologic profiles are discussed roughly in the order that they would be considered in an evaluation session. However, the sequence may be regarded as fluid and should be prioritized for the most relevant procedures in each case.

1. Postural Analysis

Static postural assessments have been a popular vehicle for clinical and experimental studies with SEMG. Testing is relatively quick and simple. Several investigators have used postural assessments and SEMG to characterize patients

with chronic pain problems or to distinguish patients from healthy control subjects.[59–62] Others have failed to find consistent SEMG differences between patients with chronic pain and control subjects.[63,64] The controversy probably exists because there have been few rigorous attempts to control patient sampling for differential pain etiologies. It seems reasonable that static postural factors are important for some patients with headache or neck or low back pain, but that the cause lies elsewhere for many others. In fact, posturally based SEMG changes vary with the type of mechanical low back pain diagnosis.[59,65] Even when there are no differences between patients with low back pain and control subjects in static posture, differences may be identified during dynamic movement tasks.[66] Therefore assessment with postural SEMG may be useful in patient classification and treatment planning, but evaluation should not be limited to such. Postural profiling should be considered a priority if the problem includes axial body pain and posture is noted to be faulty during the history intake and physical examination (level 1 assessment). Postural profiling is also indicated when symptoms are exacerbated during functional activities performed in sustained sitting or standing positions, or when symptoms cumulatively increase throughout the work day. See the box "Clinical Procedure—Postural Analysis."

It is recommended that postural assessments with SEMG be linked to visual observations of patient alignment. Simple, reliable methods of postural measurement are available.[67] A flexible ruler can be used to document spinal curves[68] and changes in alignment associated with changes in SEMG activity. In their classic book, Kendall and associates[57] discuss structural alignment as it relates to postural muscle length–strength balance. They define several postural types, how each deviates relative to ideal postural plumb lines, and which muscles are likely to be changed in length in each case. Adaptive changes in length are probably both a cause and effect of faulty postures. For example, a forward head, protracted shoulder girdle posture tends to be accompanied by shortness at the suboccipital re-

---

Clinical Procedure—Postural Analysis

1. Ask the patient to assume his or her spontaneous sitting and standing postures. For standing tests, have the patient bear equal weight with each foot placed on a separate, standard bathroom scale.
2. Comparisons are made within a single muscle site across postures and for symmetry between the left and right muscles of homologous pairs.
3. Aberrant activity observed in one position but not in others is posturally related.
4. Databases constructed from standardized recording and assessment protocols are available for some commercial brands of SEMG devices.
5. If SEMG activity appears elevated or asymmetric, experiment with postural adjustments to see whether changes can be induced. For asymmetries recorded for standing postures, instruct the subject to correct a weight-bearing asymmetry or a lateral trunk shift. Try placing a small platform or book under the short leg in an apparent leg length discrepancy, so that the iliac crests are leveled. When forward head, protracted shoulder girdles, and increased thoracic kyphosis are noted, instruct the patient to retract the head gently or lift the sternum. Experiment with a sternum lift also for lumbar problems. Cue patients with increased lumbar lordosis and relative anterior pelvic tilt in standing into a slight posterior tilt, and patients with a decreased lordosis and posterior pelvic tilt into a gentle anterior tilt. Instruct patients standing in knee recurvatum to unlock the knees slightly.
6. For asymmetries recorded for sitting postures, equalize ischial weight bearing or place a folded towel under one buttock. Consider repositioning a forward head alignment. Retest the patient in supine or prone position if a corrective position is not identified.
7. Excessive or asymmetric muscle activity due to postural effects should be dissipated with assumption of non–weight bearing. If aberrant activity persists from standing to sitting to supine to prone, the effects cannot be attributed to simple postural dysfunction, and other kinesiologic profiles must be performed. Document positions that do relieve asymmetric or excessive muscle activity in preparation for treatment. These positions should also support biomechanically efficient joint alignment.

---

gion, as well as at the pectoralis minor, pectoralis major, and latissimus muscle groups. Certain interscapular muscles may be predictably lengthened. According to Kendall and coworkers,[57] shortened muscles tend to be strong on formal manual muscle testing, and lengthened muscles tend to be weak. These findings may be a consequence of sarcomere number, test position, and each muscle's length–tension relationship.[69] Active muscle compensations are required when adaptive shortening or lengthening disturbs the mechanical alignment of joint segments. If there is less passive slack in a region, the joint segments will fail to attain their optimal passive alignment, and active tension may be generated to overcome passive stiffness. Increased tone may also result if periarticular soft tissue is excessively lengthened to the extent that a joint is inadequately stabilized. Thus it is useful to look at the overall dimensions of each body segment, how each segment seems to fit relative to the others, and how these observations correlate with results of specific tests for passive soft tissue extensibility and joint integrity.

Patients with forward head posture tend to show increased SEMG activity from the cervical paraspinal and upper trapezius muscles.[70,71] A flexion moment is generated by the position of the heavy head over the protracted cervical vertebral column. The posterior cervical muscles must remain active to hold the face level for function (Figures 2–10 and 2–11). With an increased thoracic kyphosis, however, thoracic paraspinal recordings may show relative quiescence. Even though a flexion moment is produced, the thoracic cage and associated soft tissues afford a greater level of inherent stability, and the patient may passively "hang" on the posterior ligaments. This type of patient tends to show considerable thoracic SEMG activity when attempting an erect posture. Increased activity is needed to counteract the habitual kyphotic posture and associated passive tissue elements that have adaptively shortened.

In the authors' experience, patients with pain who stand with decreased lumbar and lower thoracic lordosis in a "flat back" alignment, and those who appear to be flexed at the lumbar spine (typically accompanied by relative posterior pelvic tilt), tend to show increased paraspinal SEMG activity. Individuals with an increased lumbar lordosis combined with increased thoracic kyphosis (usually accompanied by an anterior pelvic tilt) also tend toward increased paraspinal activity on presentation. It is speculated that the lumbar paraspinal musculature is activated in this latter group to enable an erect trunk alignment, the foundation for which is an anterior pelvic inclination. Less often in this group, the paraspinal muscles are quiescent, and the lordosis is probably maintained passively by shortening of hip flexor and paraspinal myofascial elements. Patients with diminished lower lumbar lordosis but increased upper lumbar/lower thoracic lordosis—meeting Kendall and colleagues'[57] description of "sway back"—tend toward relatively decreased postural lumbar paraspinal SEMG activity. An extension moment appears to be produced at the lumbar level with this type of alignment, so presumably there is little need for extensor muscle activity.

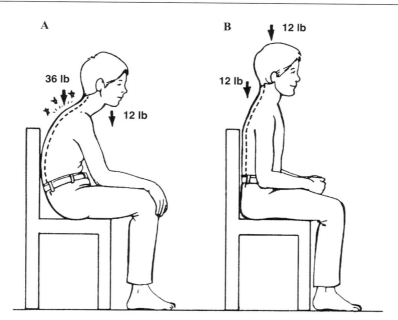

Figure 2–10 Illustration of the neck acting as a lever arm, causing development of torque at the base of the cervical spine. This force is increased with the assumption of (**A**) forward head posture compared with (**B**) retracted head posture. *Source:* Reprinted with permission from HD Saunders: *Evaluation, Treatment, and Prevention of Musculoskeletal Disorders*, p 102, © 1985, The Saunders Group, Inc.

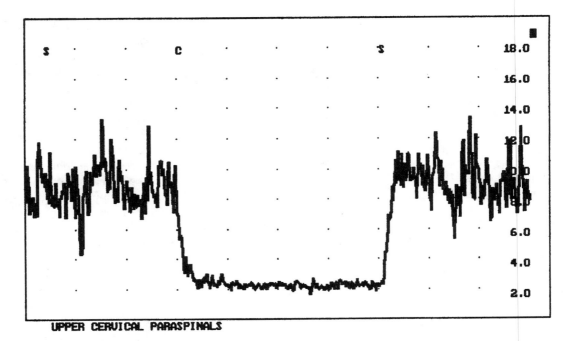

Figure 2–11 SEMG activity recorded over the upper cervical paraspinal region during assumption of spontaneous forward head posture (**S**) versus corrected retracted head posture (**C**). The forward head posture is associated with increased muscle activity, corresponding to the biomechanical model depicted in Figure 2–12.

With respect to frontal plane effects, a lateral trunk shift is usually accompanied by increased activity on the side contralateral to the direction of trunk shift. Increased SEMG activity tends to be observed on the convex side of a true scoliosis. The effects of scoliotic asymmetries, however, may vary. Curvatures can be maintained for many years after skeletal maturation or injury. Ligamentous and myofascial tissues may accommodate to varying degrees in acting as restraints of the curvature, and the balance of active and passive compensations seems to be patient specific. Not all deviations from the ideal are necessarily problematic. Some SEMG patterns clearly are not ideal but are normal for that individual. If a patient has had a scoliosis for 30 years, the clinician can expect paraspinal SEMG asymmetries and should not expect to restore perfect symmetry. Whether a finding is considered to be of clinical significance depends on the patient's symptom behavior, physical examination findings, and remainder of the SEMG profiles.

2. Active Range of Motion

Observations of active range of motion (AROM) are fundamental to the diagnosis of movement system faults. Active range of motion is the maximally available angular range of joint motion achieved by active contraction of muscles that cross the joint. During physical examination, the term is often used in contrast with passive range of motion, which is the maximally available angular range of joint motion achieved by application (usually by the clinician) of a force extrinsic to the motion segment. Both amount and quality of active motion are studied. Painful portions of the active movement arc, deviations from the normal path of movement, and faulty coordination of joint segments are noted as clues of pathologic abnormalities. SEMG profiling involves recording muscle activity as the corresponding AROM is performed. This approach has been used routinely in kinesiologic experiments and studies on the effects of specific types of exercises. Active range of motion profiling has also been used to evaluate patients with musculoskeletal pain at the trunk and extremities.[72–74] See the box "Clinical Procedure—Active Range of Motion."

During the concentric phase, the muscle shortens as it contracts. The muscle lengthens as it contracts during the eccentric phase. An agonist muscle acts in a concentric manner while moving a body part up against gravity. The body part is accelerated by the concentric contraction. The same agonist acts in an eccentric fashion to lower the body part back down. The muscle then decelerates the body part against gravity and controls descent. Greater tension is developed during maximal effort eccentric contractions, compared with maximal effort concentric contractions. The elastic properties of the tissue and contraction time differences may impart a tensile advantage while acting in an eccentric manner.[75,76] However, greater SEMG amplitude tends to be observed during the concentric phase of AROM, compared with the eccentric phase (Figure 2–12). Perhaps this is because the same load is moved at roughly the same velocity, but because that tensile advantage is absent during the concentric phase, more motor units must be recruited. Increased motor unit recruitment is then reflected by a greater SEMG amplitude. The concentric–eccentric SEMG phenomenon is sufficiently robust that it can be used to discriminate between patients with chronic low back pain and healthy control subjects by using lumbar paraspinal recordings during standing trunk flexion (eccentric) and return to a neutral position (concentric).[74] Clinical observations by the authors have shown dysfunctional patterns of motor control in patients during one phase and not the other, more often the eccentric component. By distinguishing problems during the concentric or the eccentric phase, SEMG feedback and corrective exercise programs can be better planned.

Clinical Procedure—Active Range of Motion

1. Ask the patient to move the associated joint(s) in the directions controlled by the target muscle. Include cardinal planes of movement as well as diagonal functional planes. For example, profile shoulder elevation during pure flexion and abduction as well as scaption (shoulder elevation in the plane of the glenoid fossa of the scapula—about 30 to 45 degrees of horizontal abduction). Include all planes of movement in which the target muscle acts. Profile the sternomastoid, for example, during cervical flexion/extension, side bending, and rotation. Include both agonistic and antagonistic directions. Examine the left sternomastoid during left as well as right cervical rotation, and vice versa. Investigate the motion direction that best isolates target muscle action if not already accounted for. For example, record the left sternomastoid during combined cervical extension, left side bending, and right rotation. Record the gluteus maximus during combined hip abduction, extension, and lateral rotation.

2. Observe the recordings for left/right symmetry in magnitude and timing. Limit left/right SEMG comparisons to the symmetrically available AROM. Qualitative or quantitative comparisons with standardized norms are available for some muscles and clinical problems. (Refer to Chapters 8–14 in this book and Chapter 7 of the companion book, *Introduction to Surface Electromyography*.[17]) Note any association of aberrant activity with a particular portion of the AROM arc. Distinguish SEMG activity during concentric and eccentric contraction phases. Use a metronome or verbal cues, so that the patient maintains an approximately constant speed of movement across repetitions.

**Forward Flexion—
Eccentric**

**Return from Flexion—
Concentric**

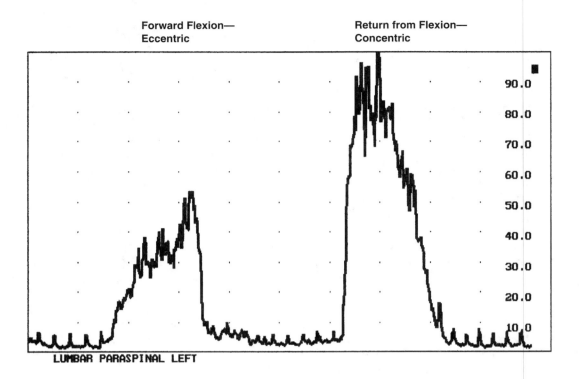

LUMBAR PARASPINAL LEFT

Figure 2–12 SEMG activity of lumbar paraspinal muscles during standing trunk flexion (eccentric contraction) and return from flexion to neutral standing (concentric contraction). Muscle activity is greater during concentric phase compared with eccentric phase of the task.

3. Isometric Contractions

Isometric contractions are contractions produced with constant muscle length. Muscle tension is generated, but gross joint movement is not produced. Isometric contractions are used with standardized manual muscle tests to assess strength and lesion location. The use of SEMG with isometric muscle contractions in populations with chronic pain has been reported most often as a reference for normalization purposes. As described previously, the peak or average microvolt score associated with some test activity is expressed as a percentage of the microvolt score associated with a maximal or standardized submaximal effort isometric contraction. Isometric contractions are included here also as a means of characterizing aberrant motor behavior. See the box "Clinical Procedure—Isometric Contractions."

In the authors' experience, subjects with unilateral involvement sometimes show symmetric SEMG activity with maximal effort, but asymmetric activity with equivalent submaximal loads. Other patients demonstrate symmetry at a very low level of resistance but generate asymmetric activity beyond that point. A variety of submaximal loads and joint angles can be used to assess the limits of symmetry and efficient return to baseline. This information is then taken into account when exercise and feedback training strategies are prescribed. Activities that are accompanied by unremarkable SEMG patterns are interpreted as safe for unsupervised home practice. Tasks that produce aberrant SEMG patterns are the focus for clinic feedback sessions

---

Clinical Procedure—Isometric Contractions

1. With the use of standardized manual muscle test positions,[56,57] ask the patient to perform a maximal volitional isometric contraction for 6 to 10 seconds. Note the average SEMG amplitude during the middle 2 to 3 seconds. Allow 30 to 60 seconds of rest between task repetitions, or longer if inconsistent results are obtained and fatigue is suspected. Assess for left/right symmetry during contraction efforts and a complete recovery to baseline magnitude during rest periods.
2. Document SEMG amplitudes during graded submaximal contractions for unilateral pain syndromes. Compare left versus right SEMG responses by using the same amount of load for each side. Use exercise weights or a dynamometer to grade the amount of load, from light to heavy. Note the amount of load required to elicit SEMG asymmetry or an incomplete recovery to baseline. Consider repeating the procedures at different joint angles.

---

with the use of equilibration and deactivation procedures.

4. Dynamic Contractions at Progressive Intensities

By profiling SEMG activity during dynamic contractions of progressive intensity, the findings from the AROM procedure can be extended. The dynamic contractions can be concentric or eccentric and are used to identify the loads that induce faulty muscle activity patterns. SEMG activity may be unremarkable in the absence of an external load, but become aberrant when objects are moved. The distinction is sig-

nificant because functional activities require subjects to lift, push, and carry articles of various weights. This profile is usually used with extremity musculature. Dynamic loading of the spine is not recommended in this way without specialized equipment and safety procedures. See the box "Clinical Procedure—Dynamic Contractions of Progressive Intensities."

The information gained from the procedure is used to guide exercise prescription and return-to-work decisions. For example, the upper trapezius on the involved side might function symmetrically with the muscle on the uninvolved side when the subject lifts 5 lb or less from table to eye

---

Clinical Procedure—Dynamic Contractions at Progressive Intensities

1. Follow the instructions in Clinical Procedure—Active Range of Motion.
2. Specify a movement plane and range of motion arc of interest. Base this decision on the patient's routine functional tasks or prior positive examination findings.
3. While allowing for adequate rest periods, ask the patient to perform at least five to six repetitions of the movement arc with a light dumbbell or cuff weight. The number of repetitions may be increased if the patient's symptoms are cumulative over a work shift. Progressively substitute increased weights.
4. Document the load range that corresponds to unremarkable SEMG activity as well as the level associated with SEMG asymmetry, varying peak values, a rising tonic amplitude level, or failure of prompt return to baseline with task cessation.
5. Allow for rest, and repeat the series to confirm findings.
6. Observe and document any changes in postural alignment, as well as in rhythm between motion segments, that correspond to the emergence of aberrant SEMG activity.

---

level. However, when he or she lifts 7 lb, the upper trapezius muscle on the involved side could display a greater peak amplitude and afterward recover to a level elevated above baseline (Figure 2–13). This patient's home exercise program would be limited to use of 5 lb or less. Supervised practice in the clinic would be directed toward reproducing the desired pattern of motor activity with greater than 7 lb. With the assumption that these findings complement the other examination procedures, the patient might be released for light duty work with a 5 lb lifting restriction.

5. Dynamic Contractions at Progressive Velocities

The intent and method of this profile are similar to those in the previous profile. The differ- ence is that external load is constant and velocity is varied. This procedure is used most often with extremity musculature, although it may be used with neck and back muscles to assess their stabilizing role during extremity movement. See the box "Clinical Procedure—Dynamic Contractions at Progressive Velocities."

The information gained from the procedure is used to guide exercise prescription, return to sport, and possibly return-to-work decisions. For example, a patient with a shoulder impingement syndrome might produce an infraspinatus SEMG recording that is unremarkable during slow abduction motions, but notable for an aberrant double peak during a painful portion of the motion arc when performed at fast speeds (Figure 2–14). Home ex-

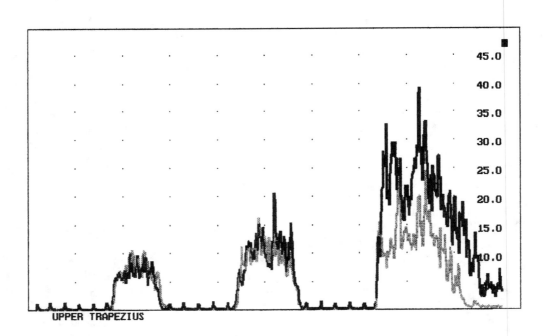

Figure 2–13 SEMG activity of left (black) and right (gray) upper trapezii during symmetric overhead lift of 3, 5, and 7 lb. Recordings were made from a patient who presented to a work conditioning program with complaints of chronic left cervical, suprascapular, and interscapular pain attributed to cumulative strain from repetitive overhead lifting at work. At the time of the recordings, rehabilitation had progressed successfully, and symptoms were resolving. It was believed that the patient might be ready to return to light duty work. Muscle activity became asymmetric with the 7-lb load, and the left side signal failed to return to baseline when movement was terminated.

Clinical Procedure—Dynamic Contractions at Progressive Velocities

1. Follow the instructions in Clinical Procedure—Active Range of Motion.
2. Specify a movement plane, range of motion arc, and load level of interest. Base this decision on the patient's routine functional tasks or prior positive examination findings.
3. While allowing for adequate rest periods, ask the subject to perform at least five to six repetitions of the movement arc at a slow velocity. Use a metronome, some other timing device, or an isokinetic (constant velocity) dynamometer to regulate the velocity of movement. Progressively increase velocity.
4. Document the velocity range that corresponds to unremarkable SEMG activity and the range associated with aberrant patterns.
5. Allow for rest, and repeat the series to confirm findings.
6. Observe and document any changes in postural alignment, as well as in rhythm between motion segments, that correspond to the emergence of aberrant SEMG activity.

ercises might be restricted to the velocities for which adequate control is displayed. Return to high-velocity sport activities that incorporate abduction motions would be approached with caution.

6. Open versus Closed Kinematic Chains

This profile is used for problems that involve the hip, knee, ankle, and foot. An open kinematic chain is a series of linked joints in which

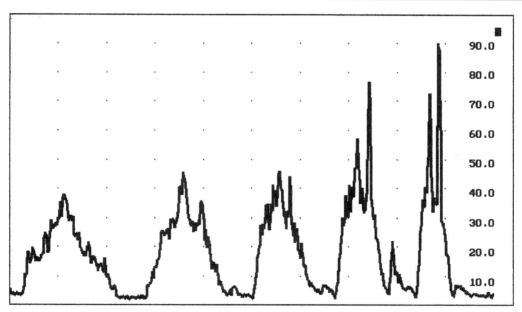

INFRASPINATUS

Figure 2–14 SEMG activity of the infraspinatus during five trials of shoulder abduction, with progressively increased velocity across trials. The recording was made from a badminton player with a chronic shoulder impingement syndrome that became symptomatic at faster movement speeds. Note the emergence of a second activity peak in the trials performed with greater velocity. This phenomenon corresponded to the development of a painful motion arc as the arm was eccentrically lowered through approximately 90 degrees of abduction.

the distal segment is free. The distal segment is fixed in a closed chain. Each joint can be moved independently of the others in an open chain, but in a closed chain, movement at one joint constrains or induces movement at the other joints.[77] Knee extension in a sitting position is an example of open chain movement. The knee can be moved without moving the hip or the ankle. Closed chain knee extension takes place when the foot is fixed on the floor, such as when arising from a squat. The knee cannot move without the ankle and the hip also moving. Joint dynamics and patterns of motor control vary across the two circumstances. SEMG has been used to demonstrate variable patterns of muscle balance between medial and lateral quadriceps components in closed versus open chains.[57,78] Lower extremity stance occurs in the closed chain,

whereas swing occurs in the open chain. Musculoskeletal problems of the lower extremity are often caused by inefficient mechanical loading in the closed chain. See the box "Clinical Procedure—Open versus Closed Kinematic Chains."

Patterns of asymmetry, elevated tonic amplitude, incomplete baseline recovery, and timing faults may be observed during both open and closed chain movement, or just in one of the two. The circumstances of occurrence are used to guide exercise prescription and SEMG feedback practice. For example, Figure 2–15 shows different activity patterns of the vastus medialis oblique and vastus lateralis during supine isometric and squat conditions. The subject does not need feedback practice with traditional open chain isometric or straight leg raising exercises. SEMG training would be focused on closed

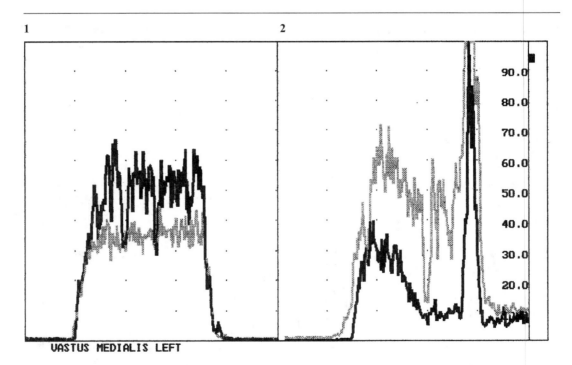

VASTUS MEDIALIS LEFT

VASTUS LATERALIS LEFT

Figure 2–15 SEMG activity of vastus medialis oblique (black) and vastus lateralis (gray) from a patient with chronic patellofemoral pain syndrome and presumed muscle imbalance, faulty patellar tracking, and inefficient dissipation of patellofemoral joint reaction force. (**1**) Activity during an isometric quadriceps contraction in the open kinematic chain. (**2**) Activity during a closed chain partial squat. Note the change in relative magnitude and timing of the two signals from open to closed chain conditions.

Clinical Procedure—Open versus Closed Kinematic Chains

1. From the intake and physical examination findings, identify functional positions that reproduce or exacerbate the patient's symptoms.
2. Assess SEMG activity from the target muscles(s) in relevant open chain positions involving supine, sitting, or standing positions.
3. Compare the results with recordings made during squat, bilateral or unilateral stance, step up, step down, or dynamic gait tasks.
4. Instruct the patient to move through the entire functional AROM arc. Examine both concentric and eccentric phases. Consider varying load and velocity.

---

chain functional tasks when the activity of the vastus medialis oblique appears poorly timed to the motion.

7. Multiple Muscle Functions

With this procedure, SEMG activity is observed as one muscle or muscle group acts to control different joint relationships and purposeful movements. Muscles that cross two joints are examined with various joint position combinations. For example, hamstring activity is assessed with isolated knee flexion, hip extension with knee flexion, and hip extension with knee extension. The rectus femoris, tensor fasciae latae, gastrocnemius, and biceps brachii, as well as the long flexors and extensors of the hand, might be analogously examined.

Uniarticular (and potentially biarticular) muscles are investigated when they have multiple roles as primary joint movers, phasic joint stabilizers, or tonic postural stabilizers. The muscles most often involved are those of the shoulder and pelvic girdle. Different patterns of activity, for instance, may be observed with a

recording site just medial to the medial scapular border at about the level of the third thoracic vertebra. SEMG activity will vary in part because there are multiple layers and closely adjacent muscles, and the site is vulnerable to volume conduction. The same interscapular electrodes detect altered patterns as different muscles are recruited to support different tasks. Different motor programs are also generated for the same muscle, depending on the movement goal. Asymmetries can sometimes be seen from the upper trapezius during scapular stabilization for shoulder movements that are distinct from tonic postural or prime scapular movement effects. See the box "Clinical Procedure—Multiple Muscle Functions."

SEMG feedback training, exercise prescription, and functional activity modification are matched to the specific circumstances associated with aberrant activity. For example, Figure 2–16 shows interscapular SEMG activity during postural maintenance, prime scapular retraction, and sustained overhead activity. These conditions vary in load, joint angle, muscle length, endurance requirements, muscle synergy, and mo-

---

Clinical Procedure—Multiple Muscle Functions

1. Consider all mechanical actions of the desired target muscle(s). Include all joints spanned and roles in postural stabilization, phasic prime movement, and phasic stabilization.
2. Ask the patient to perform representative tasks for all conditions.
3. Document those circumstances that induce aberrant SEMG activity and those that do not. Note patterns of asymmetry, elevated or erratic amplitudes during contraction, or incomplete baseline recovery.

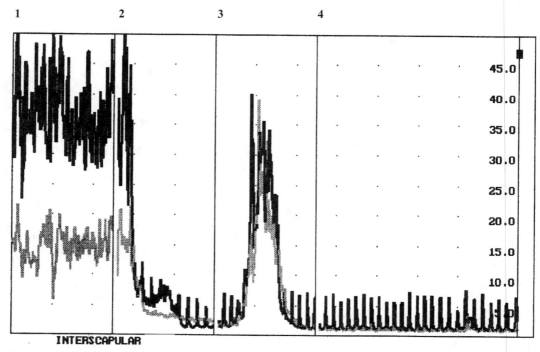

Figure 2–16 SEMG activity recorded from the left (black) and right (gray) lateral interscapular region at the level of the fourth thoracic vertebra (for the same patient as in Figure 2–13 at start of rehabilitation program). (**1**) Symmetric overhead occupational task on a ceiling. (**2**) Recovery time after cessation of **1**. (**3**) Simultaneous left/right scapular retraction with arms at sides of the trunk. (**4**) Standing with arms relaxed. Muscle activity appears asymmetric during scapular stabilization for the work task and unremarkable during the prime scapular movement and simple postural tasks.

tor goal. Asymmetries are observed during the overhead activity only, and feedback training can be so directed without a need for postural or prime movement training.

8. Tension Recognition Thresholds

This is a subjective procedure used with unilaterally involved, apparently hyperactive muscles about the head, neck, and proximal shoulder girdle. The upper trapezius and masseter are common recording targets. It was suggested in Chapter 1 that some patients with chronically elevated muscle tension might not recognize that increased muscle activity is present. Exacerbated pain is their only marker of dysfunction. The intent of this procedure is to assess whether subjects are able to recognize subtle increases in muscle activity from base-

line. See the box "Clinical Procedure—Tension Recognition Thresholds."

A patient might perceive a rise in muscle activity at a higher microvolt reading on the involved side, compared with the uninvolved side (Figure 2–17). The authors believe differences of more than about two microvolts are noteworthy when consistently reproduced. Specific SEMG feedback techniques can be selected during treatment to facilitate kinesthetic awareness.

9. SEMG Feedback Coordination Tasks

Coordination tasks are used with patients with unilateral involvement, generally with shoulder girdle, upper extremity, and facial muscles. A computer-assisted system is required that enables subjects to play a game wherein the action is controlled by the magnitude of the recorded SEMG signal. A number of game activities are

---

Clinical Procedure—Tension Recognition Thresholds

1. Turn the visual display away from the client and terminate any audio display.
2. Instruct the subject as to how the target muscle can be activated, for example, by using a shoulder shrug for the upper trapezius or a jaw clench for the masseter.
3. Begin with the uninvolved side. Ask the patient to think about contracting the target muscle and performing its associated joint action, but not actually to do it. Then ask the client to begin contracting the muscle on your command, increasing intensity as slowly as possible. Instruct the patient to say "now," or to raise a hand if jaw muscles are targeted, when he or she can *feel* an actual increase in muscle activity or joint movement above the baseline resting level.
4. Document the microvolt value at that moment.
5. Repeat the procedure on the involved side.

---

available with commercial devices. The task might involve matching an on-line SEMG tracing to a preprogrammed template line, or perhaps a sophisticated set of graphics similar to a video arcade game. These games can be quite challenging in terms of fine gradations of contraction intensity and timing. See the box "Clinical Procedure—SEMG Feedback Coordination Tasks."

A patient might score appreciably lower on the involved side, compared with the uninvolved side. The difference potentially reflects a decrement in volitional motor control on the involved side. As with the previous profile, this procedure

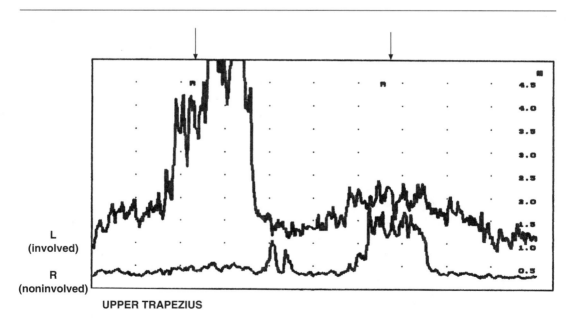

UPPER TRAPEZIUS

Figure 2–17 SEMG activity of left (**L**) and right (**R**) upper trapezius from a patient with chronic left cervical and suprascapular pain during the tension recognition thresholds procedure. Patient report of tension perception is indicated by arrows, first for the left side test and next for the right side test. The recognition point is associated with a higher microvolt value on the involved side, compared with the noninvolved side.

Clinical Procedure—SEMG Feedback Coordination Tasks

1. Instruct the patient to respond to the SEMG feedback in ways that support the goal of the available game. Have the patient perform the task for a designated time on uninvolved and then involved sides.
2. Document the game score for each side.

---

is regarded as a secondary assessment. A number of spurious factors may influence performance, and not all practitioners have equipment with these capabilities. Nevertheless, the procedure may be useful in documenting perceptual–motor limitations and planning training strategies that facilitate kinesthetic awareness. Specific feedback techniques can be selected to promote fine dynamic motor control.

10. Analysis of Agonist/Antagonist/ Synergist and Related Muscle Patterns

Muscles rarely act in isolation during the execution of purposeful movements. Agonist muscles work together with antagonists and synergists so that a movement goal is attained. This profile focuses exclusively on the relationship of an agonist relative to its antagonists and synergists.

An agonist/antagonist pair may reciprocate joint movement in opposite directions during task performance or co-contract to stabilize a joint. Synergists co-contract with peculiar timing relationships to produce force couples that control joint movement in one or more planes. The left and right sides of the lumbar paraspinal muscles function as synergists during static postural control and trunk flexion–extension motions; they function as antagonists during rotation and side-bending maneuvers. The cervical paraspinal and sternomastoid muscles on opposite sides jointly recruit to produce head rotation. During upward rotation of the scapula, the upper trapezius, lower trapezius, and lower fibers of the serratus anterior act as synergists. The vastus medialis oblique and vastus lateralis act as antagonists for control of the patella in the frontal plane, and ultimately as

synergists for efficient sagittal plane knee extension. During hip extension, the hamstrings and gluteus maximus function synergistically. Although not true synergists with the lumbar paraspinals in that they act at different joints, these muscles work together to control the body during forward bending. Thus there is interest in functionally synergistic muscle groups that participate in a kinematic chain. See the box "Clinical Procedure—Agonist/Antagonist/Synergist and Related Muscle Patterns."

This is a most challenging area for SEMG analysis. Hardware, software, and operator skill may be pushed to their limits. Guidelines for specific body regions are provided in subsequent chapters. The intent is to obtain a clear assessment of which muscles are hyperactive, are hypoactive, co-contract inappropriately, fail to co-contract appropriately, or display timing faults at particular phases of movement. When one muscle is hyperactive (relative to its homologous mate), there is usually an antagonist or synergist that is hypoactive, or vice versa. Sometimes it seems that one aberrant pattern is causal and another is compensatory. By understanding how the muscular elements of the motion segment function together, the clinician can efficiently plan treatment.

A patient with neck pain and an upper trapezius that is hyperactive during shoulder flexion could be treated with SEMG feedback downtraining (Figure 2–18). The client would repeat shoulder flexion movements while consciously trying to relax the upper trapezius. Feedback would be used to assess the success of the subject's inherent motor control strategy and direct adjustments over successive trials. By using multiple SEMG channels, the clinician might

Clinical Procedure—Agonist/Antagonist/Synergist and Related Muscle Patterns

1. On the basis of intake and physical examination findings, identify a discrete movement for study. This may be a movement that provokes symptoms on physical examination or one that is relevant to the client's functional life activities.
2. Set up for recording from all accessible muscles that subserve the target movement. If many muscles are involved, prioritize recording sites for muscles that cross the painful joint segment, muscles that stabilize proximally, or muscles that reproduce symptoms when palpated or manually tested.
3. Have the subject perform five to six repetitions of the desired movement. Vary conditions as described earlier in the first six kinesiologic profiles. Study the left and right sides individually and during bilateral simultaneous symmetric motions. Compare SEMG activity across each homologous muscle pair. Limit left/right SEMG comparisons to the symmetrically available AROM. Use normalization procedures to compare peak SEMG activity across recording sites, as well as to compare with standardized databases when available. Examine timing patterns from the left, compared with the right, side or relative to standardized activity patterns.
4. Print a hard copy of the tracings to simplify documentation.

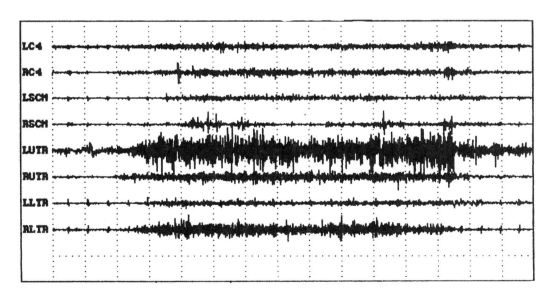

Figure 2–18 SEMG activity from left (**L**) and right (**R**) cervical paraspinal (**C4**), sternocleidomastoid (**SCM**), upper trapezius (**UTR**), and lower trapezius (**LTR**) during bilateral, symmetric shoulder flexion. Recordings were derived from a patient with chronic left cervical and periscapular pain. The left upper trapezius appears hyperactive relative to the right upper trapezius, and baseline and recovery activity appears greater on the left. During motion, the left lower trapezius appears hypoactive relative to the right lower trapezius. The combination of upper trapezius and lower trapezius asymmetry may represent an aberrant muscular synergy pattern, resulting in an inefficient force couple imparted to the scapula during upward rotation.

also identify a hypoactive lower trapezius. An option is then presented for uptraining the lower trapezius. Uptraining an apparently hypoactive muscle often seems to be easier for patient learning than downtraining a hyperactive muscle. As recruitment of one synergist is increased, the hyperactivity of another may be seen to resolve spontaneously. Taylor[79] has attributed the phenomenon to reflexive patterns of reciprocal inhibition. This may be the case for some agonist/antagonist pairs, and additional mechanisms may be responsible for some synergist relationships. When the activity of a hypoactive synergist is increased, a hyperactive muscle is mechanically unloaded to some degree. That is, its excessive work is "taken back over" by the previously hypoactive muscle. A more normal muscular force couple is produced and more normal patterns of intrinsic proprioceptive feedback are restored. Motor programs, involving both segmental reflex loops and suprasegmental systems, are probably reset to achieve the goal with an economy of effort.

11. Functional Activity Analysis

Functional activities bring with them unique mechanical and behavioral demands that may not be reproduced with the previous test procedures. The authors have evaluated many patients with unremarkable findings on SEMG examinations until they have been studied in functional contexts. This population has included keyboard operators; telephone operators; motor vehicle operators and mechanics; homemakers; athletes; performing artists; and assembly line, farm, and janitorial workers. There have been many reports on the experimental use of SEMG to study this range of functional activity.[39,80-85]

Simulation of functional activities can be straightforward or highly demanding. Complexity depends on the required equipment, activity environments, and movement loads and velocities. Functional profiles may be performed in the clinic or in the field. Portable SEMG devices can be used during a supervised visit to the workplace. Miniaturized systems with data logging ability are also commercially available. Some of these are capable of storing data over an entire work shift. Data are then downloaded directly to a printer or personal computer for processing. A fascinating example of this type of profiling can be found in the work of Sherman,[86] who has recorded SEMG activity from soldiers while performing functional military tasks. See the box "Clinical Procedure—Functional Activity Analysis."

It is an obvious advantage to be able to define the functional circumstances that induce aberrant patterns of motor activity. The findings are the basis for activity modifications and ergonomic adjustments during treatment. Figure 2–19 summarizes selection of kinesiologic profiles.

Clinical Procedure—Functional Activity Analysis

1. Identify functional activities that directly exacerbate and alleviate the patient's complaints. If these are unknown, select sustained or repetitive tasks associated with the patient's activities of daily living. Prioritize for those activities that would be expected to load the injured body region mechanically or that are known to be of high ergonomic risk.
2. Observe SEMG activity from the desired muscles as the task is performed, with as close a replication of real-life conditions as feasible. Many task repetitions may be required.
3. Document SEMG asymmetries for simultaneous symmetric activities or reciprocally symmetric activities. For all activities, document baseline recovery during intertrial intervals, inconsistent or erratic recruitment, and suspected timing faults. Also look for increasing tonic amplitude or decreasing microrest frequency during task performance. Document SEMG patterns from agonists, antagonists, synergists, and other muscles that function in a coordinated pattern. Compare with normative data if available.

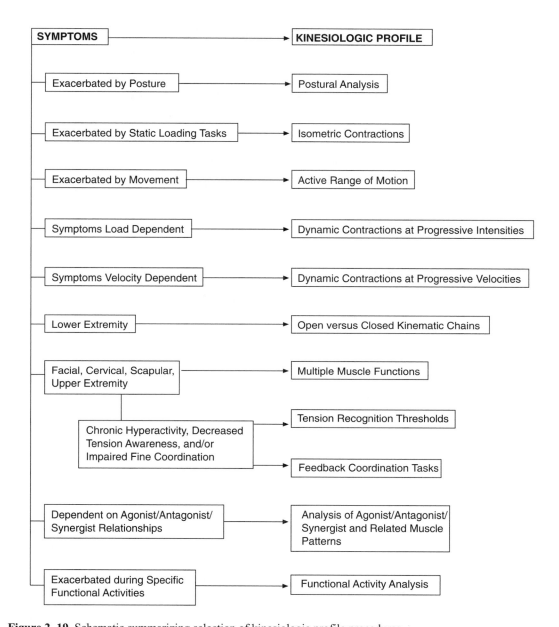

Figure 2–19 Schematic summarizing selection of kinesiologic profile procedures.

LEVEL 3 ASSESSMENT

The level 3 assessment consists of organizing the results of the evaluation procedures into a cohesive framework. There are two parts to the level 3 assessment. The first part incorporates a general model for clinical assessment. The sec-

ond part assigns a syndrome classification to the aberrant SEMG findings.

Various schemes have been proposed for interdisciplinary clinical assessment related to function and disability.[87,88] Nagi[89] has conceptualized a four-stage model that has found favor in adaptations in the physical medicine community

(Figure 2–20). Assessment is organized to delineate pathology, impairment, functional limitation, and disability. Pathology results from trauma and degeneration at the cellular level. This can be thought of as the fundamental disease process. Pathology is confirmed on the basis of laboratory study, radiographic imaging, and other test findings that are diagnostic in a basic way. Impairment refers to dysfunction at the level of tissue, organs, or physiologic or psychologic systems. Restricted AROM, weakness, hypertonicity, anxiety, and depression are examples of impairments. They are determined by clinical examination. Functional limitation is a restriction at the level of the individual person. A functional restriction involves purposeful, goal-directed activities. Decreased sitting tolerance, disrupted sleep, restricted gait, and an inability to perform specific work or household tasks in the normal manner constitute functional limita-

tions. Questionnaires and patient reports are used with clinical examination to delineate functional limitations. Finally, disability is a restriction at the social level—limitations in the ability of a person to fulfill socially expected roles. Included are problems with personal care, child care and family interaction, vocation, and recreation. Disabilities are surmised from patient self-reports and responses to questionnaire instruments. Specific tools have been recommended to sort disability issues, for example, in patients with low back pain.[1,12,90–92]

The first part of the level 3 assessment, then, is a description of the pathology, impairments, functional limitations, and disabilities. This component of the assessment is not peculiar to SEMG evaluation. It is an attempt to identify quality of life indicators and relate desired outcomes to specific impairments. Because each category of dysfunction drives the next, disabili-

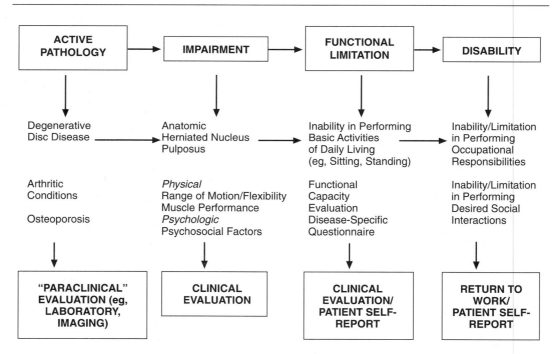

Figure 2–20 Nagi's conceptual scheme for disablement, illustrated with examples relating to low back dysfunction. The bottom portion of the figure represents the actual source of data. *Source:* Reprinted from *Physical Therapy*. Delitto A. Are Measures of Function and Disability Important in Low Back Care? 1994; Vol 74, pp 452–462, with the permission of APTA.

ties should be reduced as the functional limitations are improved. Functional limitations should be amended as the impairments are resolved, and so forth. Goals for treatment are constructed at the level of functional limitations and disabilities. Treatment techniques known to have an impact on the identified impairments are prioritized for those that achieve the goals with acceptable cost and maximal patient satisfaction. SEMG assessments help define impairments. Feedback interventions also are aimed at the impairment level. An interdisciplinary team is best equipped to provide care at every level of dysfunction for management of patients with complex chronic pain problems.

The second part of the level 3 assessment classifies muscle impairments into particular syndromes. Sorting is based directly on the assessment findings for levels 1 and 2 and is unique to SEMG evaluation. The classifications are used to type SEMG findings into clinically meaningful and practical categories. These categories direct treatment so that appropriate strategies are matched to particular impairment patterns. The syndromes are listed in Figure 2–21. Detailed discussion of the syndromes is deferred to Chapter 7, after discussion of SEMG feedback methods.

CONCLUSION

A three-level assessment scheme has been proposed for patient intake. The objectives of the level 1 assessment are to determine the appropriateness of SEMG intervention, whether additional consultations are indicated, and whether SEMG evaluation is best directed toward psychophysiologic issues, kinesiologic factors, or both. A variety of screening procedures are suggested to assist with decision making. The objective of the level 2 assessment is to determine what specific conditions evoke aberrant patterns of motor activity. Clinicians select relevant SEMG profiles from a menu of options. SEMG recordings are examined on the basis of specific amplitude and timing parameters. Interpretation is completed by the level 3 assessment, in which the SEMG findings are integrated with other aspects of psychophysiologic and musculoskeletal evaluation.

The clinician can choose to limit SEMG profiling to relatively simple procedures, or to per-

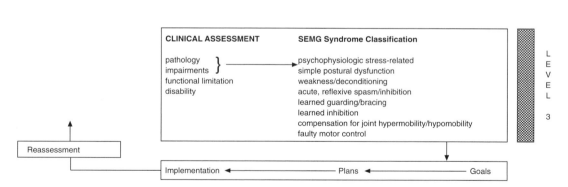

Figure 2–21 Schematic of level 3 assessment and subsequent intervention. *Source:* Reprinted with permission from GS Kasman, *Surface EMG in Physical Therapy,* © 1995, Movement Systems.

form highly complex assessments. Four- and eight-channel SEMG devices will most efficiently support certain of the profiles. Units with oscilloscope-like graphics and advanced signal processing are required for sophisticated timing analyses. However, procedures that can be performed with a broad array of commercial equipment have been emphasized. The most important point is for the operator to exercise clinical reasoning skills during assessment. After all, it is the results of evaluation that must reasonably drive the selection of treatment techniques. A seasoned perspective will enable the practitioner to exploit any SEMG system to its fullest potential.

REFERENCES

1. Delitto A, Erhard RE, Bowling RW. A treatment-based classification approach to low back syndrome: Identifying and staging patients for conservative treatment. *Phys Ther*. 1995;75:470–489.

2. Cyriax, J. *Textbook of Orthopaedic Medicine. Volume One: Diagnosis of Soft Tissue Lesions*. 8th ed. London, England: Bailliere Tindall; 1982.

3. Bigos S, Bowyer O, Braen G, et al. *Acute Low Back Problems in Adults*. Rockville, MD: Agency for Health Care Policy and Research, Public Health Service, US Dept of Health and Human Services; Clinical Practice Guideline No. 14, AHCPR publication 95-0642.

4. Boissonnault WG, Koopmeiners MB. Medical history profile: orthopedic physical therapy outpatients. *J Orthop Sports Phys Ther*. 1994;20:10–12.

5. Boissonnault WG, Bass C. Pathological origins of trunk and neck pain, part I: pelvic and abdominal visceral disorders. *J Orthop Sports Phys Ther*. 1990;12:192–207.

6. Boissonnault WG, Bass C. Pathological origins of trunk and neck pain, part II: disorders of the cardiovascular and pulmonary systems. *J Orthop Sports Phys Ther*. 1990;12:208–215.

7. Boissonnault WG, Bass C. Pathological origins of trunk and neck pain, part III: diseases of the musculoskeletal system. *J Orthop Sports Phys Ther*. 1990;12:216–221.

8. Roach KE, Brown M, Ricker E, Altenburger P, Tompkins J. The use of patient symptoms to screen for serious back problems. *J Orthop Sports Phys Ther*. 1993;21:2–6.

9. Deyo RA, Rainville J, Dent DL. What can the history and physical examination tell us about low back pain? *JAMA*. 1992;268:760–765.

10. Feuerstein M, Beattie P. Biobehavioral factors affecting pain and disability in low back pain: mechanisms and assessment. *Phys Ther*. 1995;75:267–280.

11. Cole B, Finch E, Gowland C, Mayo N, Basmajian JV, eds. *Physical Rehabilitation Outcome Measures*. Toronto: Canadian Physiotherapy Association; 1994.

12. Deyo RA. Measuring the functional status of patients with low back pain. *Arch Phys Med Rehabil*. 1988;69:1044–1053.

13. Lewis C, McNearney T. *The Functional Toolbox*. Washington, DC: Learn Publishers; 1994.

14. McDowell I, Newell C. *Measuring Health*. 2nd ed. New York: Oxford University Press; 1996.

15. Stewart D, Abeln SH. *Documenting Functional Outcomes in Physical Therapy*. St Louis, MO: Mosby–Year Book; 1993.

16. Selye H. *The Stress of Life*. New York: McGraw-Hill, 1978.

17. Cram JR, Kasman GS. *Introduction to Surface Electromyography*. Gaithersburg, MD: Aspen Publishers; 1997.

18. Gaarder KR, Montgomery PS. *Clinical Biofeedback: A Procedural Manual*. Baltimore: Williams & Wilkins; 1977.

19. Stoyva JM. Autogenic training and biofeedback combined: a reliable method for the induction of general relaxation. In: Basmajian JV, ed. *Biofeedback: Principles and Practice for Clinicians*. 3rd ed. Baltimore: Williams & Wilkins; 1989;169–186.

20. Arena JG, Hobbs SH. Reliability of psychophysiological responding as a function of trait anxiety. *Biofeedback Self Regul*. 1995;20:19–37.

21. Heath HA, Oken D, Shipman WG. Muscle tension and personality: a serious second look. *Arch Gen Psychiatry*. 1967;16:720–726.

22. Kelley D, Brown CC, Shaffer JW. A comparison of physiological and psychological measurements on anxious patients and normal controls. *Psychophysiology*. 1970;6:429–441.

23. Shellenberger R, Lewis M. Reliability of stress profiling. *Biofeedback Self Regul*. 1986;11:81–91.

24. Shipman WG, Heath HA, Oken D. Response specificity among muscular and autonomic variables. *Arch Gen Psychiatry*. 1970;22:369–374.

25. Smith RP. Frontalis muscle tension and personality. *Psychophysiology*. 1973;10:311–312.

26. Flor H, Turk DC. Psychophysiology of chronic pain: do chronic pain patients exhibit symptom-specific psychophysiological responses? *Psychol Bull*. 1989;105:215–259.

27. Sandrini G, Antonaci F, Pucci E, Bono G, Nappi G. Comparative study with EMG, pressure algometry, and manual palpation in tension-type headache and migraine. *Cephalalgia.* 1994;14:451–457.

28. Flor H, Turk DC, Birbaumer, N. Assessment of stress related psychophysiological reactions in chronic back pain patients. *J Consult Clin Psychol.* 1985;53:354–364.

29. Flor H, Birbaumer N, Schugens MM, Lutzenberger W. Symptom-specific psychophysiological responses in chronic pain patients. *Psychophysiology.* 1992;29:452–460.

30. Basmajian JV. *Biofeedback: Principles and Practice for Clinicians.* 3rd ed. Baltimore: Williams & Wilkins; 1989.

31. Fischer-Williams M, Nigl AJ, Sovine DL, eds. *A Textbook of Biological Feedback.* New York: Human Sciences Press; 1986.

32. Peper E, Ancoli S, Quinn M. *Mind/Body Integration: Essential Readings in Biofeedback.* New York: Plenum Publishing; 1979.

33. Schwartz MS, ed. *Biofeedback: A Practitioner's Guide.* 2nd ed. New York: Guilford Press; 1995.

34. White L, Tursky B, eds. *Clinical Biofeedback: Efficacy and Mechanisms.* New York: Guilford Press; 1982.

35. Hagberg M. The amplitude distribution of surface EMG in static and intermittent static muscular performance. *Eur J Appl Physiol.* 1979;40:265–272.

36. Johnsson B. The static load component in muscle work. *Eur J Appl Physiol.* 1988;57:305–310.

37. Johnsson B. Measurement and evaluation of local muscular strain in the shoulder during constrained work. *J Hum Ergol (Tokyo).* 1982;11:73–88.

38. Johnsson B. Kinesiology. With special reference to electromyographic kinesiology. *Contemp Clin Neurophysiol.* 1978;34(EEG suppl):417–428.

39. Winkel J, Westgaard, RH. Occupational and individual risk factors for shoulder–neck complaints, part II: the scientific basis (literature review) for the guide. *Int J Indust Ergon.* 1992:10:85–104.

40. Veiersted KB, Westgaard RH, Andersen P. Electromyographic evaluation of muscular work pattern as a predictor of trapezius myalgia. *Scand J Work Environ Health.* 1993;19:284–290.

41. Veiersted KB, Westgaard RH, Andersen P. Pattern of muscle activity during stereotyped work and its relation to muscle pain. *Int Arch Occup Environ Health.* 1990;62:31–41.

42. Jorgensen K, Fallentih N, Krogh-Lund C, Jensen B. Electromyography and fatigue during prolonged, low-level static contractions. *Eur J Appl Physiol.* 1988; 57:316–321.

43. Sjogaard G, Kiens B, Jorgensen K, Saltin B. Intramuscular pressure, EMG and blood flow during low-level prolonged static contraction in man. *Acta Physiol Scand.* 1986;128:475–484.

44. Bjorksten M, Johnsson B. Endurance limit of force in long term intermittent static contractions. *Scand J Work Environ Health.* 1977;3:23–27.

45. Sundelin G, Hagberg M. The effects of different pause types on neck and shoulder EMG activity during VDU work. *Ergonomics.* 1989;39:527–537.

46. Perry J. *Gait Analysis.* Thorofare, NJ: Slack; 1992; 381–411.

47. Donaldson CCS. *The Effects of Correcting Muscle Asymmetry upon Chronic Low Back Pain.* Calgary, Alberta: University of Calgary; 1989. Dissertation.

48. Middaugh SJ, Kee WG, Nicholson J, Allenback G. Right versus left muscle asymmetry in normal subjects in upper trapezius and midscapular paraspinal muscles. In: *Proceedings of the Association for Applied Psychophysiology and Biofeedback (AAPB), 27th Annual Meeting, Albuquerque, New Mexico, March 1996.* Wheat Ridge, CO: AAPB; 1996;88–89.

49. Ballantyne BT, O'Hare SJ, Paschall JL, et al. Electromyographic activity of selected shoulder muscles in commonly used therapeutic exercises. *Phys Ther.* 1993;73:668–682.

50. Knutson LM, Soderberg GL, Ballantyne BT, Clarke WR. A study of various normalization procedures for within day electromyographic data. *J Electromyogr Kinesiol.* 1994;4:47–60.

51. Redfern MS. Functional muscle: effects on electromyographic output. In: Soderberg GL, ed. *Selected Topics in Surface Electromyography for Use in the Occupational Setting: Expert Perspectives.* Rockville, MD: US Dept of Health and Human Services; 1991;104–120. National Institute for Occupational Safety and Health publication No. 91-100.

52. Soderberg GL, Cook TM. Electromyography in biomechanics. *Phys Ther.* 1984;64:1813–1820.

53. Turker KS. Electromyography: some methodological problems and issues. *Phys Ther.* 1993;73:698–710.

54. Winter DA. Pathologic gait diagnosis with computer-averaged electromyographic profiles. *Arch Phys Med Rehabil.* 1984;65:393–400.

55. Yang JF, Winter DA. Electromyographic amplitude normalization methods: improving their sensitivity as diagnostic tools in gait analysis. *Arch Phys Med Rehabil.* 1984;65:517–521.

56. Hislop HJ, Montgomery J. *Daniels and Worthingham's Muscle Testing: Techniques of Manual Examination.* 6th ed. Philadelphia: WB Saunders Co; 1995.

57. Kendall FP, McCreary EK, Provance PG. *Muscles Testing and Function.* 4th ed. Baltimore: Williams & Wilkins; 1993.

58. Souza DR, Gross MT. Comparison of vastus medialis oblique:vastus lateralis muscle integrated electromyographic ratios between healthy subjects and patients with patellofemoral pain. *Phys Ther.* 1991;71:310–320.

59. Arena JG, Sherman RA, Bruno GM, Young TR. Electromyographic recordings of 5 types of low back pain subjects and non-pain controls in different positions. *Pain.* 1989;37:57–65.

60. Cram JR. EMG muscle scanning and diagnostic manual for surface recordings. In: Cram JR, ed. *Clinical EMG for Surface Recordings.* Vol 2. Nevada City, CA: Clinical Resources; 1990;1–142.

61. Cram JR, Engstrom D. Patterns of neuromuscular activity in pain and non-pain patients. *Clin Biofeedback Health.* 1986;9:106–115.

62. Cram JR, Steger JC. EMG scanning in the diagnosis of chronic pain. *Biofeedback Self Regul.* 1983;8:229–241.

63. Cohen MJ, Swanson GA, Naliboff BD, Schnadler SL, McArthur DL. Comparison of electromyographic response patterns during posture and stress tasks in chronic low back pain patterns and control. *J Psychosom Res.* 1986;30:135–141.

64. Nouwen A, Bush C. The relationship between paraspinal EMG and chronic low back pain. *Pain.* 1984;20:109–123.

65. Arena JG, Sherman RA, Bruno GM, Young TR. Electromyographic recordings of low back pain subjects and non-pain controls in six different positions: effects of pain levels. *Pain.* 1991; 45:23–28.

66. Ahern DK, Follick MJ, Council JR, Laser-Wolston N, Litchman H. Comparison of lumbar paravertebral EMG patterns in chronic low back pain patients and non-patient controls. *Pain.* 1988;34:153–160.

67. Harrison AL, Barry-Greb T, Wojtowicz G. Clinical measurement of head and shoulder posture variables. *J Orthop Sports Phys Ther.* 1996;23:353–361.

68. Youdas JW, Suman VJ, Garrett TR. Reliability of measurements of lumbar spine sagittal mobility obtained with the flexible curve. *J Orthop Sports Phys Ther.* 1995;21:13–20.

69. Gossman MR, Sahrman SA, Rose SJ. Review of length associated changes in muscle: experimental evidence and clinical implications. *Phys Ther.* 1982;62:1799–1808.

70. Middaugh SJ, Kee WG, Nicholson JA. Muscle overuse and posture as factors in the development and maintenance of chronic musculoskeletal pain. In: Grzesiak RC, Ciccone DS, eds. *Psychological Vulnerability to Chronic Pain.* New York: Springer Publishing Co; 1994;55–89.

71. Schuldt K, Ekholm J, Harms-Ringdahl K, Nemeth G, Arborelius UP. Effects of changes in sitting work posture on static neck and shoulder muscle activity. *Ergonomics.* 1986;29:1525–1537.

72. Bagg SD, Forrest WJ. Electromyographic study of the scapular rotators during arm abduction in the scapular plane. *Am J Phys Med.* 1986;65:111–124.

73. Sczepanski TL, Gross MT, Duncan PW, Chandler JM. Effect of contraction type, angular velocity, and arc of motion on VMO:VL EMG ratio. *J Orthop Sports Phys Ther.* 1991;14:256–262.

74. Sihvonen T, Partanen J, Hanninen O, Soimakallio S. Electric behavior of low back muscles during lumbar pelvic rhythm in low back pain patients and healthy controls. *Arch Phys Med Rehab.* 1991;72:1080–1087.

75. Nordin M, Frankel VH. *Basic Biomechanics of the Musculoskeletal System.* 2nd ed. Philadelphia: Lea & Febiger; 1989.

76. Rodgers MM. Musculoskeletal considerations in production and control of movement. In: Montgomery PC, Connolly BH, eds. *Motor Control and Physical Therapy: Theoretical Frameworks and Practical Applications.* Hixson, TN: Chattanooga Group; 1991;47–60.

77. Norkin CC, Levangie PK. *Joint Structure and Function: A Comprehensive Analysis.* Philadelphia: FA Davis; 1989.

78. Cuddeford T, Williams AK, Medeiros JM. Electromyographic activity of the vastus medialis oblique and vastus lateralis muscles during selected exercises. *J Orthop Sports Phys Ther.* 1996;24:10–15.

79. Taylor W. Dynamic EMG biofeedback in assessment and treatment using a neuromuscular reeducation model. In: Cram JR, ed. *Clinical EMG for Surface Recordings:* Vol 2. Nevada City, CA: Clinical Resources; 1990;175–196.

80. Andersson GB, Schultz AB, Ortengren R. Trunk muscle forces during desk work. *Ergonomics.* 1986;29:1113–1127.

81. Arborelius UP, Nisell ER, Nemeth G, Svensson O. Shoulder load during machine milking: an electromyographic and biomechanical study. *Ergonomics.* 1986; 29:1591–1607.

82. Hosea TM, Simon SR, Delatizky J, Wong MA, Hsieh CC. Myoelectric analysis of the paraspinal musculature in relation to automobile driving. *Spine.* 1986;11:928–936.

83. MacIntyre DL, Robertson BE. Quadriceps muscle activity in women runners with and without patellofemoral pain syndrome. *Arch Phys Med Rehabil.* 1992;73:10–14.

84. Philipson L, Sorbye R, Larsson P, Kaladjev S. Muscular load levels in performing musicians as monitored by quantitative electromyography. *Med Prob Perform Art.* 1990;5:79–82.

85. Toivanen H, Helin P, Hanninen O. Impact of regular re-laxation training and psychosocial working factors on neck–shoulder tension and absenteeism in hospital cleaners. *J Occup Med*. 1993;35:1123–1130.

86. Sherman RA. Applied psychophysiological research and development in the US Army. In: *Proceedings of the Association for Applied Psychophysiology and Bio-feedback (AAPB) 25th Annual Meeting, Atlanta, Georgia, March 1994*. Wheat Ridge, CO: AAPB; 1994.

87. Heerkens YF, Brandsma JW, Lakerveld-Heyl K, van Ravensberg CD. Impairments and disabilities—the dif-ference: proposal for adjustment of the International Classification of Impairments, Disabilities and Handi-caps. *Phys Ther*. 1994;74:430–442.

88. Jette AM: Physical disablement concepts for physical therapy research and practice. *Phys Ther*. 1994;74:380–386.

89. Nagi S. Disability concepts revisited: implications for prevention. In: Pope A, Tarlov A, eds. *Disability in America: Toward a National Agenda for Prevention*. Washington, DC: National Academy Press, 1991;309–327.

90. Delitto A. Are measures of function and disability im-portant in low back care? *Phys Ther*. 1994;74:452–462.

91. Fairbanks JCT, Couper J, Davies JB, et al. The Oswestry low back pain disability questionnaire. *Physiotherapy*. 1980;66:271–273.

92. Roland M, Morris R. A study of the natural history of back pain, part I: development of a reliable and sensitive measure of disability in low back pain. *Spine*. 1983;8:145–150.

CHAPTER 3

Motor Learning with SEMG Feedback

The goal of surface electromyography (SEMG) feedback training is to manipulate an individual's movement control system, so that learning occurs and function improves. SEMG feedback is simply a motor learning tool. To optimize the feedback setup, it is useful to begin by considering the principles of motor learning and their relation to the SEMG equipment. The basic premise is that feedback regarding motor performance is a crucial aspect of motor learning. Also central is the idea that access to performance information that is typically inaccessible can aid skill acquisition. Fundamental principles of motor learning and feedback will be reviewed in this chapter. These principles include information processing, phases of motor learning, feedback structure, skill transfer, and motivation. Practical considerations for patient learning, based on these concepts, will be discussed in Chapter 4.

SEMG feedback training involves the use of machine-produced, extrinsic cues that signal the outcome or quality of a muscle response relative to an intended goal. Training assists with the development of skilled motor responses by providing nearly instantaneous, performance-contingent information. The subject gains knowledge as to the functioning of a muscle, or group of muscles, with far greater sensitivity than could be obtained from the intrinsic senses acting alone. SEMG feedback cues serve as a reference for error detection. This error reference helps the subject identify effective movement strategies and eventually contributes to the development of an independent, intrinsic reference of correctness. Patients learn to relax overly tense muscles, to activate weak muscles more effectively, and to better coordinate muscle activity among agonists, antagonists, and synergists. Various response strategies are explored during training, and the results are evaluated for those that will lead to optimally skilled behaviors.

ROLE OF MOVEMENT CONTROL AND LEARNING IN LIFE EXPERIENCE

Movement ability has been modeled as an emergent property of an organism that enables it to solve problems.[1] An organism is inevitably subjected to changing intrinsic and extrinsic environmental conditions that require adaptive responses. Movement strategies are developed as solutions to environmental problems. Humans encounter myriad problems that can be solved with an almost infinite array of movement strategies. If individuals are to execute their daily activities without clinical impairment, movement strategies must be implemented that solve the problem at hand, in a behaviorally efficient way, without overloading the musculoskeletal system.

Application of movement strategies to life tasks requires learning. Motor learning is the organization and control of perceptual, cognitive, and motor resources to effect a relatively lasting change in movement behavior.[2,3] From a practical standpoint, learning implies that the ability to retain motor plans and to generalize those plans to variable situations indeed exists. A skilled motor response is one that efficiently achieves a specific goal over time and across different functional contexts.[1]

Movement Control

A single joint rarely acts alone during functional movement. Most often, the movements of several joints are linked together in a kinematic chain. The kinematic chain, conceptually adapted from engineering for musculoskeletal systems, consists of a series of adjacent body segments that are moved simultaneously to produce a specific outcome.[4,5] Kinematic chains may be composed of a part of a limb or an entire limb and may incorporate a portion of the body axis together with an extremity (Figure 3–1). The potential individual and combined joint motions of any kinematic chain result in many degrees of freedom.[6] Movement is constrained by

exploiting the biomechanical and neuromuscular properties of the segments in coordinated ways.[7,8] Included is the use of motor programs to harmonize the actions of muscles with each other and with the intended movement goal.[6,9,10] Motor programs are goal oriented, preplanned groupings of motor commands from the central nervous system (CNS), and they vastly simplify movement control.[3,11]

Skilled responses are characterized by integrated spatial and temporal control of kinematic chains. An effective motor program must consolidate appropriate rates of force development and modulation of reflex activity over the involved joint segments. In historical models of motor control, it has been posited that a hierarchical structure exists in which spinal segmental, intersegmental, and brainstem reflex systems form the fundamental components for programming, with superimposed regulation by the cerebellum, diencephalon, basal ganglia, and cerebral cortex.[12,13] These approaches, however, do not account for the degree of complexity ob-

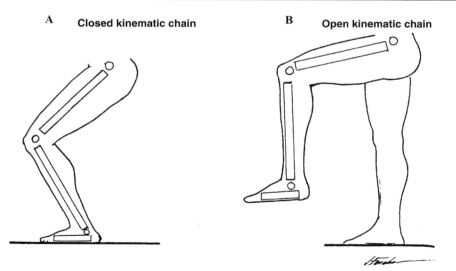

Figure 3–1 Conceptualization of the kinematic chain—a series of linked body segments that are moved simultaneously to achieve a movement outcome. (**A**) Closed kinematic chain, in which the distal segment is fixed. (**B**) Open kinematic chain, in which the distal segment is free. The two vary in biomechanical and motor control properties, but in both, the degrees of freedom of the systems are constrained by the harmonizing effect of motor programs. *Source:* Reprinted with permission from CC Norkin and PK Levangie, *Joint Structure and Function*, p 78, © 1983, FA Davis Company.

served in human motor behavior and have been largely replaced by systems models.[14,15] Systems models depart from a focus on central excitatory and inhibitory drive over reflex systems and more broadly consider the interplay of sensory, perceptual, cognitive, and command subsystems during functional movements. The remainder of this chapter will focus on the information processing aspects of movement control and learning. Basic physiologic considerations for neuromuscular systems are reviewed in Chapter 2 of the companion book, *Introduction to Surface Electromyography*,[16] and elsewhere.[3,10,15,17–19]

INFORMATION PROCESSING FOR MOVEMENT CONTROL AND LEARNING

Schmidt[3] discusses a three-phase process that occurs in the CNS between stimulus presentation and movement output. These phases are stimulus identification, response selection, and response programming (Figure 3–2).

In the first phase, an individual's sensory receptors transduce extrinsic energy into peripheral neural codes that are transmitted to the CNS. The individual perceptually processes the information, selectively attending to and sorting the stimuli, comparing stimuli to memory, and recognizing critical variables associated with stimuli.[20,21] A cognitive–motor problem is generated for which a solution must be found.[1]

During the second phase, a particular motor plan is chosen from among the many possible response patterns. Mulder[21] argues that the subject responds not so much by sorting through a CNS catalog of stimulus-specific motor engrams, but by overlaying rules of grammar on a vocabulary of potential motor patterns. Schmidt refers to these prototypical programming rules as schema.[22]

Schema theory forms the foundation for many contemporary ideas of movement control and learning.[3,22–24] Each scheme relates how variations in a generalized spatial and temporal pattern of activation will affect a goal outcome.

According to Schmidt, the temporal sequence of action steps, phasing relationships between muscles, and proportionate contraction intensities of the involved muscles are fixed. However, the overall force and speed are determined by the immediate environmental context. The motor program is modified to account for starting posture, external loads, and available response time. For example, in throwing a football overhead, the sequence of joint movements, muscles involved, and proportionate contributions and timing of each muscle are relatively preserved across different circumstances. The absolute force and velocity of the throwing motion, however, will vary with the distance to the receiver and the available time to execute the throw. Programming rules are acquired through previous experience involving repetition and evaluated by feedback from the movement with respect to the intended goal.

Once the response is selected, motor commands must be generated to implement it. Dur-

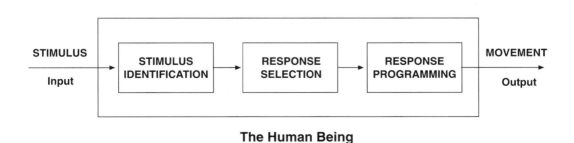

The Human Being

Figure 3–2 Schmidt's information-processing model for movement control. *Source:* Reprinted by permission from RA Schmidt, 1988, *Motor Control and Learning*, 2nd ed (Champaign, IL: Human Kinetics Publishers), 77.

ing Schmidt's third phase, response programming, the pieces of the motor plan are assembled, made coherent, and initiated.[3,20,21] Changes in postural tone may occur in anticipation of the motor response, so that a stabilized base is created for the coming movements.[25] Obviously, not all movements involve the same degree of information processing. A spinal stretch reflex is relatively "hard wired," whereas complex voluntary movements such as those involved in driving a car are highly processed.[26]

Sensory information is used to regulate movements before, during, and after motor program execution. Information derived before a movement prepares the CNS and creates a cognitive expectational set.[26,27] The expectational set is formed by abstracting the immediate sensory information with knowledge of past experiences. The results determine the ways in which the variable features of programming schema are put into play. Movement errors may be produced when the expectational set leads to program execution with an inappropriate absolute force level or velocity.[3] This happens, for example, when a door is suddenly flung open because the individual expected to encounter much greater resistance, or when a box that is thought to be heavy turns out to be light.

Information indicating the results or quality of movement is feedback. Feedback is used during certain types of tasks for regulating movement and, afterward, for learning.[28,29] Proprioceptive feedback is extracted from receptors embedded in musculotendon and periarticular structures, signaling changes in position, load, and velocity. Information is also acquired through auditory, vestibular, and visual systems. Sensory data are produced by either the effects of movement on the body itself or through observations of the consequences of movement on other objects. These are types of intrinsic feedback[28,29] (Figure 3–3). Extrinsic feedback is generated from other observers or machines. Feedback from extrinsic sources augments intrinsic feedback in skill acquisition. Cues from a SEMG machine are a type of extrinsic feedback. The feedback from a

SEMG device can be classified as artificial in that it does not occur naturally. Artificial extrinsic information from the SEMG display is combined with natural extrinsic and intrinsic cues during the individual's learning.

Some situations demand extremely rapid movement responses. These movements are generated by feedforward, or open loop, control.[21,26,30] Their execution occurs too quickly to be modified by sensory feedback and information processing. Therefore, movements performed with feedforward control do not depend on feedback for their execution, although they may be modified by sensory feedback over subsequent trials.[23,26,30] Highly practiced movements such as keyboard typing can be performed successfully with feedforward control. However, feedback, or closed loop, control is required while an individual is learning precision movements, as well as when he or she is performing slower functional tasks in a dynamic environment.[3]

In pioneering work, Adams[31] proposed that feedback cues are used to determine whether the movement under execution is being performed as was intended and to direct corrections if an error is detected. A movement reference of correctness, called a perceptual trace, is formed over many practice trials. This cognitive reference then guides the execution of motor programs. Adams' theory places a strong emphasis on feedback regulation of all types of movement. This is a point of departure from Schmidt's subsequent schema theory, which recognizes the use of concurrent feedback to help slow or novel movements play out correctly but views the regulation of open loop systems differently.[3] The components of open and closed loop systems are represented in Figure 3–4.

Information processing for movement control requires a memory interface.[20] In reviewing the influence of memory on movement planning, Schmidt[3] considers the roles of short-term sensory storage, short-term memory, and long-term memory. The short-term sensory storage accepts

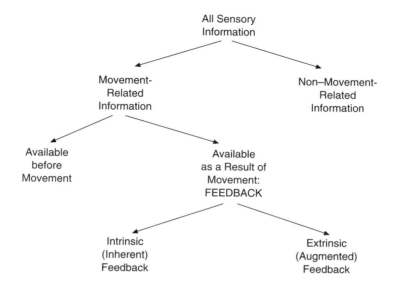

Figure 3–3 A classification of sensory information. *Source:* Reprinted with permission from RA Schmidt, 1988, *Motor Control and Learning,* 2nd ed (Champaign, IL: Human Kinetics Publishers), 424.

a large volume of stimulus information but retains it for less than 1 second. The long-term memory also holds a huge volume of information, but in highly abstracted forms and for long periods. Stimulus recognition and programming schema are stored in long-term memory. The short-term memory holds a comparatively limited amount of information for periods of seconds to minutes. Functionally, short-term memory acts as a buffer between short-term sensory storage and long-term memory, analogous to the random access memory of a personal computer.[20] When the individual is faced with a movement problem, many stimuli are presented to the short-term sensory store (Figure 3–5). Information that is selectively attended to is passed on to short-term memory, where it can be combined with other bits of information and abstracted. Data can also be retrieved from long-term memory and passed to short-term memory to recognize pivotal stimulus variables. To prepare for a motor response, programming schema are shifted from long-term memory to short-term memory and processed to meet the perceived circumstances.

PHASES OF MOTOR LEARNING

Many investigators have described a progression of skill learning.[1,3,31,32] Fitts and Posner[33] have used a three-stage model incorporating cognitive, associative, and autonomous phases. During the cognitive phase, the subject is intellectually focused, seeking basic orientation to the task. The fundamental task demands are analyzed, so that the problem and goals are understood and gross motor strategies are evaluated. Attentional demands are high during this period, and there is considerable verbal–cognitive processing. Performance scores tend to vary greatly, although rapid gains may ensue.

Next, during the associative phase, the gross motor strategies identified as effective are refined. The level of movement and task analysis becomes subtle, and the subject cultivates more efficient motor solutions. There is gradually less

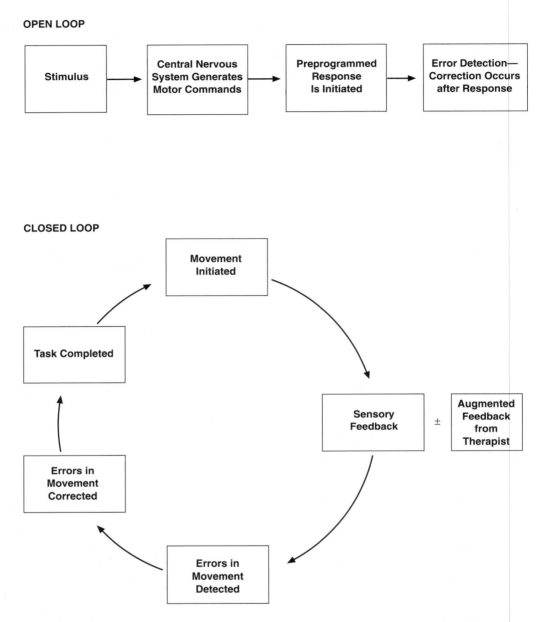

Figure 3–4 Components of open and closed loop movement control systems. *Source:* Reprinted with permission from MB Badke and RP Di Fabio, Sensory Information and Movement: Implications for Intervention, in *Motor Control and Physical Therapy: Theoretical Frameworks and Practical Applications*, PC Montgomery and BN Connolly, eds, p 100, © 1991, The Chattanooga Group.

reliance on extrinsic feedback and more on an intrinsic reference of correctness. Performance scores continue to improve and variance de-

creases, but the rate of gain tends to slow. Learning moves to the final autonomous phase with continued practice. Because the rate of gain in

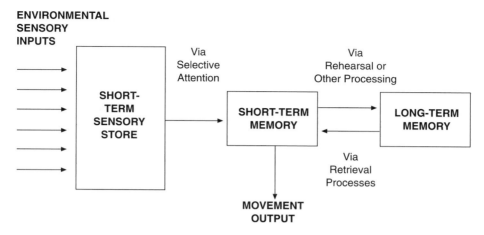

ENVIRONMENTAL SENSORY INPUTS

Figure 3–5 Relationships among memory compartments, showing processes involved in moving among them. *Source:* Reprinted with permission from RA Schmidt, 1988, *Motor Control and Learning*, 2nd ed (Champaign, IL: Human Kinetics Publishers), 91.

performance tends to be very slow at this stage, many cumulative trials may be required to reach the autonomous level. Performance is now precise, and the degree of cognitive focus is vastly reduced.

The objective for therapists is to facilitate the patient's learning experience into the autonomous phase. Patients must be independent in applying motor solutions, and their responses must be efficiently sequenced if they are to be functional. Schmidt[3] frames the cognitive phase as learning *what* to do, the associative phase as learning *how* to do it, and the autonomous phase as learning how to make the responses *automatic*. He emphasizes that learners shift across cognitive dimensions as they progress toward automaticity. The individual moves away from intellectual analysis, across different spatial and kinesthetic awareness abilities, in the direction of mature schema. By making use of cognitive structures, the individual is relieved of conscious processing demands and able to attend to other aspects of the task, or to process information about another task simultaneously. For example, the reader may have had the experience of driving a well-traveled route while being engaged in intense thought about some aspect of work or personal life, arriving at

the destination with little conscious awareness of the trip.

It is believed that automaticity is achieved by the formation of specialized networks to take care of stimulus sorting and response selection.[34,35] These networks use cognitive and neurophysiologic systems to move information efficiently among short-term sensory storage, short-term memory, and long-term memory. Processing networks are also developed to integrate afferent cues with efferent commands within short-term memory. Individuals learn to chunk serial movement steps together into unified programs[11] and build basic movement components into more complex patterns that can be preprogrammed if the tasks are very predictable.[3] In addition, subjects may develop a skill through more efficient use of reflex systems[36] as well as by learning to use the inertial and mechanical properties of the moving body parts.[1,9] Thus a gymnast might learn to use angular momentum to carry through a swinging movement, suppress or modify protective visual–motor and vestibular–motor reflexes, take advantage of muscle length–tension relationships, and pool sequences of steps into unitary movement blocks. The reader may reflect on his or her personal experience in learning how to perform some athletic task. The pattern of muscle activation may have improved, and energy consumption declined, as skill developed. The reader may also remember becoming able to recognize what to look for quickly to distinguish skilled performance, of both self and others, and how certain observations would automatically lead to complex response sequences without conscious thought.

SEMG FEEDBACK AND SKILL ACQUISITION

Mechanisms of movement control and learning have interested biofeedback practitioners from the first applications. The use of EMG feedback to retrain patients with neurologic deficits was described in the early 1960s.[37,38] During the same period, Basmajian[39] convincingly demonstrated that subjects could use EMG feedback to learn to self-regulate the activity of individual motor units. Many attempts to apply EMG feedback followed, some within the domain of physical rehabilitation[40,41] and others within the emerging realm of relaxation training.[42–45] Relaxation practice, with SEMG as well as other feedback modalities, was intended to address psychologic stress-based disorders and focused largely on establishing voluntary control of autonomic function. Training was modeled on principles of operant conditioning.[46]

From an operant conditioning perspective, feedback cues are seen as contingent reinforcers for motor behaviors.[47–49] The view is that cues indicating goal achievement are perceived as positive, whereas cues that indicate error are perceived as neutral or negative. Individuals tend to increase the frequency of positively rewarded behaviors and decrease the frequency of nonrewarded or punished behaviors.[50] In this way, subjects learn to reproduce motor behaviors that meet the favored goal. Operant conditioning principles hold for many examples of animal learning and human verbal learning, and certain variables seem relevant for human motor learning. Brucker and Bulaeva[51] believe that inclusion of an operant paradigm is a critical determinant of successful SEMG training. An operant

paradigm is supported by a goal marker on the display, verbal reinforcement of success, and contingent changes in the goal criterion value. The range of experimental observations reported over recent years, however, cannot be fully accounted for by operant theory, and many investigators have turned to an information-processing approach.

Much debate has centered on the extent to which SEMG training reflects dominance of feedforward versus feedback mechanisms. One context was set early by Brener while elaborating a closed loop model for the acquisition of autonomic control.[52–55] According to Brener, subjects use feedback cues to learn to generate new responses (ie, responses that did not exist before training). Learning takes place by repeated associations of artificial extrinsic cues from the feedback machine with natural intrinsic cues. The machine feedback cues, which are obvious, direct the subject to attend to relevant but subtle intrinsic cues. Because the machine feedback is goal contingent, the subject is led to recognize and label intrinsic afferent information that characterizes a desired response. Brener proposed that the individual forms a response image over multiple trials, similar in concept to Adams' perceptual trace.[31] The response image is a cognitive template of the desired output. During any new trial, feedback is used to compare the actual output with the response image. Thus the interaction of the response image with sensory cues is an error detection mechanism. In interpreting Brener's model within the information-processing framework discussed earlier, artificial feedback promotes formation of cognitive structures for efficient intrinsic stimulus identification. Recognition of critical afferent cues guides the development of new voluntary efferent programs. Skilled execution is accomplished through comparison of ongoing, response-contingent sensory cues with the response image. Machine-derived feedback serves as a reference of correctness until the subject develops an intrinsic reference system.

Implicit in Brener's model is the idea that subjects should progressively demonstrate conscious awareness of afferent cues. Lacroix[56] reviewed evidence for and against the role of afferent information in the development of autonomic skills as proposed by Brener, concluding that two types of information processing better account for skill acquisition. Lacroix stated that control is achieved most often by an open-loop mechanism. Learners do not develop new efferent programs; rather, they select from a pool of preexisting responses and execute them in a feedforward manner. Feedback is critical during the early stages of training in that it provides information regarding the outcome of the selected response, a type of knowledge of results (KR). Machine feedback informs the learner whether the selected response achieved the desired outcome. Over many trials, the subject uses the extrinsic feedback to narrow the range of potential responses. Responses that fail to support the feedback goal are discarded, whereas responses that achieve the goal are retained. The learner identifies progressively smaller subsets of acceptable responses until performance reaches a plateau. Machine feedback aids not so much with intrinsic stimulus identification and efferent programming as with response selection. Because the subject executes a known program, the model suggests that continuous feedback during execution is relatively unimportant. On-line knowledge of performance quality is less useful than knowledge of outcome results. Lacroix, however, went on to propose that an afferent identification role for artificial feedback and closed loop control may be operative under certain, less frequently occurring conditions. Included are times when the subject's response repertoire lacks an adequate efferent program to achieve the goal; that is, when there is no existing response to select that will solve the problem. This occurs when the desired response is not one that is normally found in the subject's natural physiologic routine. A new efferent program would also be needed if there was cognitive interference with the response selection process because of experimental manipulations or clinical impairments.

Several investigators have sought to examine these theories specifically with SEMG feedback and voluntary motor tasks. Researchers have attempted to discriminate between motor control skills and sensory awareness skills. The idea has been that if afferent awareness skills are causally linked to improvements in task motor control, then closed loop mechanisms will be invoked. If, on the other hand, awareness and control are independent of each other, then open loop systems will predominate. It once was believed that awareness of muscle tension levels was a necessary skill in the development of voluntary deep motor relaxation.[57] Results of experimental studies, however, vary in their support for[45] and against[44,58] a relationship between subjective tension awareness and SEMG scores during relaxation training.

This issue was examined in a group of subsequent reports with the use of related methodologies. Awareness skill was tested by (1) asking subjects to guess whether muscle tension increased or decreased over successive trials in resting postures,[59–61] (2) assessing the accuracy of voluntary activation to targeted SEMG magnitude levels,[62–66] (3) comparing rank on a subjective tension scale with actual SEMG levels, [67,68] and (4) evaluating subject verbal responses to structured inquiry.[69] All but one of these investigations used forehead frontal recording sites, with one group additionally recording SEMG activity from the sternocleidomastoid and posterior cervical groups[68] and two others additionally recording from the forearm.[66,67] The remaining study used masseter recording sites.[64] Subjects were trained primarily with audio cues over a small number of sessions.

Results of one study showed that continuous feedback was superior to both discrete (noncontinuous) posttrial verbal results feedback and no feedback in training relaxation responses.[59] Continuous feedback seemed to have positive effects in enhancing muscle awareness responses. Findings in other reports confirmed that SEMG feedback promoted relaxation and muscle tension awareness, as compared to findings with no feedback control groups,[60,61] and identified a correlation between performance on a SEMG magnitude production task and muscle perception.[64] However, other investigators, some of whom used refined designs of the earlier studies, have argued against muscle tension awareness being related to either relaxation ability or muscle activation procedures.[62,66,69] Also, deliberately attending to muscles did not, in itself, necessarily lead to relaxation,[67] and subjective tension rankings did not necessarily correlate with SEMG changes.[68] The application of closed loop models to SEMG feedback training was therefore questioned by several researchers, and open loop mechanisms were seen as the primary feature of motor skill acquisition.[62,66,69] Awareness of muscle tension was viewed as a less critical element. The machine feedback was believed to assist with the selection of existing, feed forward responses.

Later, Glaros and Hanson[63] reported on experimental evidence that they interpreted as supporting an awareness (closed loop) mechanism for more difficult tasks while suggesting a predominance of an open loop system for less difficult tasks. Most recently, Segreto[65] returned to the two-process model advocated by Lacroix[56] to explain experimental tests of awareness and tension magnitude discrimination.

Collectively, results of these studies suggest that SEMG feedback is effective in producing relaxation, active muscle control, and awareness, but the acquisition mechanisms and relationships among the variables are not clear. Both feedforward and feedback mechanisms may be involved, depending on the training task and learning environment. Unfortunately, none of the experimental designs included a delayed transfer task. As will be discussed, factors that improve motor skill acquisition may have positive, neutral, or negative effects when retention is assessed after no-training delays.[23] Investigations of short-term performance during feedback training may not relate to long-term learning. Whether skill acquisition takes place in clinical populations as it does with healthy subjects is also unclear. Skill acquisition in these reports was investigated almost exclusively with audio feedback. Although the use of visual feedback may not have had a differential effect on the forehead relaxation results,[58] it is not known whether currently available visual displays would have changed the results for the other tasks. Differences in stimulus–response compatibility between visual versus auditory stimuli and motor responses have been suggested.[3] Moreover, most of the experiments focused on forehead SEMG recordings. Yet one group proposed that the forearm flexors and frontalis may be controlled by different mechanisms,[66] and another group showed that trained frontalis responses do not generalize to other muscles.[68] Cram and Freeman[70] also demonstrated that forehead frontal relaxation training does not transfer to other axial body sites, nor across training postures. With a unique role in emotional expression,[71,72] the extent to which facial control mechanisms apply to other muscles is not known. Investigations that use forehead frontal recording sites and single posture relaxation training exclusively may have limited generalizability.[70] The relative importance of feedback and feedforward models may vary among relaxation training, tension discrimination training, and functional movement training, tasks that differ in context and speed.

The cognitive mechanisms of SEMG feedback learning are as yet obscure. Without evidence pointing to a peculiar set of mechanisms for SEMG training, such learning will be considered as being mediated by the same principles that underlie motor learning in general. It will be assumed that (1) both feedback and feedforward systems are operative, (2) subjects can move from one system to the other as skill is acquired, and (3) the systems operate differently for different types of movement. The amount and type of information provided by SEMG feedback are probably unique, but the mechanisms that subserve skill acquisition are likely the same as in other situations.

ADJUNCTIVE FACTORS IN MOTOR LEARNING

Patients who are engaging in motor learning are reorganizing their programming schema.[21] Several factors influence this process. Issues related to feedback, practice schedules, skill transfer, and motivation will be introduced here, with suggestions for the field deferred to Chapter 4.

Feedback Variations

Human experimental learning does not take place without feedback.[3,73,74] Feedback indicates error on a particular movement trial and helps direct correction on subsequent trials. Error detection is used over many trials to determine the usefulness of a specific movement strategy in solving a particular problem.[1] Subjects use extrinsic feedback cues as an error reference during the early stages of learning, and with practice, they substitute an intrinsic reference of correctness.[75]

For example, suppose a patient with neck and shoulder pain is being trained with SEMG feedback to improve posture and decrease activity of the upper trapezius. The functional problem is one of posturally related pain and muscle tension. To explore potential problem-solving strategies, the patient experiments with different positions for the head, trunk, and shoulders, looking for a decrease in SEMG activity. The therapist observes both the SEMG display and the patient, ensuring that the posture chosen to decrease upper trapezius activity is also satisfactory in terms of the biomechanical alignment of the spine and shoulder girdle. Thus a relaxed but forward slouched posture would be discouraged. Another posture, which shows decreased trapezius activity with an appropriately retracted head and elevated sternum, would be reinforced. The extrinsic feedback from the therapist and the SEMG machine tell the patient when the goal response (ie, erect alignment with decreased trapezius activity) has been obtained. Over several trials, these extrinsic cues are associated with intrinsic kinesthetic sensations. The patient becomes able to recognize independently both goal and faulty posture and to detect the difference between them.

Two categories of extrinsic feedback have been experimentally distinguished: (1) KR, which provides outcome information, and (2) knowledge of performance (KP), which pro-

vides information as to movement quality.[3,23,24,28,76] Knowledge of results indicates whether the goal was achieved and, oftentimes, the direction and magnitude of error from the intended goal. Knowledge of performance denotes the quality with which movement was performed. Gentile[76] states that KR answers the learner's question, "Was the goal accomplished?" Knowledge of performance answers the question, "Was the movement executed in the intended manner?"

Consider the following example. If a patient is trying to reproduce a 5 μV-level contraction of the upper trapezius without looking at the SEMG display, verbal KR from the therapist could indicate the actual average number of microvolts during the trial. If the patient actually averages 8 μV, this KR tells the patient that the goal was exceeded by 3 μV. On the next trial, the patient would know to decrease the intensity of effort. If a 4-μV output relative to the same 5-μV goal was produced, the patient would know to increase effort slightly on the next trial. A schema would be formed that relates recruitment intensity to SEMG magnitude over many trials. Suppose that this patient moves on to another task. The objective is to increase the firing of the lower fibers of the serratus anterior as the arm is raised through shoulder flexion. At the same time, recruitment of the upper trapezius is decreased. SEMG activity from each target muscle site could be shown as a tracing with oscilloscope-like graphics. Patterns of SEMG activity observed on the display would be a form of KP. The feedback would show how the movement was accomplished through the range of motion arc.

Because KR parameters are relatively easy to define and control and KR is believed to be used intuitively by subjects learning in the field, the effects of KR on motor learning have been studied extensively in the laboratory.[3,24,28] Knowledge of results has been studied primarily with healthy subjects learning novel, short-duration tasks. The consequences for functional movements are not known, but the fundamental findings have been consistently replicated and framed for those teaching new motor skills.[28,76,77] One might suppose that the KR factors that contribute to performance early in training would also lead to better retention over time. However, this does not seem to be the case, at least under the experimental conditions studied so far. By providing immediate, specific KR for every trial attempt, performance during skill acquisition is facilitated, but this tactic seems inferior to other KR regimens on retention tests. Retention scores are superior in experimental groups receiving KR on every other trial, every third trial, or less frequently.[78–81] Improved retention scores have also been produced by using summary KR for a number of previous trials,[82,83] as well as by delaying KR presentation for several seconds.[80,84] Another successful approach has been demonstrated with bandwidth KR, in which no extrinsic feedback is given—as long as the measured response falls within a range of acceptable values—but an error signal is otherwise generated.[85]

Frequent or immediate KR may promote a cognitive dependency on the extrinsic feedback, impeding the formation of an intrinsic reference for error identification.[3,24,83,84] Winstein[28] believes that intermittent and delayed KR regimens compel subjects to process intrinsic and natural extrinsic cues in comparison with the artificial KR cues. The association of the various feedback cues produces an internal reference of correctness and eventually decreases dependence on KR provided by the experimenter or feedback machine. Writing for clinicians, Winstein[28] implies caution should be used with devices intended to provide continuous feedback and suggests that astute therapists spontaneously use cues in intermittent, delayed, or bandwidth formats. Interestingly, one group of investigators has reported anecdotal subject preference for cycled periods of feedback/no feedback, rather than continuous feedback, during relaxation training monitored with SEMG.[86,87] The subjects implied that they used each no-feedback period to try to apply corrective actions, based on SEMG feedback from the

previous period, and then evaluated the results of their effort with the feedback from the following period.

Knowledge of performance variables have not been as well defined as those relating to KR. However, the traditional use of SEMG feedback has been classified as a KP variant.[3] Knowledge of performance has been characterized as vitally important in real-life settings.[3,76] SEMG feedback provides real-time information about movement quality. The machine information is exacting in terms of the spatial and temporal pattern of activated muscles. This degree of sensitivity and specificity provides unique information content relative to other types of motor feedback. By bringing forth an awareness of a muscle's recruitment subtleties through a range of motion arc or, perhaps, the coordination pattern between two muscles that would normally go undetected, additional dimensions of information processing may be brought into play. As previously described, SEMG feedback can also be used for KR, indicating the outcome of simple activation or relaxation attempts in terms of signal magnitude. In any case, the artificial error reference of the display enables rapid sorting of potential responses for those that will support goal attainment. The machine feedback serves as a reference for error detection during the preliminary stages of strategy evaluation, until the patient builds an internal reference and goal-specific schema. Because the relationship between the selected response and outflow to the muscles is so explicit, data points for schema tuning[3] are readily available. This sense of SEMG feedback, taken from the perspective of KR and KP, is generally consistent with the models of feedback skill acquisition proposed by Brener[54] and Lacroix.[56]

Practice Schedules

In learning new motor skills, the "practice makes perfect" principle has been widely taught. Indeed, task repetition is an integral part of the motor learning process. It has been argued that repetition allows not so much for the opportunity to cement a stereotypic response pattern as for the chance to explore solutions to the motor problem.[6,88] The cognitive process of learning how to solve the problem is seen as the critical element of practice. Repetition enables the subject to evaluate what does and does not work to solve the problem, and it is the resulting schema that is retained over time and used to solve problems in novel contexts.[88]

If repetition is so vital, then how practice is structured within and across sessions must also be important. A special set of considerations relates to the scheduling of practice for multiple training tasks. As is the case with feedback delivery, practice schedules that promote the rapid acquisition of performance ability are not necessarily those that optimize skill retention and transfer. Motor learning of multiple tasks has been studied by using blocked versus random schedules.[3,24,88] With a blocked schedule, a number of practice trials for one task are completed before practice on another task are initiated. For example, in knee rehabilitation a patient would learn how to generate desired SEMG patterns during weight shifting before attempting partial squats. Practice with lunges would be started once practice with squats was completed, and so forth. With a completely randomized schedule, the training sequence would randomly alternate across repetitions within each session.

Blocked practice has been shown repeatedly to produce higher scores for initial performance, but lower scores on retention and transfer tests.[24,88–92] The effect has been attributed to the cognitive dimensions of motor learning. Randomized practice may force a subject to process information in a richer manner because the motor goal changes from one trial to the next.[24,92] The learner is unable to maintain a stable expectational set. Performance on one task also may interfere with repetitious recall for another, driving the subject to try to figure out how to solve each problem each time it is presented.[88,93,94] For every random trial, the subject must recognize key stimuli variables, determine

an objective, evaluate potential responses, and execute the desired program. Blocked practice, on the other hand, may enable a subject to use short-term recall and simply repeat a response that generated positive feedback on previous trials.[93] The subject satisfies the goal by repeating a stereotypic response, without learning a programming schema. Thus subjects on a randomized schedule take longer to achieve the same performance level as those who use blocked practice. Because the subjects with randomized training learn problem-solving strategies more completely, however, they do better on retention tests. Randomized practice leads to repetition of the motor learning process, whereas blocked practice can actually obstruct learning.[3,88]

Skill Transfer

The ability to reproduce desired motor responses in real-life functional contexts must be the criterion for successful training. Patients usually come to the clinic for SEMG feedback practice. Effort must be taken to ensure transfer of skill from the feedback laboratory to each individual's daily environments.[49] Transfer is defined as a change in performance of one activity as a result of experience with another.[3] Skill transfer can involve carry over from a relatively disparate task or a nearly identical one with slightly different contextual demands. For example, a patient may achieve relaxation of the upper trapezius in a comfortable chair in a nondistracting room with a supportive therapist. The larger challenge will be to reproduce trapezius relaxation in a time- and socially pressured work setting. It is widely believed that skill with a particular task requires specific motor programs and differing conditions between practice and performance testing may impede learning.[95] According to Schmidt,[3] this is akin to the principles of state-dependent learning well known to psychologists. He argues that the acquisition and learning test conditions may differ, so long as the underlying cognitive and motor processes are similar. Schmidt recommends practice variability as a means of developing sensorimotor schema, based on a broad range of experience, that will transfer across settings. Practicing relaxation in the feedback laboratory may help the individual transfer that skill to a work setting if the same basic strategies are applicable. If, however, there is insufficient time to replicate the relaxation procedure at work, background distractions are too disruptive, or social pressures impair compliance, carry over is unlikely to be obtained. Specifically, there is experimental evidence that relaxation training transfers poorly across muscle sites and training postures.[16,68,86,87] Therefore, the clinician will need to consider the specificity of muscle training sites, as well as changes in posture and environmental context, while planning transfer progressions.

Motivation

Motivation is the set of cognitive processes that drive behavior toward goal completion.[96] Subjects become motivated to achieve goals that result in attainment of rewards or reduction of negative experiences.[97] Thoughts, feelings, and behaviors all have an impact on, and are affected by, motivational processes. These processes may involve approach to, or avoidance of, specific factors in a subject's experiential field. Motivational issues are important to the feedback therapist to the extent that they direct arousal, attention, and adherence during task performance.

Subjects structure their behavior on the basis of anticipated consequences of the event. Lewthwaite[96] describes this situational meaning as being idiosyncratic to the individual, based on personal perceptual and cognitive factors and interpersonal social relationships as discussed below. To engender positive meaning, the task must satisfy the individual's goals and be able to be performed in a way that is consistent with the person's goal orientations. Two types of goal orientations are distinguished: self-referenced and social comparison. Subjects who reference to the self to evaluate task performance tend to

focus on skill mastery. They acquire skill by seeking challenges and are largely internally driven and validated. Subjects who reference to the social judgments of others work for approval and interpersonal acceptance. Subjects with this social comparison goal orientation tend to self-select tasks of lower complexity, and they may vary in observed affect, response to failure, and persistence from subjects with a self-referenced orientation.

A person's goal orientation closely interacts with a sense of performance competence in producing motivated behaviors and effective problem solving. Individuals with perceptions of self-efficacy believe that they can produce positive outcomes in a given situation. Self-efficacy is derived from memories of similar past experiences, observations of others who are perceived as similar to the self, and contextual issues related to arousal and social reinforcement. Thus Lewthwaite[96] identifies highly motivated persons as those who have an adequate skill base and perceived self-efficacy, and who are motivated by a belief that they can attain a certain outcome that will have beneficial effects. Motivated subjects with a self-referenced goal orientation will maintain effort and positive affect during periods of failure. They will try to develop new strategies to solve the problem. Motivated individuals with a strong social comparison reference will also persist, but they may prefer to avoid complex challenges that risk error and negative social judgments. Persons who have a social comparison goal orientation and low perceptions of self-efficacy are characterized by Lewthwaite as tending toward learned helplessness. These individuals respond poorly to failure, developing anxiety and frustration. Increased arousal and enduring feelings of inadequacy tend to impede problem solving further. Such persons are prone to motivation loss and termination of program participation.

It has been known for some time that motivational issues have an impact on general feedback training experiences.[98,99] In accordance with classical biofeedback theory, contingent rewards such as reduced pain may operantly re-inforce practice.[49] Cognitions regarding self-efficacy influence both pain perception and responses to SEMG feedback training.[100,101] In addition, motivation also affects compliance with rehabilitation exercise programs.[102–104] Patient motivation is therefore likely to contribute to SEMG training outcomes in a direct way. Also, an individual's motivational level may itself be modified by feedback training. Knowledge of results has motivational aspects in addition to its informational dimension.[3,105] Motor learning feedback seems to promote interest and persistence,[106,107] attention,[108] and goal setting.[109] Thus the very act of participating in feedback sessions may be motivating to individuals, a point noted anecdotally by many therapists.

CONCLUSION

Skilled motor responses are produced so an individual can solve problems efficiently in his or her environment. Movement is controlled in part by processing information through three stages: stimulus identification, response selection, and response programming. Informational feedback is processed over repeated trials so that motor programming schema are learned. These prototypical rules harmonize the actions of muscles in achieving specific movement goals. A learner progresses through cognitive and associative learning phases to automaticity. Information processing becomes highly sophisticated at the automaticity level. The role of feedback in motor learning has been extensively studied as KR and KP variables. Learning is enhanced through the use of intermittent, delayed, and summary KR, as well as by randomization of learner tasks. Functionally significant outcomes result when skills are transferred from the clinic or laboratory to real-life environments. Motivation consists of a complex set of constructs that support the learner in achieving movement goals.

Informational cues from a SEMG display are a type of artificially produced extrinsic feedback. Both open and closed loop control systems seem to be operative during SEMG feedback learning. The feedback cues serve as an extrinsic error reference until the learner assimilates an intrinsic reference of correctness. In this way, SEMG feedback helps the learner extract intrinsic sensory cues and relate motor programming to movement results. SEMG feedback therefore helps the subject in learning programming schema. It is likely that the factors that govern motor learning in general also regulate SEMG feedback learning. The information content of the SEMG signal is, however, especially rich, and this is probably the source of its potency in augmenting the learner's experience. From a practical standpoint, the learner exploits the information to relax muscles that are too tense, increase the output of muscles that are weak, or improve coordination of multiple muscles that must work together. Participation in feedback training may be inherently motivating to the learner as he or she progresses through a motor training program. Exhibit 3–1 lists some advantages of SEMG feedback as a motor learning tool.

Exhibit 3–1 Usefulness of SEMG Feedback in Motor Learning

- Provides continuous display of muscle activity, essentially as it occurs.
- Yields precise feedback as to goal attainment.
- Provides exquisitely sensitive and accurate feedback regarding movement quality.
- Motivating; works well with patient exploration of movement strategies.
- Easily adapts to intermittent, summary, or delayed feedback schedules as the learner progresses.
- Integrates with practice in functional contexts and skill transfer progressions.
- Objectifies performance for documentation.

REFERENCES

1. Higgins S. Motor skill acquisition. *Phys Ther.* 1991; 71:123–139.

2. Fischer E. Factors affecting motor learning. *Am J Phys Med.* 1967;46:511–519.

3. Schmidt RA. *Motor Control and Learning: A Behavioral Emphasis.* 2nd ed. Champaign, IL: Human Kinetics; 1988.

4. Gowitzke BA, Milner M. *Understanding the Scientific Basis of Human Movement.* 2nd ed. Baltimore: Williams & Wilkins; 1980.

5. Norkin CC, Levangie PK. *Joint Structure and Function: A Comprehensive Analysis.* Philadelphia: FA Davis; 1989.

6. Bernstein N. *The Coordination and Regulation of Movements.* Oxford: Pergamon Press; 1967.

7. Keshner EA. Controlling stability of a complex movement system. *Phys Ther.* 1990;70:844–854.

8. Rodgers MM. Musculoskeletal considerations in production and control of movement. In: Montgomery PC, Connolly BH, eds. *Motor Control and Physical Therapy: Theoretical Frameworks and Practical Applications.* Hixson, TN: Chattanooga Group; 1991;47–60.

9. Kelso JAS, Schoner G. Self-organization of coordinative movement patterns. *Hum Movement Sci.* 1988; 7:27–46.

10. Latash, ML. *Control of Human Movement.* Champaign, IL: Human Kinetics; 1993.

11. Keel SW, Summers JJ. The structure of motor programs. In: Stelmach GE, ed. *Motor Control: Issues and Trends.* New York: Academic Press; 1976;109–142.

12. Pew RW. Acquisition of hierarchical control over the temporal organization of a skill. *J Exp Psychol.* 1966;71:764–771.

13. Phillips CG, Porter R. *Corticospinal Neurones: Their Role in Movement.* New York: Academic Press; 1977.

14. Horak FB. Assumptions underlying motor control for neurologic rehabilitation. In: *Contemporary Management of Motor Problems: Proceedings of the II Step Conference.* Alexandria, VA: Foundation for Physical Therapy; 1991;11–27.

15. Shumway-Cook A, Woollacott MH. *Motor Control: Theory and Practical Implications.* Baltimore: Williams & Wilkins; 1995.

16. Cram JR, Kasman GS. *Introduction to Surface Electromyography.* Gaithersburg, MD: Aspen Publishers; 1997.

17. Basmajian JV, De Luca CJ. *Muscles Alive: Their Functions Revealed by Electromyography.* 5th ed. Baltimore: Williams & Wilkins; 1985.

18. Enoka RM. *Neuromechanical Basis of Kinesiology.* Champaign, IL: Human Kinetics; 1988.

19. Newton RA. Neural systems underlying motor control. In: Montgomery PC, Connolly BH, eds. *Motor Control and Physical Therapy: Theoretical Frameworks and Practical Applications.* Hixson, TN: Chattanooga Group; 1991.

20. Light KE. Issues of cognition for motor control. In: Montgomery PC, Connolly BH, eds. *Motor Control and Physical Therapy: Theoretical Frameworks and Practical Applications.* Hixson, TN: Chattanooga Group; 1991.

21. Mulder T. A process-oriented model of human motor behavior: toward a theory-based rehabilitation approach. *Phys Ther.* 1991;71:157–164.

22. Schmidt RA. A schema theory of discrete motor learning. *Psychol Rev.* 1975;82:225–260.

23. Schmidt RA. *Motor Learning and Performance: From Principles to Practice.* Champaign, IL: Human Kinetics; 1991.

24. Schmidt RA. Motor learning principles for physical therapy. In: Lister MJ, ed. *Contemporary Management of Motor Control Problems.* Alexandria, VA: Foundation for Physical Therapy; 1991;49–63.

25. Lee WA. Anticipatory control of posture and task muscles during rapid arm flexion. *J Motor Behav.* 1982;12:185–196.

26. Badke MB, Di Fabio RP. Sensory information and movement: implications for intervention. In: Montgomery PC, Connolly BH, eds. *Motor Control and Physical Therapy: Theoretical Frameworks and Practical Applications.* Hixson, TN: Chattanooga Group; 1991; 99–108.

27. Nashner LM, Cordo PJ. Relation of automatic postural responses and reaction-time voluntary movements of human leg muscles. *Exp Brain Res.* 1981;43:395–405.

28. Winstein CJ. Knowledge of results and motor learning—implications for physical therapy. *Phys Ther.* 1991;71:140–149.

29. Winstein CJ, Schmidt RA. Sensorimotor feedback. In: Holding D, ed. *Human Skills.* 2nd ed. Chichester, England: John Wiley & Sons; 1989;17–47.

30. Giuliani CA. Theories of motor control: new concepts for physical therapy. In: *Contemporary Management of Motor Problems: Proceedings of the II Step Conference.* Alexandria, VA: Foundation for Physical Therapy; 1991;29–35.

31. Adams JA. A close-loop theory of motor learning. *J Mot Behav.* 1971;3:111–150.

32. Gentile AM. Skill acquisition: action, movement, and neuromotor processes. In: Carr JH, Shepherd RB, eds. *Movement Science: Foundations for Physical Therapy in Rehabilitation.* Rockville, MD: Aspen Publishers; 1987;93–154.

33. Fitts PM, Posner MI. *Human Performance.* Belmont, CA: Brooks/Cole Publishing; 1967.

34. Schneider W, Shiffrin R. Controlled and automatic human information processing, I. Detection, search, and attention. *Psychol Rev.* 1977;84:1–66.

35. Shiffrin RM, Schneider W. Controlled and automatic human information processing: II. Perceptual learning, automatic attending, and a general theory. *Psychol Rev.* 1977;84:127–190.

36. Hellebrant FA, Houtz SJ, Partrige MJ, Walters CE. Tonic reflexes in exercises of stress in man. *Am J Phys Med.* 1956;35:144–159.

37. Andrews JM. Neuromuscular re-education of hemiplegic with aid of electromyograph. *Arch Phys Med Rehabil.* 1964;45:530–532.

38. Marinacci AA, Horande M. Electromyogram in neuromuscular re-education. *Bull Los Angeles Neurol Soc.* 1960;25:57–71.

39. Basmajian JV. Conscious control of individual motor units. *Science.* 1963;141:440–441.

40. Brundy J, Grynbaum BB, Korein J. Spasmodic torticollis: treatment of feedback display of EMG. *Arch Phys Med Rehabil.* 1973;55:403–408.

41. Johnson HE, Garton WH. Muscle re-education in hemiplegia by use of electromyographic device. *Arch Phys Med Rehabil.* 1973;54:320–322.

42. Budzynski TH, Stoyva SM. An instrument for producing deep muscle relaxation by means of analog information feedback. *J Appl Behav Anal.* 1969;2:231–237.

43. Budzynski TH, Stoyva SM, Adler CS, Mullaney DJ. EMG biofeedback and tension headache: a controlled outcome study. *Psychosom Med.* 1973;35:484–496.

44. Lader MH, Matthews AH. Electromyographic studies of tension. *J Psychosom Res.* 1971;15:479–486.

45. Matthews AM, Gelder MG. Psychophysiological investigations of brief relaxation training. *J Psychosom Res.* 1969;13:1–12.

46. Fischer-Williams M, Nigl AJ, Sovine DL. *A Textbook of Biological Feedback.* New York: Human Sciences Press; 1986;21–37.

47. Black AH, Cott A, Pavloski R. The operant learning theory approach to biofeedback training. In: Schwartz GE, Beatty J, eds. *Biofeedback: Theory and Research.* New York: Academic Press; 1977;89–127.

48. Furedy JJ, Riley DM. Classical and operant conditioning in the enhancement of biofeedback: specifics and speculation. In: White L, Tursky B, eds. *Clinical Biofeedback: Efficacy and Mechanisms.* New York: Guilford Press; 1982;74–104.

49. Shapiro D, Surwit RS. Learned control of physiological function and disease. In: Peper E, Ancoli S, Quinn M, eds. *Mind/Body Integration.* New York: Plenum Publishing; 1979;7–46.

50. Thorndike EL. The law of effect. *Am J Psychol.* 1927;39:212–222.

51. Brucker BS, Bulaeva NV. Biofeedback effect on electromyography responses in patients with spinal cord injury. *Arch Phys Med Rehabil.* 1996;77:133–137.

52. Brener J. A general model of voluntary control applied to the phenomena of learned cardiovascular change. In: Obrist PA, Black AH, Brener J, DiCara LV, eds. *Cardiovascular Psychophysiology: Current Issues in Response Mechanisms, Biofeedback, and Methodology.* Chicago: Aldine; 1974;365–391.

53. Brener J. Sensory and perceptual determinants of voluntary visceral control. In: Schwartz GE, Beatty J, eds. *Biofeedback: Theory and Research.* New York: Academic Press; 1977;29–66.

54. Brener J. Psychobiological mechanisms in biofeedback. In: White L, Tursky B, eds. *Clinical Biofeedback: Efficacy and Mechanisms.* New York: Guilford Press; 1982; 24–47.

55. Brener J, Ross A, Baker J, Clemens WJ. On the relationship between cardiac discrimination and control. In: Birbaumer N, Kimmel HD, eds. *Biofeedback and Self Regulation.* Hillsdale, NJ: Lawrence Erlbaum Associates; 1979;51–70.

56. Lacroix JM. The acquisition of autonomic control through biofeedback: the case against an afferent process and a two-process alternative. *Psychophysiology.* 1981;18:573–587.

57. Jacobson E. *Progressive Relaxation.* Chicago: University of Chicago Press; 1938.

58. Alexander AB, French CA, Goodman NJ. A comparison of auditory and visual feedback in biofeedback assisted muscular relaxation training. *Psychophysiology.* 1975;12:119–123.

59. Kinsman RA, O'Banion K, Robinson S, Staudenmayer H. Continuous biofeedback and discrete posttrial verbal feedback in frontalis muscle relaxation training. *Psychophysiology.* 1975;12:30–35.

60. Sime WS, DeGood DE. Effect of EMG biofeedback and progressive muscle relaxation training on awareness of frontalis muscle tension. *Psychophysiology.* 1977; 14:522–530.

61. Staudenmayer H, Kinsman RA. Awareness during electromyographic biofeedback: of signal or process? *Biofeedback Self Regul.* 1976;1:191–199.

62. Bayles GH, Cleary PJ. The role of awareness in the control of frontalis muscle activity. *Biol Psychol.* 1986; 22:23–35.

63. Glaros AG, Hanson K. EMG biofeedback and discriminative muscle control. *Biofeedback Self Regul.* 1990;15:135–143.

64. Pollard RQ Jr, Katkin ES. Placebo effects in biofeedback and self-perception of muscle tension. *Psychophysiology.* 1984;21:47–53.

65. Segreto J. The role of EMG awareness in EMG biofeedback learning. *Biofeedback Self Regul.* 1995;20:155–167.

66. Stilson DW, Matus I, Ball G. Relaxation and subjective estimates of muscle tension: implications for a central efferent theory of muscle control. *Biofeedback Self Regul.* 1980;5:19–36.

67. Lehrer PM, Batey DM, Woolfolk RL, Remde A, Garlick T. The effect of repeated tense-release sequences on EMG and self-report of muscle tension: an evaluation of Jacobsonian and post-Jacobsonian assumptions about progressive relaxation. *Psychophysiology.* 1988;25: 562–569.

68. Shedivy DI, Kleinman KM. Lack of correlation between frontalis EMG and either neck EMG or verbal ratings of tension. *Psychophysiology.* 1977;14:182–186.

69. Dunn TG, Gillig SE, Ponsor SE, Weil N, Utz SW. The learning process in biofeedback: is it feedforward or feedback? *Biofeedback Self Regul.* 1986;11:143–156.

70. Cram JR, Freeman CW. Specificity in EMG biofeedback treatment of chronic pain patients. *Clin Biofeedback Health.* 1985;8:101–108.

71. Kall R. Emotional self regulation and facial expression muscle measurement and training. In: Cram J, ed. *Clinical EMG for Surface Recordings.* Vol 2. Nevada City, CA: Clinical Resources; 1990;371–388.

72. Schwartz GE, Fair PL, Salt P, Mandel M, Klerman GL. Facial muscle patterning to affective imagery in depressed and nondepressed subjects. *Psychosom Med.* 1976;38:337–347.

73. Bennett DM, Simmons RW. Effects of precision of knowledge of results on acquisition and retention of a simple motor skill. *Percept Mot Skills.* 1984;58:785–786.

74. Bilodeau EA, Bilodeau IM, Schumsky DA. Some effects of introducing and withdrawing knowledge of results early and late in practice. *J Exp Psychol.* 1959; 58:142–144.

75. Winstein CJ. Motor learning considerations in stroke. In: Duncan PW, Badke MB, eds. *Stroke Rehabilitation: Recovery of Motor Control.* Chicago: Yearbook Medical Publishers; 1987;109–134.

76. Gentile AM. A working model of skill acquisition with application to teaching. *Quest.* 1972;17:3–23.

77. Magill RA. Motor learning is meaningful for physical educators. *Quest.* 1990;42:126–133.

78. Baird IS, Hughes GH. Effects of frequency and specificity of information feedback on the acquisition and extinction of a positioning task. *Percept Mot Skills.* 1972;34:567–572.

79. Ho L, Shea JB. Effects of relative frequency of knowledge of results on retention of a motor skill. *Percept Mot Skills.* 1978;46:859–866.

80. Winstein CJ, Pohl PS, Cardinale C, Green A, Scholtz L, Waters CS. Learning a partial-weight-bearing skill: effectiveness of two forms of feedback. *Phys Ther.* 1996; 76:985–993.

81. Winstein CJ, Schmidt RA. Reduced frequency of knowledge of results enhances motor skill learning. *J Exp Psychol.* 1990;16:677–691.

82. Lavery JJ. Retention of simple motor skills as a function of type of knowledge of results. *Can J Psychol.* 1962;16:300–311.

83. Schmidt RA, Swinnen S, Young DE, Shapiro DC. Summary knowledge of results for skill acquisition: support for the guidance hypothesis. *J Exp Psychol.* 1989; 15:352–359.

84. Swinnen SP, Schmidt RA, Nicholson DE, Shapiro DC. Information feedback for skill acquisition: instantaneous knowledge of results degrades learning. *J Exp Psychol.* 1990;16:706–716.

85. Sherwood DE. Effect of bandwidth knowledge of results on movement consistency. *Percept Mot Skills.* 1988;66:535–542.

86. Alexander AB. An experimental test of assumptions relating to the use of electromyographic biofeedback as a general relaxation training technique. *Psychophysiology.* 1975;12:656–662.

87. Alexander AB, White PD, Wallace HM. Training and transfer effects in EMG biofeedback assisted muscular relaxation. *Psychophysiology.* 1977;14:551–559.

88. Lee TD, Swanson LR, Hall AL. What is repeated in repetition? Effects of practice conditions on motor skill acquisition. *Phys Ther.* 1991;71:150–156.

89. Goode S, Magill RA. The contextual interference effects in learning three badminton serves. *Res Q Exerc Sport.* 1986;57:308–314.

90. Hagman JD. Presentation and test trial effects on acquisition and retention of distance and location. *J Exp Psychol (Learn Mem Cogn).* 1983;9:334–345.

91. Lee TD, Magill RA. The locus of contextual interference in motor skill acquisition. *J Exp Psychol (Learn Mem Cogn).* 1983;9:730–746.

92. Shea JB, Morgan RL. Contextual interference effects on the acquisition, retention, and transfer of a motor skill. *J Exp Psychol (Hum Learn).* 1979;3:179–187.

93. Cuddy LJ, Jacoby LL. When forgetting helps memory: analysis of repetition effects. *J Verb Learn Verb Behav.* 1982;21:451–467.

94. Marteniuk RG. Information processes in movement learning: capacity and structural interference effects. *J Mot Behav.* 1986;18:55–75.

95. Barnett ML, Ross D, Schmidt RA, Todd B. Motor skills learning and the specificity of training principle. *Res Q.* 1973;44:440–447.

96. Lewthwaite R. Motivational considerations in physical activity involvement. *Phys Ther.* 1990; 70:808–819.

97. Cofer CN. The history of the concept of motivation. *J Hist Behav Sci.* 1981;17:48–53.

98. Schwartz GE. Biofeedback as therapy: some theoretical and practical issues. *Am Psychol.* 1973;28:666–673.

99. Shapiro D, Schwartz GE. Biofeedback and clinical learning. *Semin Psychiatry.* 1972;4:171–184.

100. Holroyd KA, Penzien DB, Hursey KG, et al. Change mechanisms in EMG biofeedback training: change underlying improvements in tension headaches. *J Consult Clin Psychol.* 1984;52:1039–1053.

101. Litt MD. Self-efficacy and perceived control: cognitive mediators of pain tolerance. *J Pers Soc Psychol.* 1988;54:149–160.

102. Duda JL, Smart AE, Tappe MK. Predictors of adherence in the rehabilitation of athletic injuries: an application of personal investment theory. *J Sport Exerc Psychol.* 1989;11:367–381.

103. Kaplan RM, Atkins CJ, Reinsch S. Specific efficacy expectations mediate exercise compliance in patients with COPD. *Health Psychol.* 1984;3:223–242.

104. Oldridge NB. Compliance with exercise in cardiac rehabilitation. In: Dishman RK, ed. *Exercise Adherence: Its Impact on Public Health.* Champaign, IL: Human Kinetics; 1988;283–304.

105. Payne RB, Dunman LS. Effects of classical predifferentiation on the functional properties of supplementary feedback cues. *J Mot Behav.* 1974; 6:47–52.

106. Bilodeau IM. Information feedback. In: Bilodeau EA, Bilodeau IM, eds. *Principles of Skill Acquisition.* New York: Academic Press; 1969;255–285.

107. Elwell JL, Grindley GS. The effect of knowledge of results on learning and performance. *Br J Psychol.* 1938;29:39–53.

108. Poulton EC. The effect of fatigue upon inspection work. *Appl Ergon.* 1973;4:73–83.

109. Locke EA, Cartledge N, Koeppel J. Motivational effects of knowledge of results: a goal setting phenomenon. *Psychol Bull.* 1968;70:474–485.

CHAPTER 4

Practical Considerations for SEMG Feedback Training

Fundamental principles of motor learning and surface electromyography (SEMG) feedback were surveyed in Chapter 3. On the basis of that approach, practical issues for the clinician will now be considered. The same format will be used for this discussion, emphasizing concepts related to problem solving, stimulus identification, response selection and programming, feedback, practice, skill transfer, and motivation. Although some aspects of motor learning and feedback training have been researched extensively, other areas have received little attention. Given that experimental confirmation is pending for the latter, suggestions will be offered, with the understanding that the reader is invited to tailor the training methods to meet each patient's apparent needs.

PRELIMINARY INSTRUCTIONS

If the patient has not already undergone a SEMG evaluation and is being monitored for the first time, the steps of the recording procedure should be explained in simple terms. The therapist should actively engage the patient, drawing attention to the learning task and helping create an appropriate arousal level and expectational set. Excessively low or high arousal has negative effects on motor performance,[1] and expectations regarding task difficulty can influence skill acquisition during SEMG training.[2] Patients should be told what they can expect to feel physically and what types of activities will be

included in the session. Some patients, especially those who have had electrodiagnostic studies, may worry about needles or electric shocks. Anxiety can be reduced if the patient understands that the process should be painless and the SEMG machine does not do anything to them; it merely detects their own muscle activity. Also, patients should be positioned with appropriate support for the trunk and proximal segments of any involved extremities. Supportive positions will minimize discomfort and reduce the complexity and energy of motor control at the start.

SELECTION OF GOALS AND PROBLEM SOLVING THE LEARNING TASK

Patients beginning SEMG training are confronted with a novel motor learning situation. A task analysis must be performed by patients so the movement problem can be defined.[3] Individuals seem to vary dramatically in their fluency with task analysis. The therapist may be tempted to advance the session into the motor execution stage, encouraging the patient to generate the SEMG pattern that the clinician believes is appropriate. Progress is unlikely to be obtained, however, if the patient does not fully understand the movement problem or is unsure about how to interpret the SEMG display.

There are two levels of task analysis to be performed, one relating to long-term objectives and the other relating to a series of short-term enabling goals. A patient must understand how existing motor control patterns contribute to the clinical impairments and how changes can be integrated into function. The long-term problem, then, is how to use new or modified movement strategies to resolve functional limitations. The patient can achieve this long-term objective by incrementally identifying and learning specific motor plans. With SEMG training, the patient's short-term goal is generally to learn one or a combination of three strategies: (1) downtraining, how to relax an overly tense muscle; (2) uptraining, how to increase recruitment of a weak muscle; and (3) coordination training, how to change the relative recruitment intensities or timing of two or more muscles.

Gentile[4] proposes that motor learning goals be concrete, challenging, outcome oriented, and within the patient's basic abilities. The patient should clearly be vested in goal attainment. Each short-term goal should be related explicitly to the patient's functional limitations and disabilities. The therapist can ask the patient whether he or she understands why a particular task has been selected for practice and, if appropriate, to paraphrase the rationale. Initial goals may be limited to uptraining or downtraining of a single muscle to facilitate the patient's task analysis. Comprehension of motor goals may be limited for complex tasks that require the coordinated action of several muscles, or a multistep control sequence from a single muscle. For example, a patient with neck pain might be taught to change the activation balance of the upper and lower portions of the trapezius during overhead work activities. The motor task for the patient is to downtrain upper trapezius activity while uptraining lower trapezius activity. This might be quite difficult for the patient to understand. The patient has probably never thought about muscle control in this way and is not familiar with the SEMG display. Rather than trying to achieve both objectives from the start, the patient could be instructed to perform a few trials of each task component without worrying about the other. The intent at this point is not to program complex movements but to ensure that the fundamental task components are grasped. Exhibit 4–1 lists summary considerations for patient preparation.

STIMULUS IDENTIFICATION

Training leads to skill in part by the formation of more efficient systems for information processing. The situation may be limited by problems with stimulus identification, response selection, and response programming[1] (see Figure 3–2), as well as with feedback control. Difficulties with the stimulus identification component can involve impairments in the transduction of extrinsic stimuli to neural codes. There may also be problems with selective attention, memory, and stimulus association and abstraction. The therapist can organize key stimuli to maximize clarity and recognition of patterns of related input.[1,5–7]

Stimulus Clarity

Some patients have visual or auditory impairment that limits their access to the SEMG display. Therefore the operator should ask patients whether they can see and hear the display clearly and modify the output accordingly. When using personal computer–assisted feedback devices, the operator usually has a choice of display modes and graphics. Patients with limited vision

---

Exhibit 4–1 Summary Considerations for Patient Preparation

- Treat any underlying acute musculoskeletal dysfunction.
- Begin in a nondistracting environment.
- Explain to the patient what he or she should expect to do and feel during the session.
- Obtain informed consent to continue.
- Position the patient with appropriate postural support, so that the involved body region is visible.
- Explain SEMG training goals and their relation to long-term function.

do best with a large bar graph and high contrast display colors. Audio feedback is also useful. Options may exist to vary the audio volume and base pitch, as well as to choose a continuous tone or an interrupted signal. The operator should select a feedback signal within each patient's auditory range, with adequate contrast to indicate changes in muscle activity.

Once the therapist is assured that the feedback signals are compatible with the patient's sensory function, the nature and meaning of feedback cues must be explained. Patients may not spontaneously become aware of the contingency between muscle activity and an SEMG display without an appropriate instructional set.[2,8] The therapist can ask the patient to contract the target muscle and instruct him or her to watch or listen to the display. The therapist would then point out how the visual graphic increases and decreases, or how the audio tone varies in pitch or click frequency, with muscle activation and relaxation. The patient may then be asked if he or she indeed understands how the display works. Changes in display sensitivity and smoothing functions should also be explained carefully, so the patient does not erroneously attribute display changes to variations in muscle performance. Adequate sensation and perception regarding the feedback cues should not be assumed for any patient population.

Stimulus Sorting

The patient will receive many different types of stimuli during the learning session. These include visual and auditory stimuli produced by noncontingent background activity, extrinsic feedback cues from the SEMG machine, extrinsic cues from the therapist, visual appreciation of a moving limb or a changing visual field on head or trunk movement, vestibular inputs, and kinesthetic cues. Kinesthetic cues relate to proprioceptive information received from somatosensory receptors, which signal changes in joint position and muscle function. The patient must be able to distinguish between movement-related cues and extraneous information. Infor-

mation must be abstracted and compared with memory for recognition.[1,6] Elderly patients, or patients with impairments due to neurologic disease, may have difficulty sorting the stimuli.[9,10] All patients will be required to increase their ability to attend to kinesthetic sensations related to joint position and muscular tension, as well as to associate these sensations with changes in visual and auditory stimuli on the SEMG display. A set of cognitive rules, or schema,[1] for comparison of intrinsic kinesthetic cues with extrinsic machine-generated cues must be formulated and committed to memory. The rule system needs to become sophisticated and linked also to the individual's conscious motor commands as various movement strategies are explored. Stimuli that are not directly relevant to the motor goal may distract the patient from the critical stimulus modalities and variables. Therefore, motor learning should be initiated in a quiet setting, and the therapist should direct the patient's attention to key stimuli.[4,5]

Integration of intrinsic kinesthetic cues with extrinsic machine-generated cues is fostered by having the patient work toward the goal pattern on the SEMG display while asking questions, such as

"What do you feel when the display goes up like that?"
"Where exactly do you feel a change when the display drops down?"
"In what way(s) does it feel different when the display is up compared with when it is down?"
"How much tension do you feel?"
"Can you detect a change in joint position?"

Patients should begin training in postures in which they can watch the involved body part, using a mirror if necessary. Visual processing is used to integrate important movement feedback cues.[11] The idea is to bring SEMG feedback together with kinematic visual cues and implied kinetic information pertaining to the moving body part. Kinematics refers to motion descriptors, such as position, velocity, acceleration, and time (without reference to the forces that produced them), whereas kinetics refers to the forces that act on the body part to produce changes in kinematic parameters.[12] Although SEMG amplitude is directly proportional to force only under specific, and often nonnatural conditions (see Chapter 3 in the companion book, *Introduction to Surface Electromyography*[13]), SEMG output is taken as an indicator of muscle tension. Thus patients may infer kinetic relationships. By watching a body part move, along with SEMG feedback, patients associate kinematic with kinetic information, which defines motor programming rules. The individual sees (ie, understands) the relationship between selected motor plans and actual movement outcomes.

It is also important to limit the number of SEMG display channels and to simplify the type of visual graphic. Through experience, the therapist will have formed cognitive schema for the simultaneous interpretation of multiple SEMG channels during complex movement sequences. However, the patient's experience is far less rich, and multiple-channel displays with oscilloscope-like line tracings may be overwhelming. The display should probably be limited to one or two channels until the patient has demonstrated the ability to manipulate the activity of each target muscle consistently. A bar graph visual display, perhaps with a moderate level of smoothing, tends to be easy to understand and has few distracting components. A visual or audio (or both) threshold function can be used to label key activation or relaxation contingencies and aid their sorting from less important events. Line tracings have the distinct advantage of preserving history on the screen. Thus results of several contraction attempts, or responses of a single muscle through a range of motion arc, can be inspected. When possible, the feedback display selected should be in rapport with the patient's dominant thinking characteristics. For example, an engineer with a visual, sequential thinking style might respond best to a line tracing. A performing artist could prefer a multicolored kaleidoscope, geometric graphic, or a complex auditory display with variable pitch or complex tonal patterns. Other learners, such as an athlete with a

strong kinesthetic sense, might be motivated by somatosensory feedback using SEMG-triggered electrical stimulation.

The authors recommend that a split screen be employed when two channels are used with line tracing graphics and the recorded muscles are not part of an agonist/antagonist/synergist unit. If the two muscles are not intuitively coordinated together and therefore are likely to be controlled with different cognitive schema, presenting them in separate fields eases interpretation. An example would be the use of a wide recording of the frontal region of the head together with a wide upper trapezius placement during general relaxation training (Figure 4–1). Two signal lines can be overlaid when they represent left and right sides of a homologous muscle pair (Figure 4–2). With this configuration, a more natural association of programming schema and stimulus compatibility between signals from the left and right sides are assumed. Overlaid signals also provide a single display field, one that will probably be larger than each of two separate fields. Although this may be a minor point for two-channel feedback, it grows in importance as does the number of recording channels.

Clinical devices that simultaneously record four to eight channels of SEMG activity are readily available. Multiple channels are often used to display left and right sides of several homologous muscle pairs. It may be best for the therapist to display each homologous pair of signals in one overlaid field. This way, the patient has half the number of fields to attend to, compared with a separate field for each channel. If unilateral movements are performed, the signals from the inactive side tend to be spontaneously ignored. Left–right comparisons are made more intuitively when bilateral or unilateral reciprocal movements are performed (Figure 4–3). The left–right overlays may help the patient "chunk" related bits of information, a process that can aid in short-term processing and recall.[14]

When multiple channels are used (no matter what type of graphic is selected), the display fields should be arranged from top to bottom or left to right in a way that matches the cephalad-to-caudal progression of recording sites. For ex-

A

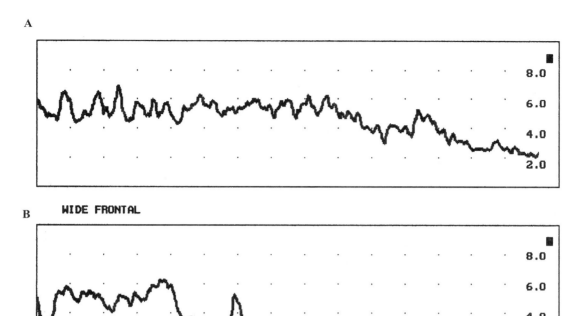

B   **WIDE FRONTAL**

WIDE TRAPEZIUS

Figure 4–1 Example of the display of SEMG activity for nonhomologous, nonsynergistic muscles in separate fields, (**A**) a wide forehead frontal recording with (**B**) a wide upper trapezius recording.

ample, a patient working on improved posture with adjunctive feedback might be receiving information from three SEMG channels, with activity derived from cervical, thoracic, and lumbar paraspinal levels. Moving line or bar graph displays would be arranged with the cervical signal at the top or left, the thoracic signal in the middle, and the lumbar signal at the bottom or right (Figure 4–4). In all likelihood, this setup will result in a more natural stimulus presentation and enhance compatibility among multiple stimuli. Similarly, when bar graphs and homologous recording pairs are used, the left side of the body should be represented on the left side of the display, the right side of the body on the right side of the display. In addition, the clinician should adopt the habit of always assigning left-body-side signals to odd-numbered channels

and right-body-side signals to even-numbered channels, or vice versa. This generally eases channel identification. If the signals are displayed on a color video monitor, all left side signals can be represented in one color and all right side signals in another color, with each homologous pair sharing a field and arranged in the top–down sequence described above (see Figure 4–3).

Overlaid moving lines also simplify visual inspection of the display when timing comparisons between channels are important. During the initial, cognitive phase of learning, patients can process only a limited amount of information. Patients use the position of the SEMG signal on the visual display to determine whether muscle activity has increased or decreased. With practice, patients extract more sophisticated infor-

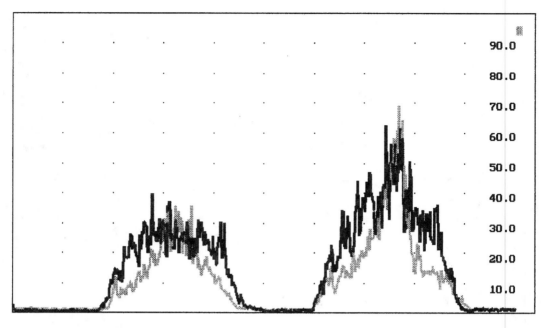

UPPER TRAPEZIUS

Figure 4–2 Example of the display of SEMG activity of a homologous muscle pair in a single field with overlaid signals, the left upper trapezius (black) with right upper trapezius (gray).

mation. In experimental studies, learners of tracking tasks draw inferences first from displacement of the signal, and later they are able to distinguish velocity and acceleration cues.[15,16] Thus patients may learn to use the rate of change of signal amplitude—the slope of a SEMG line tracing—to cue the velocity of recruitment and decruitment. The steeper the slope, the faster the recruitment or decruitment event. This progression would be unimportant for traditional relaxation in which the response latency is relatively slow. However, patients seem to use slope cues intuitively during dynamic tasks. Patients can be instructed to compare the slopes of two recording channels to look for timing relationships between two synergists, or for a stabilizing agonist–antagonist cocontraction. More efficient regulation of limb acceleration may be learned as this information is integrated with kinematic visual appreciation of the moving body part. This association can be meaningful for worker and athlete coordination training. Exhibit 4–2

lists summary considerations for feedback display setups.

RESPONSE SELECTION AND PROGRAMMING

Once the movement problem is understood and relevant stimuli are processed, the patient is ready to prepare a response. For initial training tasks, this response will involve prototypical cognitions for muscle recruitment or muscle relaxation. Further on, schema may need to be available to plan timing changes in recruitment or relaxation of one muscle relative to other muscles. The patient must choose among broad relaxation or recruitment strategies, selecting those that will satisfy contextual demands and achieve the specific training goal. For example, application of a shoulder girdle relaxation response would solve the problem of excessive upper trapezius tension and achieve the goal of decreased upper trapezius activity. This patient

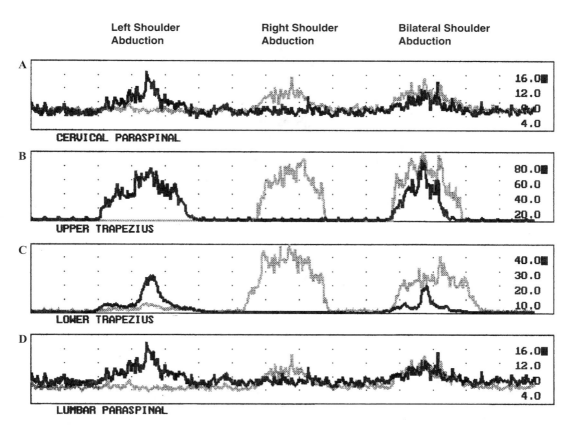

Figure 4–3 Example of the display of four homologous muscle pairs—(**A**) cervical paraspinals, (**B**) upper trapezii, (**C**) lower trapezii, and (**D**) lumbar paraspinals—for a total of eight channels. SEMG activity is shown for left shoulder abduction, right shoulder abduction, and bilateral abduction. The signals of each homologous muscle pair are overlaid in a separate display field. All left side signals are displayed with one signal identifier (black). All the right side signals are displayed with another identifier (gray). The signal pairs are arranged from top to bottom in a manner corresponding to cephalad-to-caudal location of muscle sites.

would intuitively recall a muscle relaxation strategy and program the trapezius to reproduce it.

If the patient does not have a developed prototypical rule for the task, he or she will not be able to select a correct response. Patients lacking a stored plan for relaxation will not be able to respond appropriately to a downtraining task.[17] Some patients report, "I don't know how to relax," because they cannot recall a corresponding strategy. They may never have consciously practiced motor relaxation responses over the involved body region, or they may be so aroused that recall and goal evaluation processes are impaired. To instruct this type of patient to "just relax" may be quite ineffective. In these cases, the therapist should seek verbal cues that promote recall of sensations allied with relaxation. Useful prompts include "Let the arm become loose." "Let the arm become heavy." "Let the leg become floppy." "Feel the chair supporting your back, . . . now sink into it deeper." If these types of cues fail to help, the patient will need to be instructed in a systematic relaxation technique. Even those patients who are able to initiate general relaxation will have difficulty plan-

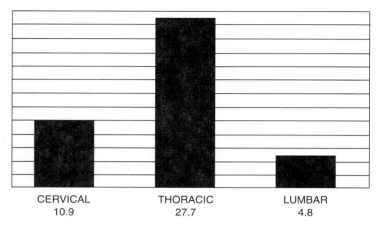

CERVICAL	THORACIC	LUMBAR
10.9	27.7	4.8

Figure 4–4 Example of bar graph display of SEMG activity from cervical, thoracic, and lumbar paraspinal muscles, arranged from left to right in a manner corresponding to the cephalad-to-caudad location of muscle sites.

ning for and programming specific muscle relaxation responses. Indeed, they would not need to be in the clinic if they could already accomplish this task. SEMG downtraining for patients who demonstrate general, but not specific, motor relaxation can be started with wide electrode placements that detect muscle activity over a large region. For this purpose, the active electrodes of a single channel could be placed at left and right suprascapular regions, over left and right masseter or temporalis regions, or at suboccipital and frontal regions (see Chapter 14 of the companion book[13]). The feasibility of using specific electrode placements and more demanding goal criteria should increase as relaxation schema are reinforced. This progression would be combined with specific relaxation and tension recognition techniques, which are detailed in Chapter 5.

Individuals also have cognitive schema for muscle activation but they may not have rules for consciously engaging the particular target muscle to achieve the desired goal. Starting with a broad motor strategy such as gross activation of the trunk or limb tends to be productive. Then, the therapist can direct the patient to perform the isolated action of the target muscle. Alternatively, the therapist could begin by performing the manual muscle test procedure for the desired muscle as the patient is instructed with the

Exhibit 4–2 Summary Considerations for Feedback Display Setup in SEMG Training

- Limit the display to one or two channels until the patient is thoroughly oriented with the training procedure.
- Consider visual feedback for one channel if it is to be the primary focus, and audio for another if it is of secondary concern.
- For visual displays, begin with a simple bar graph or line tracing.
- Ensure that the patient can see and hear the feedback display clearly.
- Demonstrate how the display operates with muscle activation and relaxation.
- Explain any changes in sensitivity/gain and smoothing.
- Use high sensitivity/gain for low-level contractions and low sensitivity/gain for strong contractions.
- Use moderate to high smoothing for downtraining and low to moderate smoothing for uptraining and coordination training.
- Use line tracing displays for timing and coordination training.
- Arrange multiple visual display fields, so that the left–right or top–down layout corresponds naturally to body site anatomy.
- Use separate visual fields for muscles with independent functions or overlaid fields for the left–right signals of homologous muscle pairs.

prompt, "Don't let me move you," and over several trials, "Notice how the display shows the correct response. Can you feel where/how you are resisting me?" By using this procedure, the therapist is helping the patient to select and program the target muscle unconsciously. Programming schema can be built by incorporating the response into functional movements over many trials, as well as by using techniques detailed in Chapters 5 and 6.

Programming may be complicated for coordination retraining tasks. Coordination requires a temporal and spatial sequence of recruitment and decruitment regulated by the recall of elaborate programs. The programs must be accompanied by anticipatory commands to postural muscles and proximal limb stabilizers. Anticipatory commands ensure that the distal segmental movements will proceed from a firm proximal foundation and that the center of mass will be maintained within the base of support.[18] Thus with coordination retraining, multiple responses must be related to each other in a coherent way. Training of coordination tasks requires a much higher level of programming integration than simple uptraining or downtraining procedures. A greater number of visits and a highly customized treatment progression may be needed. Programming may also be complicated by reflex inhibition and spasm phenomena, as discussed in Chapter 1. In these cases, conscious motor control is subordinated to avolitional patterns of activity induced by pain and effusion. It is therefore important to address the underlying pathology, working to resolve acute symptoms and signs. SEMG feedback strategies for coordination retraining are also detailed in Chapters 5 and 6. As with uptraining and downtraining techniques, coordination retraining procedures are designed to facilitate information processing and motor command systems.

FEEDBACK AND INSTRUCTIONAL CUES

The use of knowledge of results (KR) feedback in intermittent, summary, delayed, and bandwidth formats was discussed in Chapter 3.

Although a distinction is made between KR and knowledge of performance (KP), it is assumed that similar recommendations can be made for their application.[1] Thus continuous KP may work against the long-term interests of the learner in the same way as continuous KR. SEMG feedback can be used for KR and KP, and it would seem appropriate to taper access to the SEMG display as training moves away from the cognitive phase. It is suggested that a *faded* SEMG feedback regimen may be used.[17,19] With a faded schedule, feedback is initially provided on every trial and then progressively reduced over the course of training.[20,21]

As an example, consider a patient with temporomandibular joint pain and a chronic clenching habit who is learning to regulate masseter tension. A tension discrimination task is practiced wherein the patient learns to reproduce a series of specific microvolt levels with graded volitional clenches, eventually without access to the SEMG display. The goal is to anchor an internal reference system for tension awareness. Initially, continuous and immediate feedback is provided from the display. The patient uses this information to explore motor selection and programming. Basic performance skill is demonstrated when the patient can hold the target microvolt values somewhat steady on the screen. At this point, the patient has determined how to select and program the desired responses and is beginning to build schema that relate recruitment effort to outcome intensity. This might occur within 5 to 15 minutes. Next, the patient must develop an intrinsic reference for error detection, so that tension recognition can be carried over to functional situations away from the clinic. The patient is challenged by withdrawing the visual display and trying to reproduce the same muscle activity levels. Then, the audio function is turned off, and the therapist substitutes verbal KR for the machine feedback. The therapist reports the actual microvolt reading relative to an intended target value every other trial. Finally, KR can be faded progressively to every third trial, every fifth trial, and so forth, or summary KR can be provided for the outcome of every three trials.

The case described above uses a tension discrimination task to illustrate a faded feedback schedule. The same approach may be used with any sort of relaxation or activation objective. Intermittent KR or KP can be provided by using a piece of cardboard to hide or reveal the screen during selected trials. With some feedback devices a display can be enabled/disabled with a single keystroke, facilitating an easy transition between feedback and no-feedback trials. The therapist can also deliberately delay feedback, either with paused verbal reports or by hiding and freezing the screen and then displaying a visual SEMG tracing to the patient. Deferring performance of any other motor tasks should probably be deferred during the delay period.[22,23] Self-evaluation of performance can be useful in promoting learning,[24] and the therapist might ask the patient to estimate the degree of error before presenting the delayed feedback.

Other SEMG Feedback Manipulations

Most feedback systems allow cues to be set up with an audio tone linked to an SEMG threshold. Often, the audio is programmed to be off when SEMG activity is below threshold and on once the threshold is exceeded. This type of feedback is binary in that it informs the patient through silence versus audio output whether the goal has been reached (below threshold for downtraining or above threshold for uptraining). A common variation is to increase the tone or click frequency once the threshold is exceeded in a manner proportionate to the SEMG magnitude, thus indicating distance above the goal. The relaxation learner is cued as to the magnitude of error, and the activation learner is cued as to the magnitude of success. Many systems allow the relationship to be inverted, so that the audio comes on below threshold if preferred.

When two channels are used, one signal can be assigned to the visual display and the other can be assigned to the audio display. This procedure is useful if the goal is coordination training, in which one muscle is to be uptrained and the other is to be downtrained. A clinical example is increasing gluteal activity while attenuating that of the hamstring muscles during functional hip extension tasks in a patient with recurrent hamstring tendinitis. Visual feedback is used for the uptrained response, and audio feedback, linked to a threshold, is used for the downtrained response. In this way, the patient can visually focus on the uptraining task component while the audio function is interpreted as a type of alarm. Some systems allow for a more sophisticated representation of the relative activity of two muscles with a ratio display. A computer calculates the mathematical ratio of two channel amplitudes and generates a virtual feedback signal. This feedback can be presented as audio KR by having a tone emitted only when a ratio goal is achieved, or displayed for online KP with a continuous variable tone or visual graphic. Bandwidth-type feedback can be generated with devices that operate with dual threshold levels. The therapist sets a goal window between the two thresholds. Audio feedback that sounds only when the signal is maintained within (or outside) the goal window constitutes a bandwidth paradigm.

Verbal Guidance

Verbal guidance is useful to patients during the early stages of motor learning.[25] Light[10] believes that guidance during the cognitive stage should be directed toward helping the learner formulate a reference of correctness. This is the time for the therapist to provide instructions on basic movement strategies, as well as tips as to what simple things the individual should look for to see whether performance is successful. The therapist might begin by showing a photograph or drawing of the target muscle to the patient while explaining the muscle's action. Task instructions include the best starting posture for the activity and what the patient can expect to feel physically. Once the patient has tried the task for a while, questions should be asked, such as

"What do you feel; can you describe it?"
"Where do you feel it?"
"How strong is the sensation compared with what you could feel before?"

With these prompts, it is hoped that the patient will learn to attend to the relevant intrinsic kinesthetic sensations. The therapist might also help the patient interpret the SEMG display, so that machine-generated cues and intrinsic sensations are associated. Questions of the following type may help in this strategy.

> "What happens inside your body when the display goes up like that?"
> "What did you do to make the signal go down that time? Can you tell me what you did that was different?"
> "Have you changed your posture or shoulder position to change the feedback signal that way?"

The goal is for the patient to build an intrinsic error reference that will function when use of the SEMG machine is discontinued. Because cognitive demands on the learner are initially great and his or her retention capabilities are limited, the instructor should prioritize the performance elements of the task and limit verbal tips to only the most important pieces.[1]

Light[10] encourages fewer verbal cues and more self-exploration during the associative stage of motor learning. Verbal remarks should not be purely redundant with SEMG feedback cues. Instead, they should reinforce problem-solving strategies, identification of key stimuli, and motivation. The therapist might say something like

> "Good job. Note how the timing of the two muscles changed when you moved your arm that way. Now that you've got the basic idea, can you figure out how to make the response smoother and larger?"

Self-directed problem solving is probably important from both information processing and motivational standpoints. The clinician also should determine whether appropriate performance could be independently recognized[5,20] by asking questions, such as

> "Could you tell whether you were doing this correctly without the feedback machine? How?"

Roles can be reversed with a question (and follow-up queries), such as

> "If you (patient) were teaching me (therapist) how to do this task, what would you tell me to do?"
> "How would I know, without the feedback machine, whether I was doing it right?"
> "What would I feel?"

The therapist should be persistent in determining the specific descriptions or demonstrations of the patient's recognition strategy.

Mistakes arising from self-exploration are to be accepted. According to the schema theory of motor learning, mistakes are useful in that they serve as data points for rule formation between some programming parameter and movement outcome[1] (Figure 4–5). It is important for the patient to learn what does not work as well as what does work to meet the goal. The therapist may ask the patient to deliberately perform an incorrect response. This procedure will serve to contrast the movement plan and associated feedback against correct trials. For example, a patient learning to increase the activity of the lower trapezius relative to the upper trapezius during shoulder abduction could be asked to purposely do the reverse for a few trials, with guidance that the trials are being used to distinguish faulty patterns from correct movement.

Manual Guidance and Demonstrations

Manual contact of the patient by the therapist is a powerful agent in the therapeutic relationship, communicating empathy, skill, and humanistic warmth. Guidance with touch is also an effective adjunct for learning.[1] Verbal communication regarding quality of posture and movement can be difficult for the patient to grasp. The desired concept, though, may be imparted by gently positioning the patient in the optimal posture. Movement quality can be facilitated by passively displacing the limb in the appropriate plane, in a fluid manner and at a comfortable speed. The therapist can use one hand to stabilize or direct movement at the proximal component of the kinematic segment, such as the

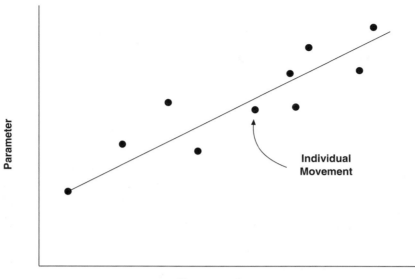

Figure 4–5 Hypothetical relationship between motor programming parameters and movement outcomes according to Schmidt. (See Chapter 3 for details.) In this view, mistakes are useful in that they serve as data points for rule formation, helping to define successful versus unsuccessful movement strategies. *Source:* Reprinted by permission from RA Schmidt, 1988, *Motor Control and Learning*, 2nd ed (Champaign, IL: Human Kinetics Publishers), 131.

scapula, and the other hand to control the distal component, such as the forearm during an overhead reaching movement. In another case, the therapist might place one hand over the lateral aspect of the patient's hip and the other hand at the patient's knee to guide a proper kinematic relationship while the patient is weight bearing. The therapist and patient can then transition to active-assisted movement, active movement by the patient alone, and, perhaps, resisted motions by using functionally indicated loads and velocities. Of course, manual contact should be practiced within each therapist's professional scope, and options are sharply limited for those within psychological disciplines.

Demonstration is a common method for teaching sporting activities and work tasks. The learner observes a skilled performer and then tries to emulate the activity. Results of experimental studies show that this type of modeling for motor tasks promotes performance and error detection.[26] Thus it may be useful for the thera-

pist to demonstrate the desired posture or movement and to exhibit it consistently throughout the session. While working on SEMG downtraining, the therapist can model relaxation by using a suitable verbal tone and pacing, breathing pattern, and open-body posturing. Considerations for feedback and instructional cues are summarized in Exhibit 4–3.

PRACTICE SCHEDULES

Patients learn at different rates. Even the most rigorously evaluated protocol will not produce the best outcome value for every member of the population. Differences in experimental motor performance and learning are attributed to diversity in spatial orientation and kinesthetic awareness skills.[1,27,28] Given that variability is the norm for most patient populations, the authors prefer the use of clinical pathways, as opposed to rigid protocols. A patient's progress can then be measured against some sort of standardized cri-

Exhibit 4-3 Summary Considerations for Feedback Structure and Instructional Cues in SEMG Training

---

- Begin with continuous SEMG feedback.
- Cue basic relaxation or activation schema. Use verbal cues, cognitive techniques, manual guidance, facilitation or inhibition techniques, and demonstration.
- Emphasize basic motor strategies to achieve the goal, as well as how to recognize goal attainment versus error.
- Use display visual and/or audio threshold markers to cue goal attainment.
- Encourage self-directed problem solving when feasible. Reinforce the utility of mistakes in learning.
- Ask about the patient's experiences by using directed questions regarding motor strategies, kinesthetic perceptions, and visual observations.
- After a preliminary period, alternate feedback trials with no-feedback trials; then, progressively fade feedback.
- Consider using a feedback delay with patient self-assessment during the delay period.

---

terion for the diagnostic grouping. Practice schedules can be set to meet the needs of individual learners. Patients who present with a high degree of chronicity or severity, or those who progress more slowly than the norm, may require a greater intensity and scope of services. Those patients who exceed pathway expectations may do well with less services. It is not difficult to specify criteria for relatively homogeneous populations (for example, for patients who have undergone surgical repair of the anterior cruciate ligament). Unfortunately, it is exceedingly difficult to construct pathways for patient populations that are inherently heterogeneous. Patients with chronic low back pain make up such a group. SEMG feedback is often used with these sorts of complex populations. Matters are made even more difficult when idiosyncratic psychosocial issues contribute to the syndrome. The emergence of managed care, though, seems to be driving the formulation of

clinical algorithms for populations with musculoskeletal pain. It is anticipated that decision rules will become available to stratify patients according to learning abilities on specific tasks. The results will likely be combined with other outcome predictors to plan the practice regimens that are most cost efficient for particular individuals. Until these criteria are defined, the following more general guidelines are recommended.

Session Frequency and Duration, Treatment Length

When SEMG training is a primary treatment focus for complex outpatients, the authors' standard is to have these patients seen at the clinic once per week for a 1-hour session. However, the entire hour may not need to be spent on SEMG feedback work. Considerable time can be devoted to psychologic counseling, exercise prescription, instruction in posture, body mechanics, activity pacing, and so forth (without SEMG feedback), or spent in the application of indicated physical agents and manual therapies. Actual time spent with SEMG feedback ranges from 20 to 50 minutes. With less complicated patients, meaningful SEMG training can be accomplished in as little as 5 minutes—for example, when SEMG feedback is used to teach correct technique during a prescribed exercise. This could be the situation when the therapist instructs optimal hamstring stretching in a patient with low back pain who has tight hamstrings and signs of adverse neural tension. Thus the length of the SEMG training component varies with patient type, stage of training, and clinician orientation.

The same is true for session frequency and total number of visits. Highly complex, hospitalized patients with chronic pain may be seen on a daily basis. The session frequency is progressively faded as the patient moves toward an outpatient setting. Visit frequency is tapered, and visit interval is lengthened, with all types of patients once the fundamental skills are in place. It is important to reassess skill at the beginning and end of every session. Consideration is given to doubling the visit interval each time carry-over of key functional components is demonstrated. Treatment is terminated when the functional objectives are achieved. In some circumstances, visits are discontinued before goals are fully met. Early visit termination is undertaken when the degree of chronicity is relatively low or the patient has displayed exceptional learning. The patient must show adequate judgment and motivation, demonstrate independence with a home program, and be objectively close to the final goal criteria. Follow-up contact can be made by telephone, and additional action can be taken if necessary.

Work:Rest Schedules

Another practice timing variable is the work:rest ratio. This parameter refers to length of time the patient performs a task trial relative to the intertrial time given to rest. A greater work:rest ratio allows for a larger number of practice trials within a limited session duration, potentially leading to more learning. However, if the rest time is insufficient, fatigue might impede performance. The work:rest schedule should vary with the inherent fatiguability of the task, but the optimum will probably be unknown. Work:rest cycle duration has been studied in motor learning experiments on the basis of classifications of massed versus distributed practice.[1,6] Massed practice occurs when trial work time is longer than intertrial rest time. Distributed practice comes about when rest time is equal to or longer than work time. Massed practice can produce decrements in acquisition performance scores, but may promote improved scores on delayed-transfer tests.[29-32] The effects tend specifically to occur with discrete tasks.[1] A discrete task is a motor activity of short duration with definable starting and ending points. In contrast, a continuous task does not have fixed starting and ending points. Massed practice might therefore be used with a patient working to increase the activity of an upper extremity muscle while reaching for and grasping an object—a discrete task.

From a practical standpoint, the number of trials that can be performed without eliciting pain

or distress should be maximized. The goal is for the patient to progress to a work:rest ratio that matches the pacing of related functional activities. The rest period should be lengthened if there is a large decrement in performance across trials or the patient is unable to effect a return of SEMG activity to the baseline amplitude as the intertrial interval begins. Consider, as an example, a patient with low back pain who is working on lumbar muscle control during repeated trials of a discrete lifting task. Longer rest periods would be given if pain is exacerbated or the intertrial SEMG amplitude—designated as tonic amplitude (see Chapter 2)—increases across trials. The situation is easily monitored by setting a visual goal marker on the screen just above the baseline average (Figure 4–6). In addition, the rest time could be lengthened if the average work or peak SEMG amplitude increases across trials (Figure 4–7). For a fixed displacement task such as lifting a box from the floor to a table, this means that greater SEMG activity is required to perform the same movement. Decreased efficiency or a compensatory motor strategy is implied.

Similar criteria are used to determine spacing and length of rest breaks for continuous training tasks. The assignment could be maintenance of upper trapezius relaxation during a stressful transactional conversation or preservation of upper trapezius activity below a threshold marker during a keyboard typing task. The patient's ability to make a full recovery to baseline SEMG levels during deliberate pauses is assessed. Rest is maintained until activity is brought back to baseline (Figure 4–8). Over time, a natural pacing is attained by progressively shortening the rest breaks.

A special note of caution is offered if one combines aggressive massed schedules with recording equipment that is designed to reject SEMG frequency components of less than 100 Hz. Although such filtering can reduce the effects of noise and artifact, it can seriously confound the information content of the SEMG signal. The frequency spectrum of the signal changes with fatigue as a greater proportion shifts below 100 Hz.[33] Thus a machine with a

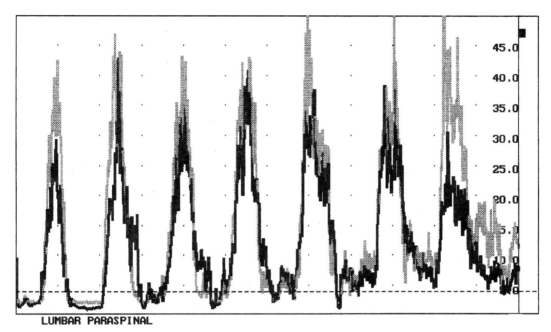

LUMBAR PARASPINAL

Figure 4–6 SEMG activity of left (black) and right (gray) lumbar paraspinals from a patient during repeated trials of lifting a crate from floor to table height. Each paired activity peak represents one lifting trial. The tonic amplitude (interlift amplitude) rises across trials, serving as an indicator to lengthen future rest periods. The dashed threshold line acts as a cue for baseline recovery.

bandpass low cutoff of 100 Hz could register a decrease in display amplitude that would not reflect true muscle activity. (See Chapter 3 of the companion publication of this book.[13]) The resulting feedback would be variably inaccurate across trials and might mislead both patient and clinician.

Randomized Practice of Multiple Tasks

A patient is usually given several different tasks to work on during a training session. In Chapter 3 randomized practice of different training tasks was distinguished from blocked practice. A blocked schedule involves completing all repetitions for one task before another task is initiated. Blocked practice produces higher acquisition scores but is experimentally inferior to a randomized schedule for long-term learning.[1,20,34] Randomized practice is thought to limit the learner's ability to become dependent on extrinsic feedback. Randomized practice assists

the learner in forming problem-solving schema instead of repeating rote responses. These effects have been studied primarily with healthy subjects and novel experimental, nonfunctional activities. Although the effects with clinical populations is unconfirmed, it is recommended that blocked practice be used when a new activity is introduced. The training sequence should be randomized as soon as base proficiency is demonstrated with each task.

As an example, a patient with back pain could be instructed to minimize paraspinal SEMG activity during routine functional activities—such as sit to stand, walking, reaching, or lifting maneuvers—and to return the SEMG amplitude to baseline quickly between movement trials. A sensible way to begin would be to have the patient practice each movement for several trials in a blocked pattern. The desired response is similar for all tasks, and it should be feasible to randomize the sequence early in training. However, too early a progression to a randomized se-

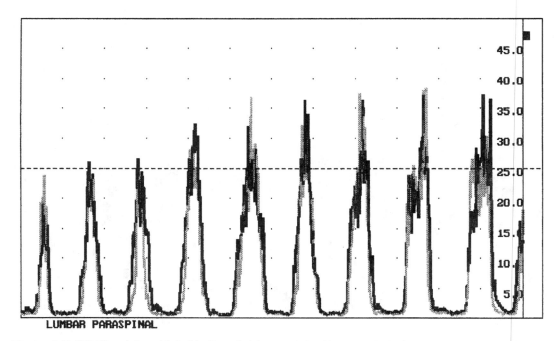

Figure 4–7 SEMG activity of left (black) and right (gray) lumbar paraspinals from a patient during repeated trials of lifting a crate from floor to table height. Each paired activity peak represents one lifting trial. Peak activity tends to rise across trials, serving as an indicator to lengthen future rest periods. The dashed threshold line acts as a cue for peak consistency.

quence would be counterproductive. One can envision an aversion to training being developed if the task is changed before the patient can "get it." Each task may pose a degree of contextual interference for the other tasks,[34] so a randomized sequence of disparate tasks could overwhelm the novice. There would be insufficient opportunity to explore problem-solving strategies by integrating feedback cues with error detection and memory. Therefore it is recommended that blocked practice be continued longer if the tasks are complex or substantially different from each other. This would allow confirmation that the patient is oriented to the correct responses. The intent is to use a blocked schedule during the cognitive learning phase and a randomized series during the associative stage and on into the automaticity stage. Exhibit 4–4 summarizes considerations for practice schedules.

SKILL TRANSFER

Ultimately, whether a patient can control the signals on the SEMG display is insignificant. The ability to transfer problem-solving strategies to functional contexts is the only training outcome that matters. Transfer, the change in performance of one activity as a result of experience with another, tends to be very small between nonidentical tasks.[1] The therapist should not assume that the skill displayed with SEMG in the laboratory will carry over to the patient's activities of daily living. Practice during functional or simulated functional activities should be included in every session.

Functional Practice and Simulations

Practice in the clinic should be as functionally accurate as possible. For example, a clinic with a

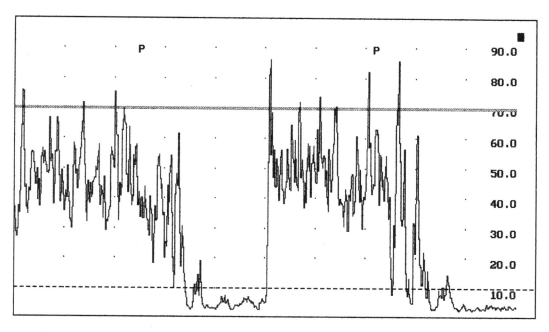

RIGHT UPPER TRAPEZIUS

Figure 4–8 Feedback training of the upper trapezius during a typing task. The learner attempts to maintain peak activity below the solid threshold marker. At random intervals, a therapist instructs the patient to pause typing (**P**). The patient then endeavors with each pause in typing to promptly reduce SEMG activity below the dashed threshold marker.

large number of patients with repetitive strain injuries related to computer work can have a simulated work station set up. This should include an operative computer system with adjustable platforms, chairs, a telephone, a document holder, and an adjustable desk surface. Patients can bring in a photograph of their actual work station and critical height or depth measurements for replication by the therapist. Other work stations may be set up with the assistance of occupational therapists, physical therapists, vocational counselors, and ergonomists. Also, patients can bring in key implements or significant other persons. Thus SEMG feedback training can be performed in the clinic while patients swing golf clubs, practice with musical instruments, use hand-held work tools, or perform child care activities. Skill for such inherently variable tasks is best derived with practice under variable conditions. When practice circum-

stances within a session are modified, skill transfer to novel settings is superior.[35,36] Therefore, clinicians should try to predict how a desired pattern of motor control might be threatened under functional conditions and stratify practice accordingly. A violinist could use SEMG feedback to practice control of scapular muscles while playing at different tempos, fingering styles, and emotional ranges within a session. A golfer would swing with different clubs, at different slope inclinations, and with different force levels during the same session. The goal is for the patient to learn programming rules that will transfer to real-world conditions.

Patients can also be given assignments with physical or cognitive exercises to be performed in the home, workplace, gym, athletic field, or other functional setting. Each assignment is adapted from a successful training technique in the feedback laboratory. Written or taped instructions

Exhibit 4–4 Summary Considerations for Practice Schedules

- Determine optimal session duration and frequency to begin with. Consider acuity, severity, co-morbidities, clinical pathways or protocols, patient scheduling needs, cost efficiencies, and capitation rates.
- Taper the visit frequency as progress ensues.
- Within each session, maximize the number of practice trials performed, without causing inappropriate symptom exacerbation or progressive performance decrements.
- If there are multiple training tasks, begin with blocked trials.
- Randomize practice tasks once the patient is oriented to each activity.
- Discontinue training when the goal outcome is attained.
- Consider early discharge with a detailed home program and telephone follow-up for competent learners.

should be provided. Because neither the SEMG display nor the therapist will be available for feedback, the patient must have a developed intrinsic reference of correctness for the activities. It is recommended that home practice be set up to meet individual time frames. A common schedule involves 10- to 20-minute periods once or twice per day. In addition, practice with high priority motor responses for 30- to 60-second periods, 6 to 10 times per day, is encouraged. As an example, a patient with excessive upper trapezius tension would practice recognition of muscle tension throughout the day, along with postural correction and an abbreviated cognitive relaxation and stretching technique, all within 1 minute or so. This implies that the patient pauses from whatever activity is happening, so that the desired responses are generalized to many settings. Training can be cued throughout the day by associating practice with regularly occurring events, using an hourly alarm on an inexpensive wristwatch, or posting brightly colored stickers where they will be intermittently seen.

Another technique with broad applicability is mental rehearsal. Mental rehearsal involves visualizing a desired response in a functional context. The process is thought to help patients cognitively evaluate response strategies—or to involve execution of a motor program at very low amplitude—and it has been shown to be effective in motor task transfer.[1,37,38] Thus, patients being trained with SEMG feedback could visualize relaxing or activating their muscles in workplace, home, car, athletic, or recreational contexts.

Transfer of motor skills may be optimally promoted through on-site functional practice with portable SEMG devices. These machines are user friendly, low cost, battery powered, single or dual channel units. The equipment may be operated under the supervision of a therapist who is making a site visit, or a system can be dispensed to a patient for independent use. Either approach involves additional expense, but the total cost of the case may be substantially reduced. An independent unit allows for daily SEMG training with fewer clinic sessions. Rental fees may be more than offset by lower clinic charges, while allowing for more frequent practice under more functional circumstances. The expense of a site visit by a therapist also may be more than made up if learning is enhanced and recidivism is reduced. A site visit should be considered when the patient's impairments are disruptive of high priority function in a setting that cannot be duplicated in the clinic. The patient's problem should be recurrent over many months and clearly exacerbated by activities at that site. An early intervention strategy is warranted when extensive workplace or athletic technique changes need to be made, or when there are fundamental safety concerns. Such criteria should be reviewed with the patient's referral source and payer case manager to secure preapproval for site visits or independent trainer devices. Specific goals and timelines should be established in conjunction with the health care team.

Part-Whole Practice

Instructors commonly break complex movements down into component pieces, which is referred to as part-whole training. Training with a part-whole paradigm can be used to simplify information-processing requirements and support motivation. The part-whole method is a transfer technique in that the skill established with each of the parts will be integrated into a new whole. Experimentally, positive results have been produced when several subtasks must be chained together in a series.[39,40] In working with a patient with elevated upper trapezius tension and neck pain, an example would be training conscious discrimination of muscle tension levels, followed by postural correction, upper trapezius stretching, and a diaphragmatic breathing technique. Each component would be learned individually, and then the series would be assembled into an integrated program to be completed within 1 minute or so.

Part-whole training has been less effective with laboratory learning of movements of very short duration[41] or high complexity in which the component pieces are performed simultaneously.[42] When continuous coordination of the parts is critical to the movement whole, part practice probably does not facilitate the learner in developing an integrated movement strategy.[1] As an example, patients with neck and shoulder pain can be trained to alter the balance of recruitment of the upper and lower portions of the trapezius. This often involves feedback downtraining of the upper trapezius and uptraining of the lower trapezius during arm elevation activities. By using a part-whole method, each component can be practiced in isolation and then put together for simultaneous performance. Many patients do quite well, or maybe better, by focusing practice on the integrated task immediately after orientation to the SEMG machine. Thus, the authors recommend using part practice for orientation, transitioning quickly to whole practice during coordination training of multiple muscles. Part-whole methods can be used more extensively for serial tasks.

Other Transfer Techniques

Other "lead up" transfer methods demand progressively greater accuracy, add more steps, and make the environmental setting more com-

plex.[1,43] These techniques can be adapted for patients learning SEMG downtraining procedures. Several methods are detailed in Chapter 5, but they are introduced here as examples of general transfer procedures.

A downtraining goal criterion can be made more difficult by progressively lowering the display threshold value, shaping the response in the desired direction. If relaxation training has been initiated with the patient in a supportive chair with few distractions, practice can be progressed by moving into a less supportive chair or perhaps to a standing position. Results of laboratory studies of motor learning have showed improved transfer by forcing subjects to engage simultaneously in unrelated cognitive tasks.[44] The patient who is receiving SEMG feedback training can be challenged to maintain a suitable relaxation response in the presence of background noise, while engaging in reading or conversation, or while using the contralateral extremity. Such a progression has been traditionally recommended for SEMG training with spasticity[45] and may be useful in learning for patients with musculoskeletal pain as well. In addition, the patient learning relaxation techniques can be asked to sustain a low SEMG amplitude while visualizing progressively charged emotional situations.[46]

Uptraining and coordination responses may be similarly advanced by using threshold shaping and distractions. Training also can be promoted by progressing skill through different joint positions and attendant muscle length–tension, tendon angle, and neurophysiologic relationships; building to simultaneous control of multiple joint segments; and shifting to diagonal movement planes.[47] Load, contraction intensity, and velocity can each be increased, working through isometric, concentric, and eccentric tasks as appropriate to the functional goal movements. Lower extremity training should incorporate closed kinematic chain activities; that is, when the foot is fixed and weight bearing on the ground. For the upper extremities, training may be initiated with unilateral movements and progressed to bilateral simultaneously symmetric movements; bilateral reciprocal symmetric movements; bilateral reciprocal asymmetric movements; and, finally, bilateral simultaneous-asymmetric movements. The situation can be made most difficult by asking for coordinated control of multiple body parts during performance of tasks with low response-response compatibility. Such responses differ fundamentally in their programming and are not related to each other in an intuitive way—as in the example of rubbing in a circular pattern over one's head while patting one's stomach.[10]

Earlier in this chapter, ways of maximizing display stimulus clarity and formatting the visual fields in the most natural way were discussed. Some computer-assisted systems allow for complex, nonintuitive graphics or video games in which the action is controlled by the SEMG amplitude. The games require high-level abstractions of SEMG feedback and motor activity, and they are a way of decreasing the stimulus–response compatibility[1] between the SEMG display and motor responses.

Integration of Transfer Methods

In designing a progressive transfer sequence, the best strategy may be to examine the functional goal response and work backward. Gentile[4] has classified tasks, among other dimensions, on the basis of the amount of intertrial variability, whether the task is internally or externally paced, and whether the task demands are predictable or relatively unpredictable. A SEMG training task can be distinguished further on the basis of starting posture, specific muscles involved, and whether each must be uptrained or downtrained in sequence or through simultaneous coordination (Figure 4–9). Thus the basic task demands as well as the essential spatial and temporal pattern of motor activity can be defined. These core features should be introduced in the training sequence as early as possible. If the key postures, muscles, contraction types, and sequences differ greatly from practice to function, it is unlikely that appropriate programming schema will be formed. Transfer would be expected to be poor. Consequently, the therapist should attempt to include these elements from

the start and then increase load, velocity, and behavioral demands in an incremental manner.

Exhibit 4–5 lists salient observations of the SEMG display for every stage of training. Satisfaction of the criteria, as appropriate to the particular task, is the therapist's cue to advance the patient to the next level of a progression. Each new task is explained or demonstrated, and the patient is asked to describe how he or she will satisfy the goal.[5] At the same time, discontinuous feedback and randomized practice sequences are introduced.

Consider the following example. A patient with chronic patellofemoral pain has insufficient recruitment of the vastus medialis oblique portion of the quadriceps relative to the vastus lateralis. The patient has difficulty playing soccer and working the clutch of her car while traveling for sales calls. Her symptoms are reproduced in the clinic during the descent phase of squatting or lunging, when the leg is used to lower the body down from a step, and when pressure on a mechanized foot pedal is released. Each of these situations involves eccentric control with the lower extremity loaded. Uptraining of the vastus medialis oblique is initiated with seated isometrics to orient the patient to the SEMG machine. After a brief period, she performs training with the foot on the ground or by pushing the pedal. The patient next begins work in standing with isometrics and then performs partial squats with limited weight bearing and trunk support leaning against a wall. This is done in blocked trials, alternating with the pedal pushing task. Continuous SEMG feedback is given. As control develops, feedback is delayed, then reduced to every second trial and, finally, reduced to every third trial. Progressively more weight is borne through the involved extremity and more force applied to the pedal. Dynamic, full weight–shifting activities follow. Lunges and step-down activities are introduced, first in blocked trials and then incorporated into randomized sequences. Continuous feedback is resumed with each new activity the patient undertakes but with the same sort of faded schedule. Greater force and velocity are used, and the working range of motion is increased for each

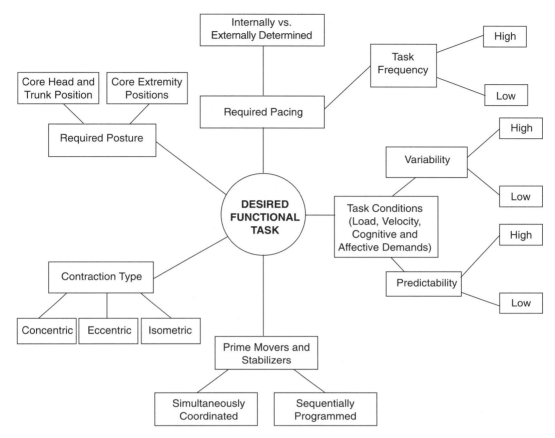

Figure 4–9 Key elements to consider in planning skill transfer progressions.

task. The patient builds to simulated soccer motions in which multiple joint segments are controlled in unpredictable combinations, with variable velocities. Home exercise and mental rehearsal for soccer are encouraged. Carry over of skill to her actual clutch pedal is practiced with a portable SEMG device in the clinic parking lot, after a day of driving. Methods of promoting skill transfer—many of which were described in this example—are summarized in Exhibit 4–6.

MOTIVATION

The therapist can outreach to the patient with chronic musculoskeletal pain to facilitate motivational processes. Included are ways in which training tasks are set up and sequenced, ways in

which machine and verbal performance feedback are given, and the therapist's willingness to engage the patient on terms that can be comfortably managed. Therapists intuitively assess motivational set toward SEMG training during the initial session. Patients who have requested a feedback training referral from their physician are likely to be highly motivated. Individuals who already participate in exercise programs, relaxation training, or mind–body integration training of one type or another should be favorably predisposed toward self-regulation practice. Presumably, these persons have a reasonably positive body image, a belief that training programs can be beneficial, and a conviction that they can achieve positive results by investing energy in practice. Adults who do not regularly participate in exercise, do not express a de-

Exhibit 4–5 SEMG Performance Criteria

- Prompt activation on command to contract.
- Prompt deactivation on command to relax.
- Complete recovery to baseline during rest periods.
- Approximate left–right symmetry for symmetric tasks.
- Appropriate activation and temporal sequencing of agonist, antagonist, and synergist musculature.
- Approximate response consistency across trials.

Exhibit 4–6 Summary Considerations To Promote Skill Transfer in SEMG Training

- Define requisite postures, muscular synergies, movement sequences, and performance demands for function. Integrate these into training as soon as possible.
- Use part–whole training to build to a skill pattern of chained subtasks.
- Train with all skill components simultaneously for continuous coordination tasks.
- Assess skill carry-over at the beginning and end of each session.
- Progressively move display thresholds up or down to shape responses in desired direction.
- Use more complex, less natural SEMG feedback displays if available.
- Progress to busy environments with background activity, functional lighting or terrain, and interruptions.
- Add simultaneous emotional stimuli, or distractor reasoning tasks or physical activities.
- Progressively withdraw postural support. Build toward simultaneous control of multiple joint segments.
- As appropriate to function, work through increased range of motion; load; velocity; open and closed kinematic chains; and isometric, concentric, and eccentric conditions.
- Provide home assignments to practice development of motor skills. Include both full practice periods and abbreviated methods that are performed throughout the day.
- Use mental rehearsal to imagine skills in functional contexts.
- Move from predictable variations in task pacing and performance to unpredictable variations.
- Replicate or simulate functional tasks every session.
- Consider the potential cost-effectiveness of a SEMG home trainer or therapist site visit.

sire to use relaxation skills, or otherwise do not seem to manifest an interest in conscious self-regulation may be less motivated.

Therapists also intuitively take into account the patient's compliance during the examination, as well as the level of enthusiasm displayed during an introduction to SEMG training, discussion of goals and plans, and receptivity to an adjunctive home program. It is critical that the therapist explain the rationale for SEMG training early in the session and explicitly ask the patient about his or her impressions. Discussion of what will happen during the feedback session will enable the patient to make an informed commitment to participate, as well as help ameliorate anxiety related to the instrumentation or the unknown nature of training. A patient's sense of ownership over the goals is important to optimize outcome.[4,48,49] The act of setting goals directly facilitates motor performance,[50] and having the patient begin with easily achievable training tasks is prudent for motivation. Individuals with a low sense of self-efficacy will build a perception of competence by succeeding early on. Persons with a social comparison goal orientation will respond to the therapist's verbal reinforcement during component tasks and, it is hoped, move toward an intrinsic reference basis.

Patients who are not highly motivated toward training may not believe in the program outcomes in general, or they may lack a sense of self-efficacy in skill development.[48] The former

may be addressed by reviewing relevant scientific outcomes, similar case experiences, and physiologic rationale in an understandable way. Patients probably will not learn much if they believe the training is ineffective or irrelevant. Problems with self-efficacy may be subtle and require careful attention throughout the course of training. Many patients begin SEMG training at the suggestion of a trusted physician or therapist. They likely will reserve judgment regarding treatment efficacy and self-efficacy for several sessions. A number of questionnaire instruments are available to judge self-efficacy, coping, and pain beliefs that potentially influence compliance.[51] At the conclusion of the first visit, reasonable options for treatment and scheduling frequency can be offered. The patient and therapist may then arrive at a mutually acceptable plan. Progress toward measurable goals should be frankly reviewed each week, with patient agreement secured for any changes. Motivation is inferred across subsequent sessions by the patient's apparent enthusiasm, scheduling compliance, adherence to home exercises and self-regulation assignments, and verbalizations regarding treatment outcomes.

Display Features

The provision of feedback is itself motivational for motor learning.[52] This process can be maximized by taking advantage of the setup options for the SEMG display. Threshold levels for uptraining and downtraining should be challenging but within a range that is reinforcing. For uptraining, it is recommended that the goal be set initially to a level that the patient can attain in about 80% of attempts. The goal can be moved progressively higher when it is met with ease in nearly all attempts. For downtraining, the goal can be set about 20% below the baseline average amplitude.[53] A more sophisticated approach is to use a computer to adjust the goal automatically to maintain a level one standard deviation (or some percentage) above or below a running 20- to 30-second amplitude average.[54] It is suggested that the display sensitivity be adjusted so the SEMG signal associated with uptraining efforts reaches the top one-third of the visual graphic. During downtraining, the sensitivity should be adjusted, so

that relaxation responses reach the bottom third of the visual graphic. Simply put, a large deflection of the graphic is more reinforcing than a response that barely seems to register (Figure 4–10). Downtraining should be performed with a high level of display smoothing, so that feedback is relatively stable and transient increases do not distract the patient or discourage self-efficacy perceptions (Figure 4–11). A low to moderate level of smoothing should be used with uptraining and coordination training. This will produce a prompt change in the SEMG amplitude with changes in recruitment effort.

If computer-assisted feedback devices are used, a number of creative graphics may be available to retain the patient's attention. Some machines have games in which the action is controlled by the patient's SEMG amplitude. The difficulty level can usually be set to match ability. The therapist should exercise caution when working with patients with a strong social comparison goal orientation. Those patients may become focused on their scores and how they rank relative to the scores of other patients. Certain systems allow a threshold-controlled signal that relays to peripheral devices, such as audiocassette tape players, toys, and the like, for motivational purposes.

Patients can get involved in tracking their progress by recording a chart of SEMG results pertaining to some goal. A visual threshold marker can be used to indicate the magnitude of response improvement from start to conclusion of a session, or from initial to current visits. Patients often seem surprised by the degree of change and are reinforced by the objective confirmation of progress. Sophisticated systems have functions for replay of earlier SEMG recordings during coordination training. More simply, a printout of an earlier session can be saved to demonstrate advancement during later treatment.

Verbal Interaction

The therapist verbally interacts with the patient in a number of ways to promote self-effi-

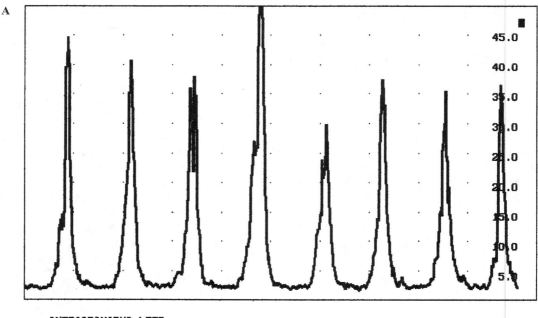

INFRASPINATUS LEFT

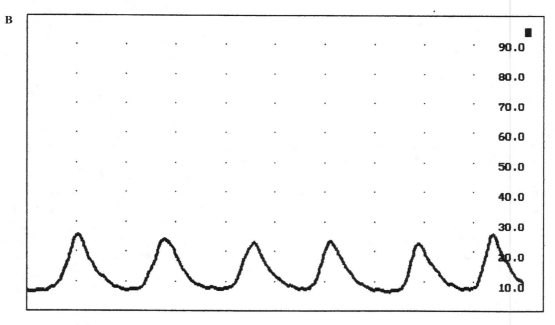

INFRASPINATUS LEFT

Figure 4–10 Uptraining is supported with (**A**) a higher sensitivity/gain and a lesser level of signal smoothing, compared with (**B**) a lower sensitivity/gain and a greater level of signal smoothing. The prompt, greater signal deflection seen in **A** is likely to be more motivating for the learner.

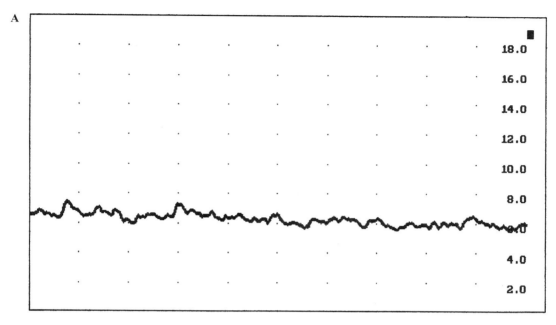

RIGHT UPPER TRAPEZIUS

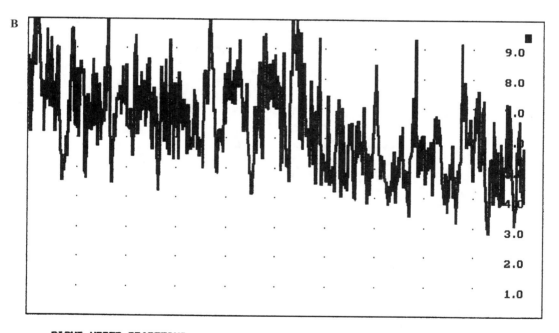

RIGHT UPPER TRAPEZIUS

Figure 4–11 Downtraining is supported with (**A**) a lower sensitivity/gain and a greater level of signal smoothing, compared with (**B**) a higher sensitivity/gain and a lesser level of signal smoothing. The stable, lower signal deflection seen in **A** is likely to be more motivating for the learner.

cacy cognitions. Verbal encouragement and reassurance, provided in a nonpatronizing way, can be helpful. The patient may be reminded to begin slowly and explore different strategies, as well as that it is permissible to make mistakes. A desired pattern of motor control may not be intuitive. The nervous system is not "wired" for fine volitional control of all muscles, and pain may lead to involuntary or unconscious muscle responses. By trying different patterns of motor activity, the patient will come to identify what it is that he or she can do, or what it is that he or she should not do, to feel better. The patient need not be victimized by pain, but active involvement is necessary to move down the road to recovery. Some persons attach negative affective labels to exertional sensations.[55] Those types of patients can be advised that pain does not necessarily imply tissue damage. Patients can be told that the sensations associated with muscle contraction and joint movement are perceived by many as pleasurable,[48] and that these sensations can be regarded as pieces of information that point to pathways to health.

Patients who verbalize excessively negative comments about their performance can be advised that the SEMG machine does not judge them. The feedback device is an impersonal, neutral entity. SEMG cues are merely an extension of one's intrinsic senses. Patients who have difficulty manipulating the SEMG display in the desired way can attempt the task on another muscle that is easier to control volitionally. The forearm serves this purpose well.[53] Unilaterally symptomatic patients first can perform the activity with the noninvolved homologous muscle. Response selection, motor programming, and feedback management may be easier with an uninvolved muscle. Success can work toward confidence and skill transfer to the involved muscle site. The process may be accompanied by verbal recognition of goal achievement on the easier task, as well as by encouragement that others who also experienced difficulty have been able to attain results. It may be useful to have the patient acknowledge a correct response by asking

"How do you think that repetition was compared with the previous one?"
"You did something to make that happen. What was it?"
"If you got it once, you can figure out how to do it again. . . . It will come."

Rather than dictating the patient's behavior, the therapist should encourage independent problem solving. That is, the therapist can ask the patient to figure out how to perform the task, provide gentle cues, and reinforce the gains.

Training Sequences

In an earlier section of this chapter, it was suggested that patients be progressed to discontinuous feedback and randomized practice of component tasks as soon as fundamental skill acquisition is evidenced. However, premature withdrawal of feedback may be demotivating for patients, especially those with a social comparison goal orientation or a low sense of self-efficacy. The same result is likely with premature task randomization. A greater number of repetitions with continuous feedback and blocked trials may help build the patient's self-confidence while allowing for extended reinforcement by the therapist. During any training task, the therapist should observe for signs of performance anxiety or frustration and modify the task accordingly. A simpler task should be selected if an individual's motivation seems to be fading because of frustration. If the patient is no longer challenged, obviously a more complex or otherwise novel goal can be attempted. A balance must be found between providing an adequate number of repetitions to explore motor strategies and integrate responses, and ensuring a periodic change of training venue that sustains interest. Also, each session can start and end by having the patient review tasks for which competency has been demonstrated. This tactic reinforces self-efficacy and allows for an assessment of intersession skill retention.

Several approaches can be used when patients seem to be sincere but unable to muster the motivation to comply with home programs. Although patients are expected to invest time and energy in their rehabilitation, limitations related to family, work, and recreational issues must be respected. As a home program is constructed, the therapist can estimate how much time will be required and ask the patient whether this will be acceptable. The therapist will find that keeping home programs to a few simple mental or physical exercises for which competence has been demonstrated will be more productive than overwhelming learners with a complex training sequence. Explicitly asking patients if they feel capable of performing the program is further advisable.[51] Therapists can emphasize to patients that it is ridiculous for them to try to work harder than patients do themselves for their own recovery. Assignment of a daily diary, with indicators of symptom level, medication usage, exercise performance, functional activity levels, and perhaps perceived tension or recruitment levels may help (Exhibit 4–7). Sometimes the better part of a session can be spent working through an action plan (Exhibit 4–8). Patients define their status with respect to posture, body mechanics skills, work station ergonomic setup, activity pacing, body weight, exercise needs, diet and nutrition, stress management, and any other indicated issues. The therapist guides the patient in rational interpretation of perceptions, as well as coaches the patient in formulating his or her own goals and plans. The patient is asked to sign the sheet as a contract with himself or herself.

Verbal encouragement, role modeling, and the opportunity to engage in social relationships all contribute in a positive way to motivation.[29,48,56] Accordingly, the therapist can ask the patient to select from techniques available in psychologic and motivational self-help publications.[57–60] These center on

- linking compliance to rewards and noncompliance to negative reinforcers
- identifying covert barriers

- clarifying values
- learning time management skills
- distinguishing social support systems
- reframing perceptions of physical sensations
- refuting irrational ideas
- developing coping skills
- creating affirmative self-talk

(The interested reader is referred to Schwartz,[61] who has detailed numerous additional procedures to foster compliance during psychophysiologic feedback training.)

A quota system is suggested for compliance problems associated with exercise or functional activity retraining programs.[62] An index card is labeled for each task in the training regimen, with parameters for resistance levels, duration, and any other technique particulars. The number of repetitions per day is indicated by marks on a graph (Figure 4–12). Quota levels are initially set by allowing patients to exercise to a self-limited number of repetitions, stopping due to pain or fatigue, under the direct supervision of a physical or occupational therapist. Performance levels over several sessions are averaged and used as the starting point for each task. Quota levels are then advanced incrementally. Once established, patients are instructed to do their best to meet the indicated levels each practice day. They are encouraged not to exceed a quota even if it seems to be a "good" day and to meet the target even if it is a "bad" day. Patients are asked to draw a line from the actual performance level to the bottom of the graph as the exercise is completed. The idea is to avoid performance swings and keep to a steady challenge that promotes tissue conditioning without overload. In this way, patients who behaviorally limit their exercise performance can be brought closer to physiologic tolerance. All patients can progressively condition their musculoskeletal system with low injury risk and maintain an objective record of goals and accomplishments. Exhibit 4–9 summarizes considerations for patient motivation.

Exhibit 4–7 A Sample Symptom Diary in SEMG Training

Name _____

Patient number _____

Week of _____

Symptoms _____

This diary is for recording your daily symptoms, activities, and medication usage. For each day list the date; then record a pain rating for your symptoms. Pain ratings are from 0 (no pain) to 5 (intolerable). Also list corresponding activities (eg, work, exercise, rest), any medications that you use and their dosage, and relaxation techniques or physical exercises that you perform. These recordings should be done for the morning, afternoon, evening, and night of each day. Space is provided for any additional comments that you feel are important.

Date:

	Pain Rating 0 1 2 3 4 5	Major Activities	Medications (what & how much)	Practice Relaxation or Exercise
Morning				
Afternoon				
Evening				
Night				
	Comments:			

Date:

	Pain Rating 0 1 2 3 4 5	Major Activities	Medications (what & how much)	Practice Relaxation or Exercise
Morning				
Afternoon				
Evening				
Night				
	Comments:			

Date:

	Pain Rating 0 1 2 3 4 5	Major Activities	Medications (what & how much)	Practice Relaxation or Exercise
Morning				
Afternoon				
Evening				
Night				
	Comments:			

Courtesy of Virginia Mason Medical Center, Seattle, Washington.

Exhibit 4–8 An "Action Plan" Form Used To Help Patients with Chronic Back and Neck Pain Address Compliance Issues

BACK AND NECK CARE ACTION PLAN

NAME:	SELF-RATING (mark date)			GOALS	PLANS
	More Than Satisfactory	Satisfactory	Needs Improvement	Long Term Short Term (Include Dates)	(Be Specific)
POSTURE					
BODY MECHANICS					
WORK STATION					
ACTIVITY PACING					
BODY WEIGHT					
EXERCISE					
Stretching					
Strengthening					
Aerobic Fitness					
DIET					
STRESS MANAGEMENT					

OTHER CONCERNS:

Courtesy of Virginia Mason Medical Center, Seattle, Washington.

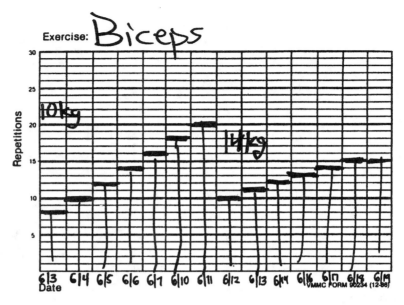

Figure 4–12 A sample exercise quota card. A separate card is used for each exercise task (elbow flexor strengthening in the example shown). Date is indicated along the bottom of the graph. Each day's quota level is designated by the therapist with a horizontal mark. A vertical mark is placed in each column by the patient once that day's quota is met. Courtesy of Virginia Mason Medical Center, Seattle, Washington.

Exhibit 4–9 Summary Considerations for Patient Motivation in SEMG Training

- Assess initial motivational set toward SEMG training.
- Secure agreement for initial patient and therapist responsibilities, and with any significant changes.
- Guide the patient in setting self-determined functional goals.
- Begin with easily achievable SEMG display thresholds and uptraining or downtraining goals.
- For uptraining and coordination training, select a display sensitivity and smoothing level that support a large, prompt signal deflection.
- For downtraining, select a sensitivity and smoothing level that supports a stable, low amplitude deflection of the graphic.
- Consider demonstrating desired SEMG responses with an uninvolved, contralateral side, or by achieving a similar goal with another muscle with easier voluntary control.
- Consider motivational SEMG computer graphics, games, or relays to toys, tape players.

- Periodically question the patient about perceptions of self-efficacy and coping.
- Reinforce an internal locus of control, self-exploration, and a rational interpretation of physical sensations.
- Encourage the patient to focus on long-term function, rather than on short-term variations in pain intensity.
- Reinforce gains verbally, with performance charts or printouts of SEMG scores, and by repeating tasks for which competence has been established.
- Keep home programs simple and within the patient's realistic lifestyle expectations.
- Explicitly ask if the patient feels able and is willing to execute the home program.
- Identify and help problem solve barriers, such as educational deficits, fear of pain, time management issues, or lack of family support.

REFERENCES

1. Schmidt RA. *Motor Control and Learning: A Behavioral Emphasis.* Champaign, IL: Human Kinetics; 1988.

2. Kotses H, Segreto-Bures J. Subject expectancy effects in frontal EMG conditioning. *Biol Psychol.* 1983;17:97–104.

3. Higgins S. Motor skill acquisition. *Phys Ther.* 1991; 71:123–139.

4. Gentile AM. Skill acquisition: action, movement, and neuromotor processes. In: Carr JH, Shepherd RB, eds. *Movement Science: Foundations for Physical Therapy in Rehabilitation.* Rockville, MD: Aspen Publishers; 1987;93–154.

5. Held JM. Theories and principles of therapeutic intervention based on contemporary models of motor control. In: Myers RS, ed. *Saunders Manual of Physical Therapy Practice.* Philadelphia: WB Saunders Co; 1995;325–332.

6. Marteniuk RG. Motor skill performance and learning: considerations for rehabilitation. *Physiother Can.* 1979;31:187–202.

7. Mulder T. A process-oriented model of human motor behavior: toward a theory-based rehabilitation approach. *Phys Ther.* 1991;71:157–164.

8. Segreto-Bures J, Kotses H. Experimenter expectancy effects in frontal EMG conditioning. *Psychophysiology.* 1982;19:467–471.

9. Light KE. Information processing for motor performance in aging adults. *Phys Ther.* 1990;70:820–826.

10. Light KE. Issues of cognition for motor control. In: Montgomery PC, Connolly BH, eds. *Motor Control and Physical Therapy: Theoretical Frameworks and Practical Applications.* Hixson, TN: Chattanooga Group; 1991:85–96.

11. Latash M. *Control of Human Movement.* Champaign, IL: Human Kinetics; 1993.

12. Rodgers MM. Musculoskeletal considerations in production and control of movement. In: Montgomery PC, Connolly BH, eds. *Motor Control and Physical Therapy: Theoretical Frameworks and Practical Applications.* Hixson, TN: Chattanooga Group; 1991:47–60.

13. Cram JR, Kasman GS. *Introduction to Surface Electromyography.* Gaithersburg, MD: Aspen Publishers; 1997.

14. Miller GA. The magic number seven, plus or minus two: some limits on our capacity for processing information. *Psychol Rev.* 1956;63:81–97.

15. Fuchs AH. The progression-regression hypothesis in perceptual-motor skill learning. *J Exp Psychol.* 1962; 63:177–182.

16. Jagacinski RJ, Hah S. Progression-regression effects in tracking repeated patterns. *J Exp Psychol (Hum Percept).* 1988;14:77–88.

17. Stilson DW, Matus I, Ball G. Relaxation and subjective estimates of muscle tension: implications for a central efferent theory of muscle control. *Biofeedback Self Regul.* 1980;5:19–36.

18. Corcos DM. Strategies underlying the control of disordered movement. *Phys Ther.* 1991;71:25–38.

19. Hefferline RF, Bruno LJJ. The psychophysiology of private events. In: Jacobs A, Sachs LB, eds. *The Psychology of Private Events.* New York: Academic Press; 1971:334–345.

20. Schmidt RA. Motor learning principles for physical therapy. In: Lister MJ, ed. *Contemporary Management of Motor Control Problems.* Alexandria, VA: Foundation for Physical Therapy; 1991;49–63.

21. Winstein CJ, Schmidt RA. Reduced frequency of knowledge of results enhances motor skill learning. *J Exp Psychol.* 1990;16:677–691.

22. Marteniuk RG. Information processes in movement learning: capacity and structural interference effects. *J Mot Behav.* 1986;18:55–75.

23. Shea JB, Upton G. The effects on skill acquisition of an interpolated motor short-term memory task during the KR-delay interval. *J Mot Behav.* 1976;8:277–281.

24. Hogan JC, Yanowitz BA. The role of verbal estimates of movement error in ballistic skill acquisition. *J Mot Behav.* 1978;10:133–138.

25. Holding DH, Macrae AW. Guidance, restriction, and knowledge of results. *Ergonomics.* 1964;7:289–295.

26. Landers DM. Observational learning of a motor skill: temporal spacing of demonstrations and audience presence. *J Mot Behav.* 1975;7:281–287.

27. Fleishman EA, Rich S. Role of kinesthetic and spatial-visual abilities in perceptual motor learning. *J Exp Psychol.* 1963;66:6–11.

28. Segreto J. The role of EMG awareness in EMG biofeedback learning. *Biofeedback Self Regul.* 1995;20:155–167.

29. Carron AV, Widmeyer WN, Brawley LR. Group cohesion and individual adherence to physical activity. *J Sport Exerc Psychol.* 1988;10:127–138.

30. Lee TD, Genovesee E. Distribution of practice in motor skill acquisition: different effects and continuous tasks. *Res Q Exerc Sport.* 1982;54:340–345.

31. Marteniuk RG, Carron AV. Efficiency of learning as a function of practice schedule and initial ability. *J Mot Behav.* 1970;2:140–148.

32. Stelmach GE. Efficiency of motor learning as a function of intertrial rest. *Res Q.* 1969;40:682–686.

33. Basmajian JV, De Luca CJ. *Muscles Alive: Their Functions Revealed by Electromyography.* 5th ed. Baltimore: Williams & Wilkins; 1985.

34. Lee TD, Swanson LR, Hall AL. What is repeated in repetition? Effects of practice conditions on motor skill acquisition. *Phys Ther.* 1991;71:150–156.

35. Catalano JF, Kleiner BM. Distant transfer and practice variability. *Percept Mot Skills.* 1984;58:851–856.

36. Kerr R, Booth B. Specific and varied practice of motor skill. *Percept Mot Skills.* 1978;46:395–401.

37. Feltz DL, Landers DM. The effects of mental practice on motor skill learning and performance: a meta analysis. *J Sport Psychol.* 1983;5:25–57.

38. Roland PE. Metabolic mapping of sensorimotor integration in the human brain. In: *Motor Areas of the Cerebral Cortex (Ciba Foundation Symposium).* New York: John Wiley & Sons; 1987.

39. Adams JA, Hufford LE. Contributions of a part-task trainer to the learning and relearning of a time-shared flight maneuver. *Hum Factors.* 1962;4:159–170.

40. Wrightman DC, Lintern G. Part-task training for tracking and manual control. *Hum Factors.* 1985;27:267–283.

41. Lersten KC. Retention of skill on the rho apparatus after one year. *Res Q.* 1969;40:418–419.

42. Briggs GE, Waters LK. Training and transfer as a function of component interaction. *J Exp Psychol.* 1958;56:492–500.

43. Hoberman M, et al. The use of lead up functional exercises to supplement mat work. *Phys Ther Rev.* 1951;31:1–11.

44. Battig WF. Facilitation and inference. In: Bilodeau EA, ed. *Acquisition of Skill.* New York: Academic Press; 1966.

45. DeBacher G. Biofeedback in spasticity control. In: Basmajian JV, ed. *Biofeedback: Principles and Practice for Clinicians.* 3rd ed. Baltimore: Williams & Wilkins; 1989;141–152.

46. Norris P. Clinical psychoneuroimmunology: strategies for self-regulation of immune system responding. In: Basmajian JV, ed. *Biofeedback: Principles and Practice for Clinicians.* 3rd ed. Baltimore: Williams & Wilkins; 1989:57–66.

47. Alders SS, Beckers D, Buck M. *PNF in Practice.* Heidelberg, Germany: Springer-Verlag; 1993.

48. Lewthwaite R. Motivational considerations in physical activity involvement. *Phys Ther.* 1990;70:808–819.

49. Singer RN, Pease D. Effect of guided versus discovery learning strategies on learning, retention, and transfer of a serial motor task. *Res Q.* 1976;47:788–796.

50. Locke EA, Latham GP. The application of goal setting to sports. *Sports Psychol.* 1985;7:205–222.

51. Feurstein M, Beattie P. Biobehavioral factors affecting pain and disability in low back pain: mechanisms and assessment. *Phys Ther.* 1995;75:267–280.

52. Payne RB, Dunman LS. Effects of classical predifferentiation on the functional properties of supplementary feedback cues. *J Mot Behav.* 1974;6:47–52.

53. Gaarder KR, Montgomery PS. *Clinical Biofeedback: A Procedural Manual.* Baltimore: Williams & Wilkins; 1977.

54. Brucker BS, Bulaeva NV. Biofeedback effect on electromyography responses in patients with spinal cord injury. *Arch Phys Med Rehabil.* 1996;77:133–137.

55. Hardy CJ, Rejeski WJ. Not what, but how one feels: the measurement of affect during exercise. *J Sport Exerc Psychol.* 1989;11:304–317.

56. Gill DL. *Psychological Dynamics of Sport.* Champaign, IL: Human Kinetics; 1986.

57. Davis M, Robbins Eshelman E, McKay M. *The Relaxation & Stress Reduction Workbook.* Oakland, CA: New Harbinger Publications; 1982.

58. Helmstetter S. *The Self-Talk Solution.* New York: Pocket Books; 1987.

59. McKay M, Davis, M, Fanning P. *Thoughts and Feelings: The Art of Cognitive Stress Intervention.* Richland, CA: New Harbinger Publications; 1981.

60. Robbins A. *Unlimited Power.* New York: Fawcett Columbine; 1986.

61. Schwartz MS. Compliance. In: Schwartz MS, ed. *Biofeedback: A Practitioner's Guide.* 2nd ed. New York: Guilford Press; 1995;184–210.

62. Fordyce WE. *Behavioral Methods for Chronic Pain and Illness.* St Louis, MO: CV Mosby; 1976.

CHAPTER 5

SEMG Feedback Training Techniques

Treatment of chronic musculoskeletal pain syndromes calls for a comprehensive approach to physiologic, biomechanic, and psychologic dysfunction. Surface electromyography (SEMG) training is only one part of the treatment process. SEMG methods should be integrated in ways that enhance each practitioner's existing treatment scope. Feedback techniques with SEMG can be used by individual practitioners or integrated into highly structured, formal pain management programs.[1] An interdisciplinary approach is recommended for patients with complex problems.

The guiding principle of treatment is to restore normal patterns of muscle activity under the circumstances, identified during evaluation, that provoked aberrant patterns. Patients are encouraged to determine what it is that they do, or do not do, that makes them feel worse, as well as what they can do to feel better. The desired result is the development of self-responsibility for the pain problem and underlying issues. Accountability leads to self-directed change, enabled by compassionate, holistic, and resolute clinical support. General treatment principles for therapists will be discussed next, followed by consideration of specific feedback strategies.

COMPREHENSIVE TREATMENT AND SEMG FEEDBACK TRAINING

Exhibit 5–1 lists treatment categories that are applicable to most patients with chronic muscu-

loskeletal pain, with or without adjunctive SEMG feedback. Postural training entails identification and reinforcement of optimal static biomechanical alignment for a particular individual. Body mechanics training involves learning efficient biomechanical principles for lifting, carrying, stooping, and other functional activities. Postural and body mechanics training may be performed concomitantly with ergonomic adjustment of equipment. Instruction in appropriate activity pacing implies analysis of functional tasks and alternating periods of light and heavy tasks, or interposition of physical rest, cognitive relaxation, or exercise periods between work bouts. Pacing can be accomplished on an individual basis or with job rotations in a group setting. Dietary education emphasizes basic nutritional principles for health and body weight management. If medically indicated, patients may be referred to a registered dietitian for counseling. Moderate use of caffeinated beverages and tobacco products is also encouraged, as appropriate to the individual. Goals are set for each relevant category and monitored throughout the therapy course.

Psychologic intervention ranges from a peripheral concern to the therapeutic center point, depending on a patient's level of impairment. Patients are educated as to their available health care options, as well as to the utility of fostering an internal health locus of control. Patients with chronic pain tend to see their problems as enduring, mysterious, and, oftentimes, quite out of

Exhibit 5–1 Common Conservative Interventions for Chronic Musculoskeletal Pain Syndromes

- postural training
- body mechanics training/ergonomic modifications
- training improved activity pacing
- dietary and nutritional education
- education for rational perceptions, attributions, and anticipated consequences regarding pain
- establishment of an internal health locus of control
- drug abuse management—prescribed, licit, illicit
- relaxation training
- stress management
- facilitation of sleep hygiene
- cognitive/behavioral psychotherapy
- manual therapies
- electrical/thermal/other physical agents
- exercise prescription/movement re-education
- pharmacologic agents
- restoration of functional activities of daily living
- vocational rehabilitation
- SEMG feedback training

their control.[2–5] Thus treatment objectives include reducing psychologic distress and facilitating self-responsibility for change. Active involvement enhances rehabilitative outcomes.[6–8] Therefore, as much as possible, patients are given a directive role in the therapeutic process. They are counseled to work toward a rational interpretation of pain and to be able to tell the difference between serious warning symptoms and benign discomfort associated, for example, with stretching shortened muscles. It is important that they come to understand that discomfort does not always mean tissue is being damaged.

Coping skills are taught. They include rational problem solving, identification and alteration of negative thoughts, distraction or focusing techniques, time management (for compliance with home programs), and relaxation techniques. Counseling is provided for sleep hygiene, so that the patient has regular bedtime and awakening schedules, uses comfortable positioning with pillows, is in bed only for sleep, avoids ingesting or imbibing stimulants after a certain time each evening, and uses relaxation techniques. A sense of self-efficacy is promoted in which cognition and behavior are used to prevent symptoms, promote healing, and control symptoms when they do occur. Ultimately, each patient constructs a toolbox of techniques that can be self-managed (Figure 5–1).

Other elements may be brought into play, including manual therapies for myofascial and joint dysfunction, thermal and electrical modalities, and pharmacologic agents administered in oral or injectable forms or through iontophoretic vehicles. Passive manual therapies, physical agents, and medications are used with special caution when copious pain behaviors are displayed, lest they reinforce an external health locus of control. All patients with musculoskeletal impairments are prescribed formal exercise programs of one type or another. Typically, this involves specific stretching exercises for tissues found to be tight on physical examination. Exercises for neuromuscular re-education, strength, power, and endurance are also provided as indicated. Aerobic conditioning is specifically recommended[9] and can be taught with target heart rate monitoring for greater exercise precision.

The efficacy of any procedures intended to have an impact on muscle function can be assessed readily with SEMG recording. For example, the therapist can examine the facilitatory effect of a neuromuscular electrical stimulation protocol or the inhibitory effect of a soft tissue mobilization technique by comparing SEMG activity before and after treatment application. The impact of an orthosis or taping technique on muscle function can be similarly assessed. In the psychologic domain, the efficacy of a particular muscle relaxation method becomes obvious with SEMG monitoring. SEMG offers a type and degree of objective confirmation not otherwise found in the clinic. Treatment processing

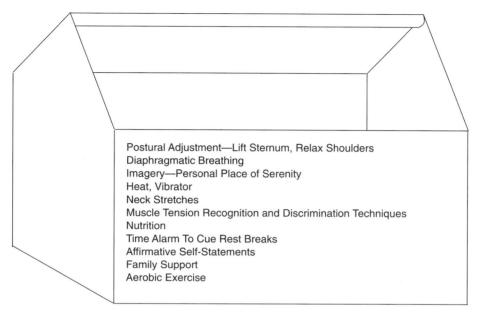

Figure 5–1 A set of patient self-management techniques illustrated as a toolbox. Different tools are selected to address particular aspects of each patient's musculoskeletal and psychologic impairments.

with SEMG helps provide each patient with a unique set of techniques to facilitate recovery.

All patients receive a home program designed to support the treatment objectives. Superficial heat and cold treatments, simple manual techniques, and straightforward electrotherapeutic programs can be performed in the home on a cost-effective basis. Written descriptions and diagrams are provided for all prescribed home exercises, along with dosing instructions for load, repetitions, and hold times. Handouts are given to the patient, describing and/or illustrating postural alignment, body mechanics techniques, activity pacing, and nutritional fundamentals. Excellent publications are available for lay readers to learn relaxation techniques, behavioral strategies for pain control, techniques for modification of cognitive appraisal of stressful events, and wellness principles.[10–13] Additional strategies to enhance motor learning and home program compliance were discussed in Chapter 4. Homework assignments that complement particular SEMG training procedures are discussed later.

SEMG TRAINING STRATEGIES

Patients with aberrant patterns of motor activity at the time of evaluation may advance to SEMG feedback training. Candidacy, display setups, and session structure for SEMG feedback training are discussed in Chapters 3 and 4 with the aim of enhancing motor learning. The goal of feedback training with SEMG is always to learn one or a combination of three strategies: downtraining, how to relax an overly tense muscle; uptraining, how to increase recruitment of a weak muscle; and coordination training, how to change the relative recruitment intensities or timing of two or more muscles. A menu of specific treatment procedures to achieve these objectives is shown in Exhibit 5–2. Practitioners are urged to select those methods that are relevant for the case at-hand and omit the others. The procedures are addressed individually next, and they have been extracted and grouped by their relevancy to general impairment syndromes discussed in Chapter 7 and to specific clinical applications discussed in Chapters 8

Exhibit 5–2 SEMG Training Technique Menu

- isolation of target muscle activity
- relaxation-based downtraining
- threshold-based uptraining/downtraining
- tension recognition threshold training
- tension discrimination training
- deactivation training
- generalization to progressively dynamic movement
- SEMG–triggered neuromuscular electrical stimulation
- left/right equilibration training
- motor copy training
- promotion of correct muscle synergies and related coordination patterns
- postural training with SEMG feedback
- body mechanics instruction with SEMG feedback
- therapeutic exercises with SEMG feedback
- functional activity performance with SEMG feedback

through 14. Procedures are discussed in roughly the order they are considered in training, but the sequence should be regarded as fluid.

1. Isolation of Target Muscle Activity

SEMG training almost always begins with muscle activation and isolation practice. The goal is for the patient to "find" the target muscle; that is to activate it distinctly, without co-activation of neighboring muscles or the contralateral homologous muscle. The technique can be used as both an orientation to feedback training and as a primary training method for patients with inappropriate muscle co-contraction. See the box "Clinical Procedure—Isolation of Target Muscle Activity."

An example of this technique is illustrated in Figure 5–2. This patient displayed apparent upper trapezius hyperactivity and initially had difficulty isolating the left upper trapezius from the right upper trapezius. The patient was then asked to perform pure shoulder shrugs on the left and raise the corresponding left SEMG signal while observing the feedback display for maintenance

of the right upper trapezius signal at baseline, and vice versa.

Another patient, whose SEMG activity is displayed in Figure 5–3, was attempting to uptrain the right lower trapezius without co-activating the upper trapezius. He was instructed to watch the display as he brought the right scapula down and back into scapular retraction and depression. The patient was then taught to distinguish the lower trapezius from the upper trapezius by repeating the "down and back" movement in contrast to a shoulder shrug.

2. Relaxation-Based Downtraining

This procedure involves traditional methods of SEMG–assisted relaxation training. The use of SEMG feedback to facilitate relaxation has been reviewed for many years and produced positive outcomes in controlled studies of chronic musculoskeletal pain.[16–22] Activity from an apparently hyperactive muscle is displayed while the subject is trained with some relaxation technique. Relaxation training with SEMG feedback is indicated by a positive finding on the psychophysiologic stress profile or other evidence of elevated tension responses linked to emotional arousal. The objective is to decouple muscle tension responses from triggering events. A step-by-step guide for selected relaxation techniques is included in Chapter 9 of the companion publication, *Introduction to Surface Electromyography.*[23] See the box "Clinical Procedure—Relaxation-Based Downtraining."

Information is gleaned from the subjective intake and psychophysiologic stress profile to judge the patient's preferred learning and thinking styles.[25] For example, an electrical engineer may prefer a logical, sequential technique such as Jacobsen's progressive contract/relax method[26] or perhaps counting backward from 10 to 1 with deepening relaxation with each digit. Another patient, such as an artistic painter, might do better with guided visual imagery.[27,28] A patient with strong kinesthetic orientation might prefer autogenics[29,30] or breathing methods.[31–35]

Figure 5–4 depicts SEMG results during a sample relaxation session. The lowest average

---

Clinical Procedure—Isolation of Target Muscle Activity

1. Select an intermediate display sensitivity and smoothing level.
2. Ask the patient to perform the isolated dynamic action or an isolated isometric contraction for the target muscle. If necessary, assist the patient by passively moving the body segments in the desired directions and then transitioning to active-assisted and active movement, or by using gently resisted manual muscle testing positions.[14,15]
3. Ask the patient to observe the SEMG display as the muscle is activated, so that the feedback relationship becomes clear. Also cue the patient to attend to the intrinsic kinesthetic sensations associated with muscle activation and observe the related body segment, so that he or she understands the role of the target muscle in movement.
4. Use additional SEMG channels to monitor muscles that may be inappropriately co-contracted.
5. Instruct the patient to activate the target muscle while seeking to inhibit or limit signal activation from another site.
6. Select a simple dual channel visual display, or combine visual feedback for the muscle to be activated with audio feedback for the muscle to be inhibited.
7. Perform several consecutive repetitions with attempted isolation of one muscle and then the other. As proficiency is gained, alternate the goal muscle on each repetition and then randomize the activation order. Consider the use of deliberate co-contractions as a contrast to isolated control.
8. Document the average peak microvolt value for each channel during three to five trials at the beginning and end of practice. Observe for increased output from the primary channel and decreased output from the secondary channel(s).
9. Alternatively, generate a representative printout of an attempt at isolation at the beginning and end of the session.

---

microvolt score was produced with the imagery method. Imagery techniques were then adapted for home practice. Therapists who regularly work in this realm are encouraged to develop a wide personal repertoire of relaxation skills. Resources may be identified from formal relaxation and stress management classes, community classes relating to meditation and mind–body work, or many tapes and books found in catalogs or the self-help or psychology sections of bookstores.

In the physical medicine setting, one approach is to explore basic relaxation strategies for one to three sessions. The goal is to identify optimal relaxation strategies and provide enough supervised training so the patient can continue to practice at home. Competence can be assessed by patient report of performance abilities in functional settings, confirmation of a decrease in baseline SEMG activity over subsequent visits, and demonstrations during psychophysiologic challenge. Should progress fail to be obtained, the therapist can return the focus to basic training and re-examine the strategies. Relaxation technique practice, however, is a patient's home responsibility. Additional sessions are used to integrate relaxation training with transfer techniques as well as other SEMG feedback procedures.

Perhaps the most difficult aspect of relaxation training is generalization of the response to actual functional contexts. Patients may become classically conditioned to relax in a quiet training room, but be unable to carry over the response to the workplace. Therefore the emphasis is on promoting quick reproduction of a relaxation response without complex "mental gymnastics." One method is to have the patient practice induction of deep relaxation by any fa-

A

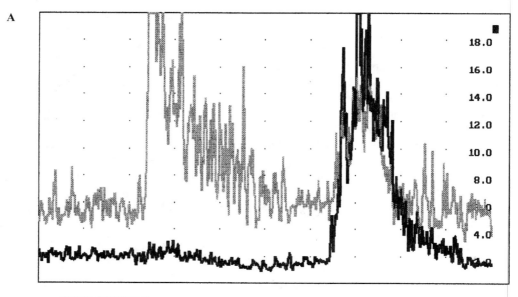

UPPER TRAPEZIUS

B

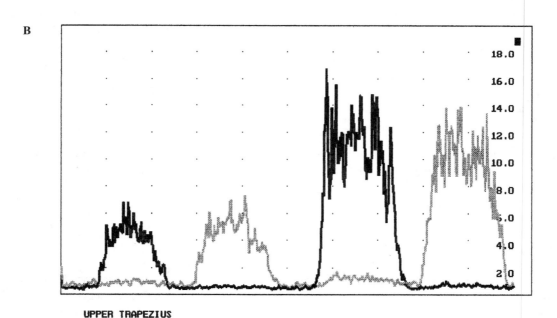

UPPER TRAPEZIUS

Figure 5–2 Isolation training with use of SEMG feedback from the left (black) and right (gray) upper trapezius muscles of a patient with chronic right cervical and suprascapular pain. (**A**) Results of a right unilateral shoulder shrug followed by a left unilateral shoulder shrug. Note elevated right side baseline and relatively erratic decruitment back to baseline after a right shrug. As would be expected, the left side signal is quiescent during the right shrug. However, the right side inappropriately co-activates during the left shrug. (**B**) Results of left and right shoulder shrugs at low and moderate intensity, respectively, from the same patient at the conclusion of therapy. Signals from the left and right are now isolated and reciprocally symmetric.

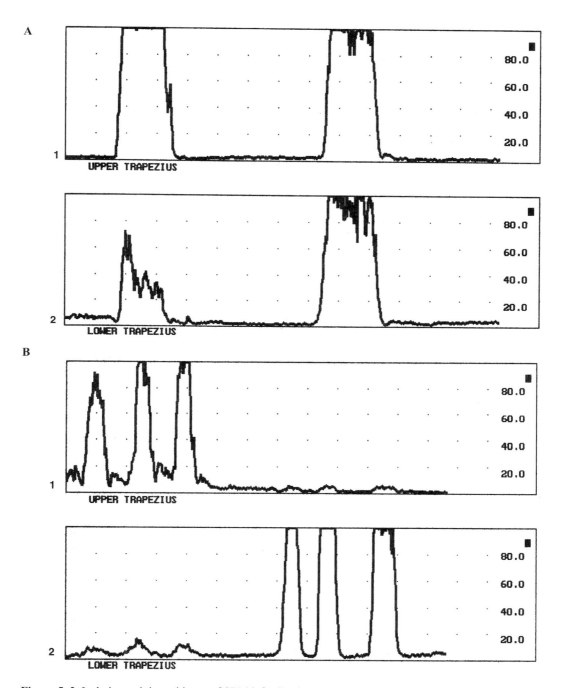

Figure 5–3 Isolation training with use of SEMG feedback from the involved side (**A1, B1**) upper trapezius and (**A2, B2**) lower trapezius muscles of a patient with chronic periscapular pain. (**A**) Initiation of therapy: Attempted isolation and uptraining of the lower trapezius. Experimenting with scapular movements and conscious control, the patient is unable to activate the lower trapezius without also activating the upper trapezius. (**B**) Later in the therapy course: the patient can now use a pure shoulder shrug to isolate the activity of the upper trapezius, and scapular retraction/depression to isolate the activity of the lower trapezius.

Clinical Procedure—Relaxation-Based Downtraining

1. Select a simple display with moderate sensitivity and high level of display smoothing.

2. Position the patient with support in upright sitting position with appropriate postural alignment. Recumbent postures may be used, but they tend to be less functional.

3. Select one to three relaxation techniques for practice over a 15- to 30-minute period. Verbally cue the client to "relax," "soften," and "let the limbs be 'loose, floppy, heavy.'"

4. Instruct the patient in the relaxation technique(s) while observing the effects at the SEMG display. Use audio feedback if the subject wishes to close his or her eyes, or only visual feedback to minimize distractions.

5. As muscle relaxation is achieved, direct the patient to attend to changes in muscle tension sensations and joint position. Assist the patient by asking questions, such as "What do you feel now?" "How is this different?" "What words describe the change in what you can feel?" "Where exactly do you feel it?" "How much has changed?" Reinforce the patient's success to facilitate a sense of self-efficacy in controlling aberrant muscle tension. Point out that he or she successfully managed the excessive tension and that the procedure can be repeated independently whenever it is needed.

6. If multiple techniques are attempted, select the method that produces the greatest reduction in activity for continued practice. Consider shifting the session focus to an educational topic, and solicit the patient's remarks to facilitate return of arousal to a normal, interactive level. Observe for changes in the SEMG display. Then repeat the favored relaxation technique and reexamine the SEMG amplitude. The most definitive results are obtained when a deep reduction of the SEMG magnitude is time-locked to performance of a specific technique.

7. Document the average microvolt value for a 1- to 3-minute baseline period and the lowest 1- to 3-minute average during practice with each technique.

8. Once the ability to induce a relaxation response is established, challenge the patient by having him or her maintain desired SEMG responses while engaging in complex problem-solving tasks, distracting conversation, or use of noninvolved body parts.

9. Withdraw postural support, add distracting background activity, or train in a busy, natural environment with a portable SEMG unit.

10. Pair key "trigger" words or hand positions with relaxation induction, so that skills can be quickly called on (see later discussion).

11. Use a hierarchical progression of stress-related imagery to practice associating muscle relaxation with different life situations.

12. Identify an abbreviated form of the relaxation method for practice throughout the day.

13. Support home practice with an audiocassette tape that directs full as well as abbreviated relaxation methods.[24] Use a prerecorded tape. Better yet, record a successful live session with the patient and give the tape to the patient for home use.

14. Teach the patient to use the abbreviated form for about 1 minute, six to eight times per day, along with postural correction and key therapeutic exercises.

15. Make home and workplace instructions as specific as possible. Assign the instructions in writing, and ensure that the patient has expressly agreed with the instructions.

A   **Mid-Lower
Cervical Paraspinal**

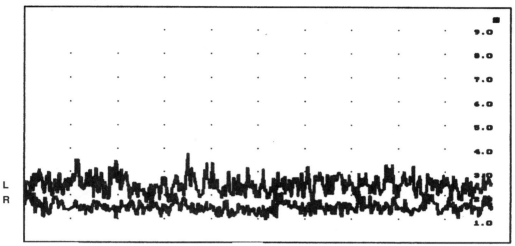

Autogenics

B   **Mid-Lower
Cervical Paraspinal**

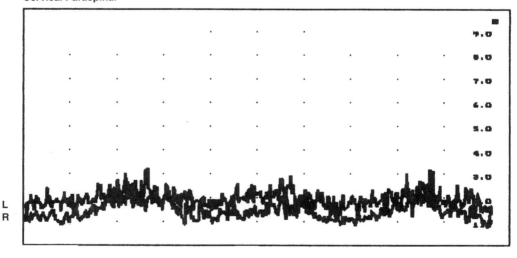

Diaphragmatic Breathing

continues

Figure 5–4 Relaxation-based downtraining with SEMG feedback from the middle-lower (left, **L**, and right, **R**) cervical paraspinals of a patient with chronic, left greater than right, neck pain. Four sample 15-second plots of activity are shown, each taken from a 7- to 10-minute instruction period in a specific relaxation technique: (**A**) Autogenics; (**B**) diaphragmatic breathing; (**C**) imagery; and (**D**) contract/relax. All training was completed within a single session. The lowest activity magnitude and greatest level of symmetry are seen in **C**, with use of imagery techniques, which were selected as the relaxation method of choice for home practice.

Figure 5–4 continued

C   **Mid-Lower**
         Cervical Paraspinal

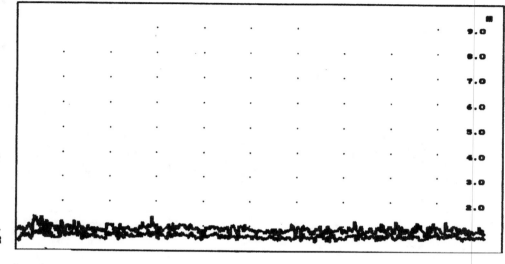

Imagery

D   **Mid-Lower**
         Cervical Paraspinal

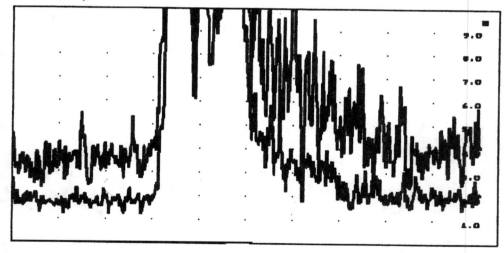

Contract/Relax

vored method and then maintain the relaxed state while slowly repeating a key "trigger word" or holding a peculiar finger position. The intent is for the key word and hand position to become classically conditioned with the relaxation response over a period of several weeks and then serve as induction aids in demanding situations.

Generalization of relaxation responses may also be facilitated by combining SEMG training and home practice with systematic desensitization or stress inoculation procedures.[36–41] First, the patient learns to induce relaxation. Then, a hierarchy of stressful situations is listed in writing, either related to a particular phobic theme or a variety of life circumstances (Exhibit 5–3). Each item is visualized as the patient maintains relaxation and periodically attends to the feedback display. Should a sense of emotional arousal become strong or the SEMG display indicate an aberrant rise in muscle tension, the image is temporarily abandoned while the individual returns to the relaxation method. Once muscle tension is reduced, the patient resumes with a less-threatening visualization and continues through the hierarchy. The procedure is aided by self-talk for positive coping skills and self-efficacy.[11]

General relaxation practice may also be facilitated by thermal feedback training.[42,43] The patient's objective is to learn to self-regulate peripheral skin temperature. A small thermistor bead is taped over the volar aspect of the index finger of the dominant hand. The thermistor connects to a processing system and display for feedback. The patient attempts to raise hand temperature while practicing relaxation techniques. Increased skin temperature is associated with peripheral superficial vasodilation, changes in autonomic tone, and decreased psychophysiologic arousal. Training can be accomplished with stand-alone thermal feedback devices, or with feedback systems with modular thermal components in conjunction with SEMG. Battery-powered temperature devices for home thermal feedback practice are sold through electronics stores and sales catalogs of companies that specialize in this type of equipment. These units incorporate a thermistor-lead wire assembly that can be taped to a finger as described above. They are simple to use, responsive, and inexpensive. Each session's starting and ending temperatures (with the use of a consistent ambient room temperature) can be charted to document progress.

Patients may also benefit from other cognitive and behavioral therapy methods, and recognizing the need for skilled psychotherapy is critical. Many subjects can be assisted with an "over-the-counter" relaxation approach, but others require

---

Exhibit 5–3 Statements Composed by a Patient, 6 Months after a Motor Vehicle Accident, with Persistent Cervical Muscle Tension and Pain When Driving

1. sitting in car; feel safe and comfortable
2. driving through neighborhoods on Bainbridge Island; feel fairly comfortable
3. city streets at regular speed, non–rush hour traffic
4. city streets at rush hour
5. two-lane highway on Bainbridge, where speed is fast
6. state highway, not much traffic, big trucks present, but slow speed (state = 4 lane)
7. interstate, not much traffic, big trucks present, but slow speed (interstate = 6–8 lanes)
8. state highway, lots of traffic, especially trucks, but slow speed
9. interstate, lots of traffic, especially trucks, but slow speed
10. on state highway or interstate, not much traffic, no trucks, but going fast
11. on state highway or interstate, lots of traffic, no trucks, going fast
12. on 6- to 8-lane freeway/interstate, with lots of traffic, no trucks, but going fast
13. on a 4-lane state highway, with lots of traffic, trucks present, going fast
14. on an interstate (6–9 lanes) with lots of traffic, especially large trucks, all going fast

---

Note: Statements are arranged in a patient-perceived hierarchy from least to most associated stress. Guided imagery related to each statement was used with relaxation techniques and electromyographic feedback from the cervical paraspinals and upper trapezius to facilitate systematic desensitization.

specific evaluation and treatment procedures that address core psychologic issues. For patients with chronic musculoskeletal pain problems, this is best provided by practitioners in psychology or psychiatry with training in rehabilitation and chronic pain management.

Another point to be emphasized is that the objective of relaxation training is not to teach patients to eliminate muscle tone, nor to produce a state of lethargy. Minds need to be alert to interact with the environment, and muscles must generate tension to subserve skeletal movement. The idea is to produce the most efficient muscle response for a functional posture or movement. Traditional relaxation training for musculoskeletal problems is rarely an end in itself, but must be followed by other training methods.

3. Threshold-Based Uptraining/ Downtraining

This procedure is another classical training paradigm in which a particular goal level in microvolts is prescribed. The patient then attempts to manipulate the active SEMG signal above or below that level.[18,44–46] Goals are cued by a marker line across a video display, by a specially colored light on a light bar display, or by onset or offset of an audio signal yoked to the threshold amplitude. Threshold-based downtraining is used with hyperactive muscles to enhance relaxation learning. The procedure is performed as described above for relaxation training, with the addition of the display goal. Threshold-based uptraining is used with poorly recruited muscles to increase activation. Uptraining consists of a series of phasic activation attempts with goal-oriented feedback. See the box "Clinical Procedure—Threshold-Based Uptraining/Downtraining."

As an example, Figure 5–5 displays the results of uptraining a weak quadriceps in a patient with chronic pain and weakness after total knee replacement. He was instructed to try to bring his activity above a 10-μV threshold line, which also turned on an audio tone that signaled goal attainment. The goal was raised as recruitment ability increased. Figure 5–6 shows SEMG ac-

tivity from a patient after a motor vehicle accident. The patient had an overly active upper trapezius averaging about 15 μV in quiet sitting. She was instructed to relax and bring her activity below a 12-μV threshold line, which also caused an audio signal to terminate. When this was achieved, the threshold was lowered to 10 μV, and so on.

4. Tension Recognition Threshold Training

This technique is used with patients who show focally elevated muscle activity with poor subjective recognition of tension sensations. These persons inappropriately tense muscles without being aware of it. Onset or exacerbation of pain is the only indication that something is wrong. Training is designed to facilitate kinesthetic awareness of tension at an initial change from the baseline level. It is hoped that these patients will be alerted to rising tension during life tasks. Using relaxation methods, they can then abort the tension event before pain increases (Figure 5–7). This procedure is recommended as a treatment strategy for patients who show poor responses on the Tension Recognition Thresholds evaluation procedure discussed in Chapter 2. See the box "Clinical Procedure—Tension Recognition Threshold Training."

Patients frequently will begin training by overshooting the goal and may report, "I can see (from the feedback display) that I tensed the muscle, but I can't feel any difference." After repeated trials, the threshold comes to be reliably matched and accompanied by a response, such as "Now I can feel myself tensing the muscle; I'm aware that it's different from a full rest." (See Figure 5–8.)

5. Tension Discrimination Training

This procedure is another method of facilitating recognition of muscle tension and graded muscle control. The training is used with hyperactive muscles and downtraining objectives, as well as with hypoactive muscles and uptraining objectives, or coordination training. The procedure is considered a core feedback task. A target

Clinical Procedure—Threshold-Based Uptraining/Downtraining

Uptraining:

1. Use Clinical Procedure—Isolation of Target Muscle Activity as a foundation for uptraining.
2. Set a low level of display smoothing. Adjust the sensitivity so that recruitment attempts activate the display to its maximal one third.
3. Instruct the patient to perform a few repetitions without a goal marker, and observe recruitment ability.
4. Select a goal value that is estimated to be attainable about 80% of attempts. Instruct the patient to recruit the target muscle maximally and try to exceed the goal. Allow adequate intertrial rest periods, and monitor for fatigue or pain provocation.
5. Progress the training by asking for graded isometric, concentric, and eccentric contractions. Consider use of quick stretch, isometric hold to quick concentric contraction, manual tapping, rapid reversal of agonist/antagonist contraction, or other facilitatory techniques.[47-49]
6. Beware of recording movement artifact. Avoid contacting the patient directly over the electrodes, sudden skin stretching, and erratic lead wire motions.
7. Document the average maximal microvolt value during three to five baseline contraction attempts and the maximal reproducible goal value obtained during practice.
8. Alternatively, document the number of times a goal value was reached relative to the number of attempts.

Downtraining:

1. Use Procedure—Relaxation-Based Downtraining as a precursor.
2. Select a high level of display smoothing and a sensitivity such that muscle activity tracks along the bottom third of the visual display. Set a threshold at about 20%, or a few microvolts, below the baseline average.
3. Provide adequate support for the patient's trunk and limb segments, and position joint segments to their points of least hypertonicity (usually with muscles in a relatively lengthened position).
4. Have the subject perform a favored relaxation technique to bring SEMG activity below the goal.
5. Document the average microvolt value for a 1- to 3-minute baseline period and the lowest 1- to 3-minute average during practice, or the lowest threshold value the patient can consistently maintain.
6. Alternatively, document the baseline average and the latency to decrease activity below a designated threshold.

Uptraining and Downtraining:

Once the uptraining or downtraining criterion is consistently met, move the threshold progressively higher or lower to shape the response in the desired direction.

A

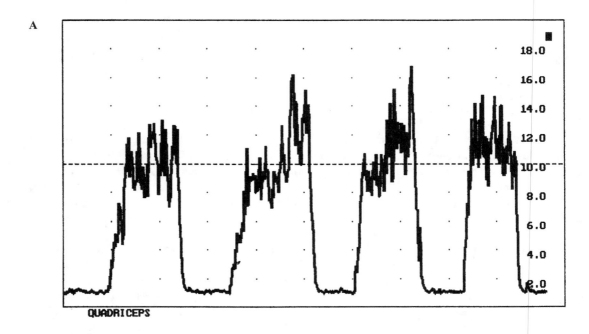

QUADRICEPS

B

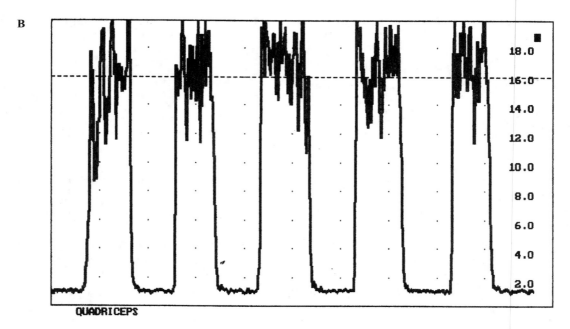

QUADRICEPS

Figure 5–5 Threshold-based uptraining with use of SEMG feedback from the quadriceps of a patient with chronic pain and weakness after total knee replacement. The patient was instructed to contract the quadriceps isometrically and bring the muscle activity signal above the dashed threshold marker. When the goal level (shown in **A**) was easily exceeded, the goal was raised to a higher value (shown in **B**). Progressively higher goals were set, and the desired response was shaped upward.

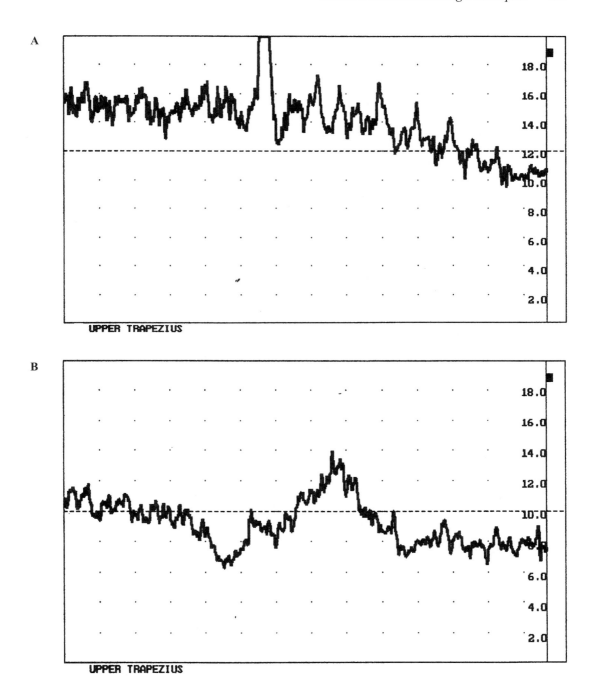

Figure 5–6 Threshold-based downtraining with use of SEMG feedback from the upper trapezius of a patient with muscle hyperactivity and pain after motor vehicle accident. The dashed threshold marker serves as a relaxation goal. When the goal level (shown in **A**) was met, the goal was lowered (shown in **B**). Progressively lower goals were set, and the desired response was shaped downward.

Clinical Procedure—Tension Recognition Threshold Training

1. Select a moderate level of display smoothing and very high sensitivity. Set a visual and auditory goal at a small value (eg, 0.5–1.0 µV RMS) above the resting baseline.
2. With the use of the isolated action of the target muscle, instruct the patient to recruit just enough activity that the SEMG signal reaches the threshold. Instruct the patient to maintain this activity level for 5 to 10 seconds. Then have the patient rest for 5 to 10 seconds, and repeat.
3. Cue the patient to attend to associated internal sensations relating to joint position and tension. Contrast activation with sensations perceived during rest. Ask questions, such as "What did you do to move the signal like that?" "What do you feel now?" "How is this different from rest?" "What words describe the change in what you can feel?" "Where exactly do you feel it?" "How much has changed?" "How would you know if your muscle was activated to this level if the feedback was disconnected?"
4. When the SEMG activity level can be reliably matched to the threshold and the patient reports that he or she can detect associated intrinsic kinesthetic cues, repeat the procedure with the display turned away (or with patient's eyes closed) and the audio turned off. If the patient can reproduce the threshold value without extrinsic feedback, decrease the criterion closer to baseline. Repeat the series until the smallest increment of change that can be detected is identified.
5. Document the resting baseline, which may drift lower during the session, as well as the lowest threshold value that is used.
6. Progress to Clinical Procedure—Tension Discrimination Training.

---

muscle is activated to a preselected threshold criterion as awareness is drawn to both extrinsic SEMG feedback and intrinsic kinesthetic feedback. The task is similar to that in Clinical Procedure—Tension Recognition Threshold Training, except that multiple goal criteria are used and at higher amplitude values. The purpose is for patients to internalize cognizance of the microvolt scale. Patients learn to judge relative SEMG intensity with feedback and then transfer recognition skills as the machine cues are removed. In this way, patients acquire skill at independently discriminating muscle tension levels. Relaxation tools can then be used to reduce muscle activity before it builds to high intensity and volitional control is lost. Through the patient's practicing of finely graded recruitment and intrinsic recognition, the method also extends basic uptraining and acts as a precursor to dynamic coordination training. Variants of discrimination training tasks have been used to test awareness skills under experimental learning conditions.[50–54] Performance on discrimination tasks is also impaired in patients with chronic low back and temporomandibular joint pain.[55] See the box "Clinical Procedure—Tension Discrimination Training."

Many patients demonstrate basic skill with these procedures within a single 15- to 20-minute practice session, although some require several sessions before proficiency is attained. Whether patients can discriminate target SEMG values with exact precision is not the main concern. A rough estimating ability is adequate, so long as it can be transferred to a variety of functional settings.

The therapist may observe that the patient has greater difficulty in goal matching on an involved side, compared with an uninvolved side. Recruitment on the uninvolved side tends to be more easily graduated in fine increments. Patients with unilateral hypertonicity commonly

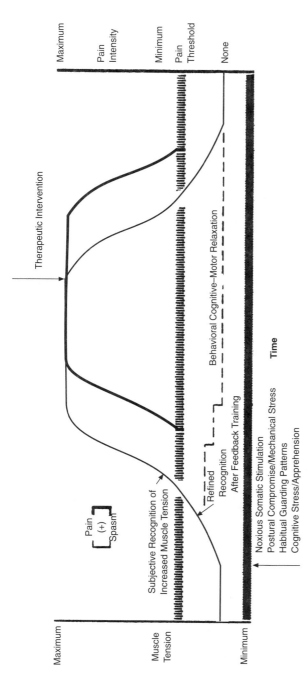

Figure 5–7 Model relating muscle tension, pain, time, and patient perception. Pain follows as a consequence of an aberrant muscle tension dosage (result of both magnitude and duration of tension). Patients with chronic muscle tension may not become aware of increasing muscle activity until pain has increased significantly. EMG feedback training procedures are used to facilitate earlier awareness of muscle tension, before symptoms become severe or hamper the patient's ability to cope successfully. Relaxation downtraining techniques are then used to abort the aberrant muscle tension cycle. *Source:* Reprinted with permission from JR Cram, *Clinical EMG for Surface Recordings,* Vol 2, © 1990, Clinical Resources, Inc.

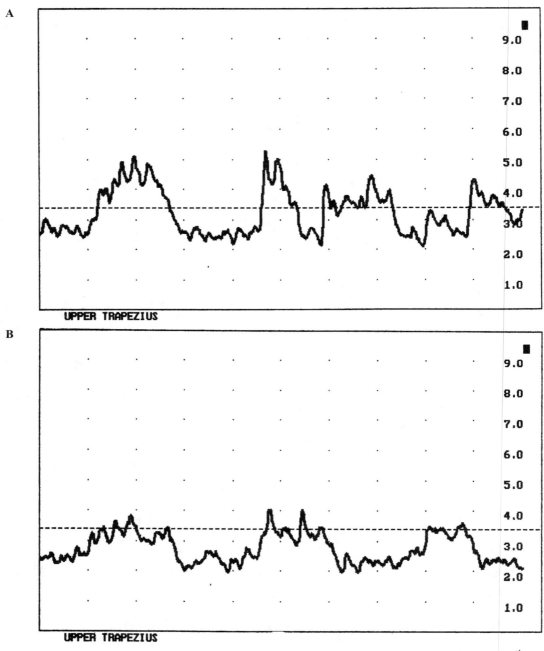

continues

Figure 5–8 Tension recognition threshold training with use of SEMG feedback from the upper trapezius of a patient with chronic muscle hyperactivity and neck pain. A dashed threshold marker is set slightly above the baseline activity level. The ability to activate the trapezius signal just to the threshold is demonstrated progressively (across **A–C**), each recorded at successive intervals. Muscle control is accompanied by increased subjective awareness of subtle tension sensations.

Figure 5–8 continued

C

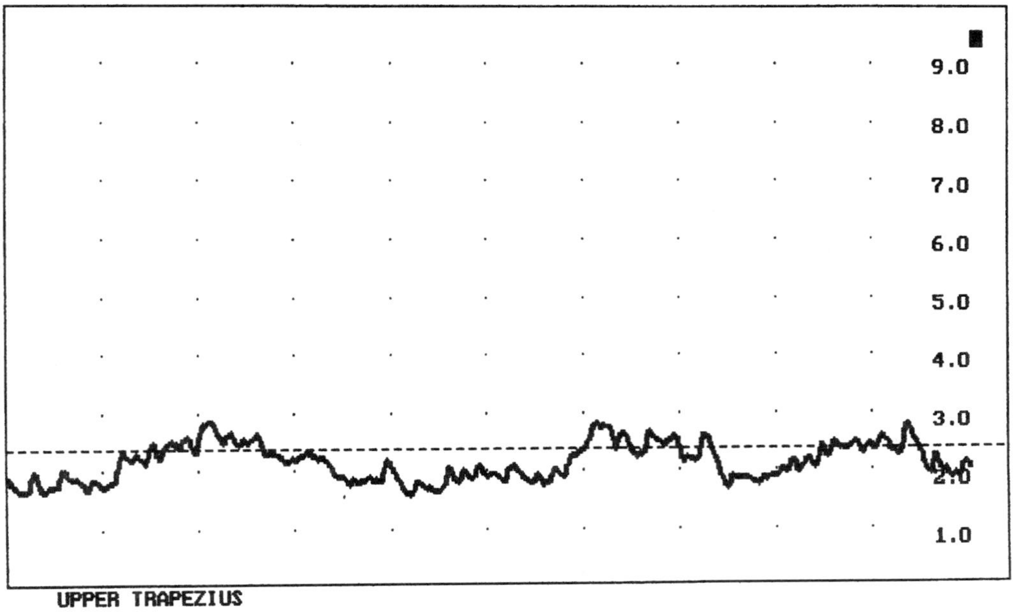

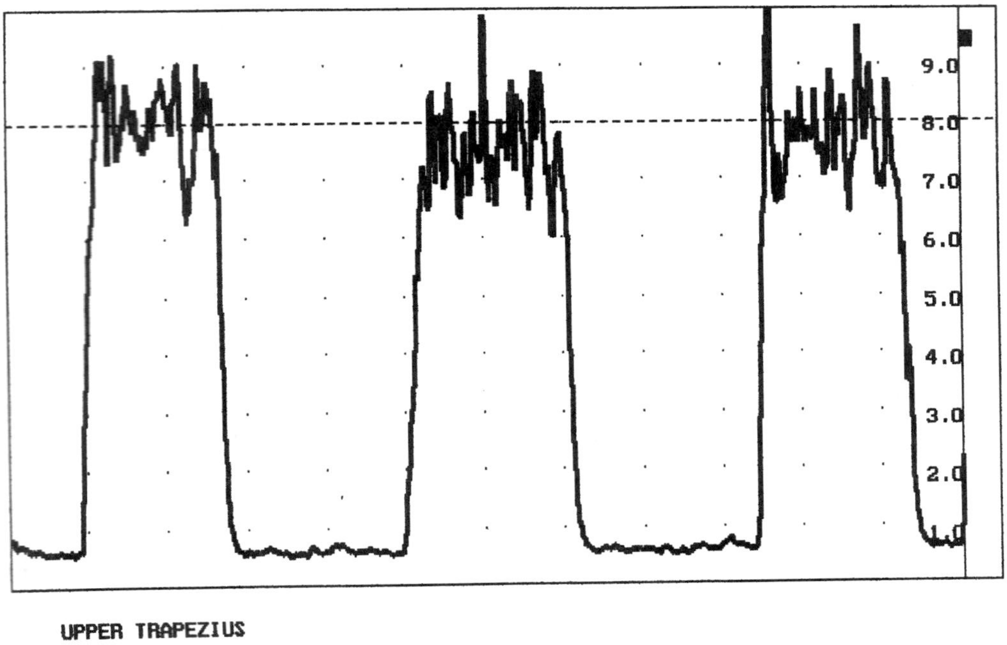

UPPER TRAPEZIUS

UPPER TRAPEZIUS

Figure 5–9 Tension discrimination training with use of SEMG feedback from the upper trapezius. The dashed threshold marker shows the target activation level.

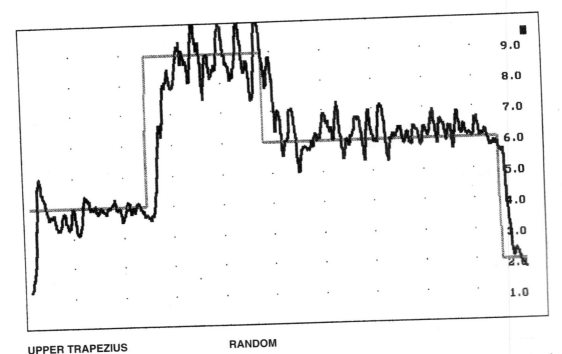

UPPER TRAPEZIUS   **RANDOM**

Figure 5–11 Progression of the tension discrimination training technique initiated as shown in Figures 5–9 and 5–10. Now the target values are selected randomly by a computer, for variable durations. The template therefore follows an unpredictable sequence.

report that they perceive greater muscular effort on the uninvolved side for the same goal value. They remark that the involved side "just goes," whereas the uninvolved side must be consciously exerted. Advanced patients may attempt simultaneous discrimination of the same or different target values from two different recording sites (Figure 5–12).

6. Deactivation Training

Deactivation training is the practice of turning muscles off. Some patients with musculoskeletal pain syndromes have difficulty relaxing their muscles to baseline on task completion or during brief pauses in work activities of long duration.[56-62] Excessive recruitment during muscle work periods may be a problem, but the salient point is that muscles are not sufficiently deactivated during rest periods. Muscle tension persists when there is no task to be performed. Ex-

pression of the phenomenon is assessed with SEMG during kinesiologic profiling (described in Chapter 2). The therapist observes for a prompt return to baseline SEMG activity on movement cessation or examines gaps in a rectified line tracing of continual SEMG activity.

Deactivation training has two main objectives: a prompt drop in SEMG activity when movement is stopped and a complete recovery to baseline SEMG magnitude (Figure 5–13). A third goal can be set for continuous tasks of long duration; that is, the production of transient rest periods. Microrests are brief respites in SEMG activity ranging from 0.2 second to several seconds. They are associated with low mechanical work and are interspersed throughout a continuous task. These reductions in muscle activity are produced at natural points in task cycling. Triggers for microrests include low demand phases of an industrial task, pauses in a typing assignment to read text, or perhaps a phasic rest during

A
B

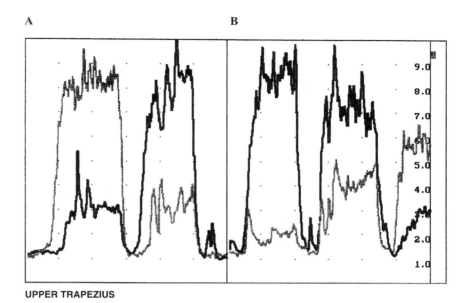

UPPER TRAPEZIUS

Figure 5–12 Successful tension discrimination training with use of SEMG feedback from the left (gray) and right (black) upper trapezius. (**A**) While using shoulder shrugs, the patient is cued to hold 8 μV on the left and simultaneously maintain 3 μV on the right (first set of peaks). The targets are then reciprocated (second set of peaks). (**B**) Three trials with randomly designated targets are performed: 2 μV left, 9 μV right (first set of peaks); 4 μV left, 7 μV right (second set of peaks); 6 μV left, 3 μV right (third set of peaks).

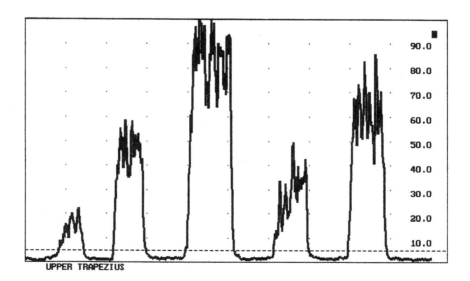

UPPER TRAPEZIUS

Figure 5–13 Deactivation training with use of SEMG feedback from the upper trapezius associated with trials of variable range shoulder flexion, performed well. For each contraction, deactivation is prompt and complete. Baseline recovery is cued by the dashed threshold marker.

an out-of-bounds call during sport performance. Healthy persons produce microrests without conscious planning. Patients require practice—practice that is initiated with regular, deliberate pauses cued by the therapist and that builds toward more functional timing. See "Clinical Procedure—Deactivation Training."

The steps involved in retraining purposeful task behavior with SEMG feedback are outlined later in this chapter in Clinical Procedure—Functional Activity Performance with SEMG Feedback. However, considerations for interspersed microrests are reviewed here as a progression of the core procedure just described. See the box "Clinical Procedure—Training for the Production of Interspersed Microrests."

Ettare and Ettare[63] have described a similar approach to training with a variety of muscle sites during practical tasks. They call the method "Muscle Learning Therapy" and have applied it to patients with cumulative trauma disorders. A primary aspect of the program is training for prompt deactivation between repetitions of sit to stand, stand to sit, walking, typing, and picking up or putting down objects. Ettare and Ettare be-

lieve that this type of feedback training enhances the patient's proprioceptive awareness and ability to regulate muscle activity in complex work environments.

7. Generalization to Progressively Dynamic Movement

The techniques discussed so far are mostly performed with the patient attempting to manipulate the SEMG display under static conditions or other relatively artificial circumstances. Whether an individual can control an SEMG tracing on a video display screen is unimportant. What matters is the ability to transfer learning to purposeful activity.

The training sequences described in this section represent a progression in motor skill complexity. The uptrained, downtrained, or coordination response is produced and maintained as the associated body parts are moved, and challenges are provided for more sophisticated patterns of motor control. See the box "Clinical Procedure—Generalization to Progressively Dynamic Movement."

Clinical Procedure—Deactivation Training

1. Position the patient in supported sitting or standing with appropriate postural alignment.
2. Select a relatively high display sensitivity and a minimal level of smoothing. Set a goal marker about 0.5–1.0 μV above the resting baseline.
3. Instruct the patient to activate the target muscle to 30% to 50% of maximum intensity and hold that level for about 3 seconds.
4. Then cue the patient to let go promptly, so that the SEMG signal falls below the threshold marker. Observe for a sharp slope in the decline of an SEMG line tracing graphic or a rapid decrease in the height of a bar graph.
5. Instruct the subject to rest for 5 to 10 seconds and continue trials until proficiency is demonstrated.
6. Repeat randomly with low-, moderate-, and high-intensity contractions.
7. Gradually withdraw continuous feedback, and assess the patient's ability to reproduce the desired response. Also withdraw extrinsic postural support.
8. Document the approximate number of seconds to baseline recovery and the average recovery amplitude, as well as conditions that evoke a delayed recovery latency or elevated recovery amplitude.

Clinical Procedure—Training for the Production of Interspersed Microrests

1. Have the patient perform a problematic repetitive activity with as realistic a functional set-up as possible.
2. Instruct him or her to concentrate on prompt, complete deactivation on your command.
3. Say "pause" every 20 to 30 seconds of practice. Direct the patient to pause long enough to maintain activity below the threshold marker for at least 5 seconds (Figure 5–14). Activity should not be resumed until the goal is attained.
4. Check for adequate posture and ergonomic arrangement.
5. Integrate the task with abbreviated relaxation methods, such as deep breathing, cognitive techniques, stretching, contract-relax maneuvers, or antagonist activation, if needed.
6. Progress by shortening rest periods to 0.5 second to 2 seconds, increasing task speed and distractions, and withdrawing continuous feedback.
7. Ask the patient to practice the procedure independently (with a portable SEMG trainer or without SEMG feedback) at his or her work station or other functional site. The patient should strive to maintain conscious practice for 3 to 5 minutes, six to eight times per day, as appropriate, until the microrests occur naturally.

Clinical Procedure—Generalization to Progressively Dynamic Movement

1. Use the first six clinical procedures to establish fundamental training proficiency, as indicated.
2. Select a low level of display smoothing, and reproduce the desired pattern of motor activity while working from
   - isometric to concentric to eccentric control.
   - small to progressively larger movement arcs.
   - supported single joint movement to unsupported simultaneous control of multiple joints, an entire body segment, or the entire body.
   - movement in cardinal planes to diagonal functional planes—for example, proprioceptive neuromuscular facilitation diagonals 1 and 2 for upper and lower extremity.[47–49]
   - slow to fast speed.
   - light to heavy external load.
   - open to closed kinematic chain (for the lower extremity).
   - unilateral movement to bilateral simultaneous symmetric movement to bilateral reciprocal movement to bilateral simultaneous asymmetric movement.
   - predictable tasks to unpredictable tasks, in which the movement goal, load, velocity, base posture, and environmental conditions are randomly varied.
3. Document conditions for which satisfactory motor control is demonstrated versus those for which it is not.

A

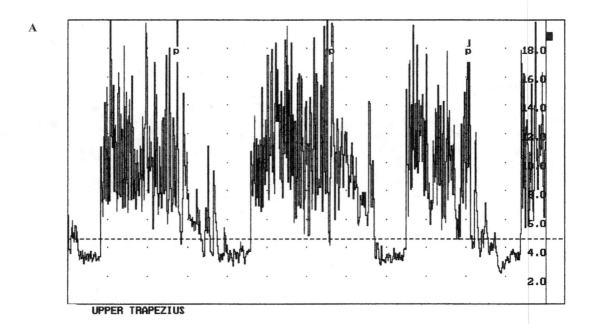

UPPER TRAPEZIUS

B

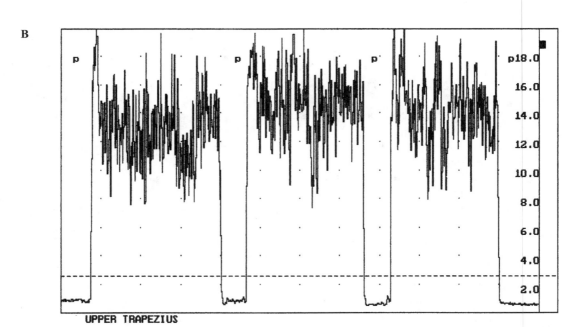

UPPER TRAPEZIUS

Figure 5–14 Deactivation training with use of SEMG feedback from the upper trapezius while a patient performs a typing task. A pause (**p**) is verbally called by the therapist periodically, at which time the patient attempts to relax and promptly restore activity to the baseline level cued by the dashed threshold marker. (**A**) Initiation of training. Note the time lag between each pause cue and baseline recovery. (**B**) Training at a later date with the same patient. Baseline recovery is now immediately linked to each pause command.

8. SEMG-Triggered Neuromuscular Electrical Stimulation

SEMG-triggered neuromuscular electrical stimulation is used for uptraining and for coordination training. The technique requires specialized equipment and skill and is discussed in detail in Chapter 6.

9. Left/Right Equilibration Training

Equilibration training is performed when the left and right sides of a homologous muscle pair act differently during a symmetric task. This could involve a static posture, a simultaneous symmetric motion, or a reciprocally symmetric motion. For example, the left upper trapezius may average 9 µV and the right upper trapezius 2 µV during quiet sitting, or a similar magnitude of asymmetry may be seen with alternating left/

right shoulder flexion to 180 degrees. There are several training options, depending on the nature of the asymmetry. See the box "Clinical Procedure—Specific Left/Right Equilibration Training."

When a patient displays asymmetric SEMG activity and bilateral symptoms, it may not be clear whether the high side amplitude is too high or the low amplitude side is too low. Judgments are also difficult when there are no normative standards available to guide interpretation or when complex compensatory motor behaviors are suspected. In addition, hyperactive responses are sometimes resistant to the downtraining and equilibration procedures described. Because of these factors, some clinicians have taken the approach of always uptraining the low amplitude side. No judgment is made as to which side is excessive. The perspective is simply that the two sides are unbalanced.[64] The method has been used

---

Clinical Procedure—Specific Left/Right Equilibration Training

Asymmetry in which the high amplitude side is painful and judged to be hypertonic— SEMG recordings from the symptomatic side show a failure to recover to baseline levels upon activity cessation, or excessive activity relative to expected normative values, whereas the other side seems unremarkable:

1. Use the first seven clinical procedures to establish proficiency with isolation, downtraining, and dynamic control tasks as indicated.
2. Monitor both sides, and step through the tasks, alternating use of left and right sides while cueing the patient toward symmetric SEMG patterns.
3. Progress to Clinical Procedure—Motor Copy Training for high-level dynamic symmetry training.
4. Consider frequent, brief pauses to perform stretching exercises specific to the involved side muscle.
5. Document training procedures and movement conditions that result in symmetry.

Asymmetry in which the low side is painful and judged to be hypotonic—SEMG recordings from the symptomatic side appear underrecruited relative to the contralateral side:

1. Use the first eight clinical procedures to establish proficiency with isolation, uptraining, and dynamic control tasks as indicated.
2. Monitor both sides and step through the tasks, alternating use of left and right sides while cueing the patient toward symmetric SEMG patterns.
3. Progress to Clinical Procedure—Motor Copy Training for high-level dynamic symmetry training.
4. Document training procedures and movement conditions that result in symmetry.

with a specific protocol to address asymmetries of the sternomastoid muscle in patients with carpal tunnel syndrome,[65] as well as with lumbar paraspinal muscle asymmetries in patients with low back pain.[66] See the box "Clinical Procedure—Nonspecific Left/Right Equilibration Training."

Clinically, it seems that high side activity spontaneously decreases as low side activity is uptrained. A similar phenomenon can be observed when retraining balanced actions between muscles acting in a synergistic relationship (see Clinical Procedure—Promotion of Correct Muscle Synergies and Related Coordination Patterns [described later]). Although downtraining hyperactivity is reasonable, success often comes faster by uptraining a related muscle that displays hypoactivity.

10. Motor Copy Training

This is a coordination training procedure. With the use of a line tracing graphic, a template of desired SEMG activity is derived and then retained on the screen. A template is recorded from the noninvolved side for patients with unilateral problems, or from an exceptional repetition with an involved muscle for patients with bilateral impairments. The training objective is to overlay the template with an active line trac-

ing recorded from the involved muscle site (Figure 5–16).

A patient attempts to match the dynamic pattern of SEMG activity over many repetitions. The amplitude of the active signal must be varied with a timing peculiar to the template. Wolf and associates[67] have used this procedure to promote rehabilitation in patients with neurologic disorders. The authors believe that this procedure is appropriate for patients with musculoskeletal pain as well. The template serves as a reference of correctness for any movement task. This reference provides robust knowledge of performance feedback during purposeful movement. The template is also useful to the clinician in determining a normative reference for unilaterally involved patients when population standards are unavailable.

The motor copy procedure, as described above, is a specialized feature of some commercial SEMG devices. Terminology and setup particulars vary from unit to unit. See the box "Clinical Procedure—Motor Copy Training."

11. Promotion of Correct Muscle Synergies and Related Coordination Patterns

With this procedure, the training emphasis shifts to the relationships between different muscles. Muscles work together to produce re-

---

Clinical Procedure—Nonspecific Left/Right Equilibration Training

The following instructions are adapted from the methods of Donaldson and Donaldson,[64] Donaldson and coworkers,[66] and Skubick and associates.[65]

1. Identify an isometric contraction procedure that produces increased, isolated SEMG activity from the low amplitude side. For example, Skubick and associates[65] used contralateral head rotation combined with cervical extension in working with the sternocleidomastoid. Manual muscle test positions[14,15] can be easily adapted for these purposes.
2. Once the target contraction method is identified, instruct the patient to activate the low amplitude side, so that its SEMG activity is equal to, or greater than, that of the high amplitude side, without causing the high side amplitude to increase any further (Figure 5–15).
3. Cue the patient to hold the contraction for about 10 seconds, followed by a rest period of 30 to 60 seconds, and repeat the cycle 6 to 10 times consecutively. In their studies, the investigators cited above further instructed patients to practice the series without SEMG feedback at home, 6 tc 10 times per day.

A   B

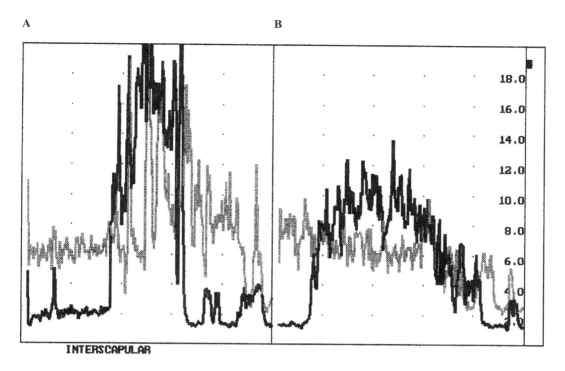

INTERSCAPULAR

Figure 5–15 Equilibration training with use of SEMG feedback from the left (black) and right (gray) interscapular muscles at level of the second thoracic vertebra, recorded from a patient with right greater than left signal asymmetry. (**A**) The "low" (baseline) left side is activated too much and is associated with a further increase in the amplitude of the "high" (baseline) right side. (**B**) The procedure is performed correctly: the low left side is activated so that its signal magnitude exceeds that of the high right side, without causing the right side to increase any further.

sultant force couples that effect movement at one joint, or to coordinate motion at adjacent joint segments. It can be appropriate to display feedback simultaneously from two or more synergists, or a particular agonist with its antagonist, and practice training the relationships between them. For example, a patient with shoulder pain could be instructed to work simultaneously on downtraining the upper trapezius while uptraining the lower trapezius during shoulder abduction. Another patient with patellofemoral dysfunction might work toward increasing activity of the vastus medialis oblique relative to the vastus lateralis while extending the knee. A patient with an insufficient anterior cruciate ligament could train for hamstring/quadriceps co-

activation. Still another patient might practice gluteal uptraining with lower lumbar paraspinal muscle recruitment during lifting. See the box "Clinical Procedure—Promotion of Correct Muscle Synergies and Related Coordination Patterns."

As an example, Figure 5–17 shows activity recorded from a patient with suprascapular and subacromial pain as a consequence of repetitive overhead work tasks. During bilateral and reciprocal shoulder flexion, activity of the upper trapezius was greater on the involved side as compared to the uninvolved side, whereas activity from the lower fibers of the serratus anterior appeared to be depressed. It was believed that the upper trapezius on the involved side was over-

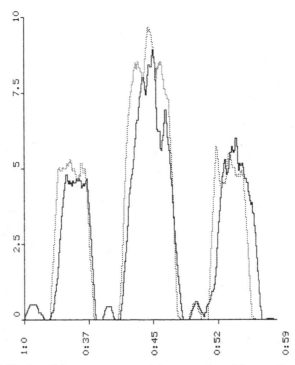

Figure 5–16 Sample SEMG plot of the motor copy training procedure. The template (dotted line) is first recorded from the asymptomatic side of a homologous muscle pair with unilateral dysfunction. Several repetitions or variations of a functional task are performed by the patient to generate the template. The template remains on the display screen over successive sweeps, while a live signal (solid line) is recorded from the same muscle site on the symptomatic side and the corresponding contralateral movement is performed. The patient attempts to match the symptomatic side signal to the asymptomatic side template. Courtesy of Verimed International, Inc., Coral Springs, Florida.

used and the serratus anterior was underused, resulting in inefficient scapular control and disturbed shoulder girdle mechanics. As activation of the serratus anterior was increased, recruitment of the upper trapezius was considerably decreased, even though there was no conscious attempt to affect the trapezius. The subject reported that she accomplished the task "by engaging the muscle just under my armpit and pulling the shoulder blade forward from there." When combined with pectoralis stretching, postural, and pacing techniques, she became able to complete her work shift without discomfort.

12. Postural Training with SEMG Feedback

Postural training is a comparatively straightforward area for SEMG feedback work. Training is indicated when aberrant muscle activity is linked to specific postures that exacerbate the patient's symptoms. The procedure is used in direct follow-up to the SEMG postural evaluation process.

Postural correction is made along standard lines. The effects are observed at the SEMG display to determine the key corrections. It is assumed that patient compliance will be greater if results are immediately visible, as opposed to when correct posture is just indicated to the patient through verbal instruction. The objective is to enhance an internal locus of control; that is, to reinforce a confident sense of what to do and what not to do, so that muscle (and joint) function is optimized. See the box "Clinical Procedure—Postural Training with SEMG Feedback."

Clinical Procedure—Motor Copy Training

Primary method:

1. Program the SEMG system for a motor copy mode.
2. Use a low level of display smoothing and a sensitivity that clearly registers the patient's muscle activity.
3. Choose a relevant functional movement, and record the template. Use the noninvolved contralateral muscle for a patient with unilateral involvement. In a patient with bilateral involvement, repeat the movement and template acquisition process until a satisfactory tracing is obtained. Save the desired template for display.
4. Instruct the patient to repeat the goal movement while attempting to match the pattern with a live signal from the involved muscle.
5. Document progress by printing a representative hard copy of a pattern match at the beginning and the end of each session. Some systems allow the template to be saved for future sessions. Certain devices average the match tracings or give a type of score to quantify performance over repeated trials.

Alternative method no. 1—used with unilaterally involved patients if the SEMG unit does not have a motor copy mode. A video monitor and line tracing graphic display, however, are required.

1. Record from the noninvolved side, and freeze the line at the end of the sweep.
2. Tape a piece of overhead transparency plastic over the display, and trace over the line by using a soft, fine marker.
3. Disconnect the involved side signal, and record from the involved side to match the pattern.

Alternative method no. 2—used with unilaterally involved patients and a dual channel feedback unit that does not have a motor copy mode or a line tracing display.

1. Set up to show independent activity from left and right sides of a homologous muscle pair.
2. Instruct the patient to perform bilateral simultaneous symmetric motions while striving for symmetric SEMG patterns.

Note: The first method is the most precise and probably preferred from a motor learning perspective. However, either of the two alternative techniques can be used as a practical compromise when needed.

Patients seem to accept the concept of postural improvement readily after seeing the outcome on the SEMG display. Exercise prescription or manual therapies may be needed to enable individuals to achieve a corrected alignment with ease. Use of a postural orthotic device, placement of tape along the dorsum of the back, or modified brassiere support may also be helpful. The effects of these techniques on muscle activity can be easily evaluated with

SEMG. Most of the time, simple corrections can be learned in the clinic. Preexisting postural habits seem to be difficult to change, though, when the patient returns to activities of daily living. Patients often return to the clinic reporting that they perform corrections, only to revert quickly back to their old habits, and that they forget to monitor themselves with sufficient frequency. Additional remarks about this recidivism are warranted, not because they are related to

Clinical Procedure—Promotion of Correct Muscle Synergies and Related Coordination Patterns

1. Use the first 10 clinical procedures to establish proficiency with isolation, downtraining, uptraining, and dynamic control tasks for each muscle as indicated.
2. Set up the feedback display to capture sufficient information for multichannel recordings, without being so complex that the patient becomes confused. Usually this means limiting feedback to two target muscles.
3. Use bar graphs as a simple way to convey the magnitude relationship between two recording sites. Combine with visual and auditory thresholds if desired. An alternative is to yoke an audio tone to the ratio of one channel's activity relative to the other. The use of the left and right sides of each of two homologous muscle pairs (total of four channels) may be optimal for display. Left versus right comparisons can then be made easily. Use moving line tracings for retraining of timing relationships and display of more than two SEMG channels. Overlay left and right signals for each target muscle of homologous pairs (see Chapter 4).
4. Select a low level of display smoothing and any sensitivity that is appropriate for the desired movement task.
5. Use movement tasks that were identified as exacerbating or alleviating symptoms during the evaluation. Emphasize those movements that are components of functional activities. Consider the biomechanical group of muscles that subserve the movement. Consult Chapters 8 through 14 for specific clinical practices.
6. If published standards are not available, compare activity on the involved side to that of the uninvolved contralateral side. When the subject has bilateral involvement, experiment with activation of antagonists and synergists for effects on agonist activity, or for those that produce symptomatic relief.
7. Instruct the patient to deliberately increase recruitment of one muscle by emphasizing its particular action.[14,15,68] Both magnitude and timing changes may be produced at other recording sites.
8. Document muscle activation procedures that evoke changes in SEMG patterns and symptom behavior.

SEMG feedback per se, but because postural training is among the most universal of interventions provided by practitioners who use SEMG.

As with all training procedures, the kinesthetic sensations associated with the desired tactic, in contrast to those associated with the uncorrected maneuver, should be emphasized. Helpful prompts include "Tune into what you can feel at your neck, your sternum, and your back now—the position of the joints, the amount of slack or tension in the soft tissues. You will want to consciously reproduce this posture and these feelings at least six to eight times throughout the day."

Postural correction should be simplified as much as possible. To promote a more erect carriage, complex maneuvers or an assumption of "military" posture should be discouraged. Instead, therapists can ask patients to raise their arms above their heads and feel the sternum naturally lift. The arms are then lowered, but the sternum is maintained in the lifted posture. Alternatively, patients can be asked to imagine a string from the ceiling helping to lift the sternum. This imagery generally improves sagittal alignment along the head, neck, trunk, and pelvic girdle. Subjects should adopt the practice of checking their posture whenever they get into their cars (eg, by using the rear view mirror as a guide), whenever they arrive to sit down at their desks, or every time they enter or leave a certain

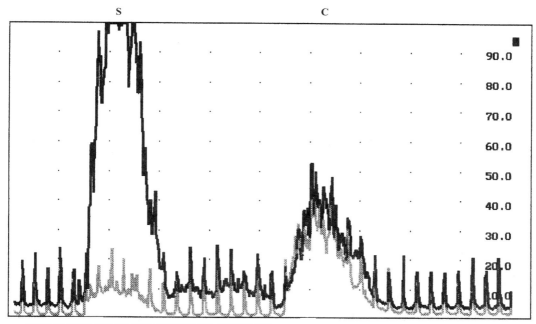

UPPER TRAPEZIUS AND SERRATUS ANTERIOR

Figure 5–17 Changing a muscle synergy pattern with use of SEMG activity of the upper trapezius (black) and the lower portion of the serratus anterior (gray), recorded from a patient with suprascapular and subacromial pain associated with repetitive overhead work. Cardiac artifact is seen in both signals as a series of repetitive baseline spikes. The first volitional contraction (**S**) corresponds to a spontaneous overhead shoulder flexion motion of the type used by the patient before training. The second volitional contraction (**C**) is associated with a shoulder flexion through the same range of motion arc, but with deliberate activation of the serratus anterior according to a learned feedback training strategy. Note the increase in serratus anterior activity and corresponding decrease in upper trapezius activity.

---

room. Some patients like to post colored reminder dots on the telephone, by a mirror, or along a door frame. Others do well by using a watch or computer signal that sounds on the hour as a reminder.

Sometimes SEMG feedback is used as an adjunct to postural training in the absence of aberrant muscle activity. Stress on articular structures is assumed to be the cause of the patient's discomfort. Because SEMG is noninvasive and quick to set up, and because many clinics do not have equipment to monitor spinal kinematics or kinetics with comparable ease, SEMG feedback may be helpful. Increased lumbar paraspinal SEMG activity is associated with increased intradiscal loads during Valsalva's maneuver.[69]

Clinically, pathologic lumbar and cervical loads are presumed to co-vary with SEMG amplitude. Decreased cervical and lumbar SEMG amplitudes are sought during training. When recordings are made simultaneously from cervical, thoracic, and lumbar levels, correction at one region frequently induces changes at other levels. In fact, increased thoracic SEMG activity may be accepted over the short term in exchange for lower activity at cervical or lumbar sites. This process helps the subject extinguish the habit of passively hanging on posterior thoracic ligaments in a position of forward head and increased thoracic kyphosis. Exercises or manual therapies can then be prescribed to restore optimal long-term alignment.

Clinical Procedure—Postural Training with SEMG Feedback

1. Instruct the patient to assume his or her spontaneous standing and sitting postures.
2. Model appropriate posture, and with the use of anatomic charts, explain the effects of inefficient static loading on joint alignment and soft tissue structures.
3. For SEMG asymmetries in standing position, instruct the subject to correct a weight bearing asymmetry or a lateral trunk shift. Try placing a small platform or book under the short leg with an apparent leg length discrepancy, so that iliac crests are leveled. Consider having the patient stand with one foot each on a standard bathroom scale for weight distribution feedback.
4. When forward head, protracted shoulder girdles, increased thoracic kyphosis, or decreased lumbar lordosis is noted, instruct the patient to retract the head gently or lift the sternum.
5. Cue a patient with a decreased lordosis and posterior pelvic tilt, or forward trunk lean, into a gentle anterior pelvic tilt.
6. Instruct a patient standing in knee recurvatum to unlock the knees slightly.
7. For seated SEMG asymmetries, equalize ischial weight bearing or place a folded towel under one buttock. Modify the seat height, seat pan depth and angle of inclination, type and location of lumbar support, or use of armrests, and so forth.
8. Document positions that relieve asymmetric or excessive muscle activity. These positions should also support biomechanically efficient joint alignment.

An analogy of paying for a commodity can be used to make a point during postural training. Consider an example of a patient with headache who displays about 3 μV of SEMG activity from the upper cervical paraspinal region when the sternum is lifted and the head gently retracted, versus 9 μV in her spontaneous slouched posture (Figure 5–18). The therapist could ask the patient to consider that she would not pay five dollars for a gallon of gasoline if she had to pay only one dollar, and it may not be in her best interest to sustain 9 μV for head posture when only 3 μV is needed. Just as a sizable expense would accumulate by filling the gas tank at five dollars per gallon over the course of a year, so might there be a cumulative strain from faulty spinal alignment. The therapist could stress that the patient now has the choice to reduce needless expenditure of energy.

13. Body Mechanics Instruction with SEMG Feedback

This procedure entails practice with standard body mechanics training while SEMG activity is displayed. The task is inherently similar to that in postural training with SEMG feedback. Now, however, the maneuvers are more dynamic, involving lifting, carrying, reaching, pushing, and pulling. The objectives are twofold: (1) identify biomechanically efficient techniques and (2) demonstrate the effects to the patient. Potentially, any patient with spinal dysfunction is a candidate. Aberrant muscle activity is not a prerequisite if SEMG feedback is likely to reinforce learning. The patient's understanding and compliance should be increased if he or she can observe the effects of body mechanics techniques on his or her own body. See the box "Clinical Procedure—Body Mechanics Instruction with SEMG Feedback."

Use of proper body mechanics will not necessarily produce a decrease in SEMG activity. Intervertebral alignment must be taken into account. A lift performed in a certain way may result in less SEMG activity but greater intradiscal pressure or ligamentous strain. For example, a box lifted from the floor with deliberate maintenance of lumbar kyphosis and posterior pelvic tilt is accompanied by decreased lum-

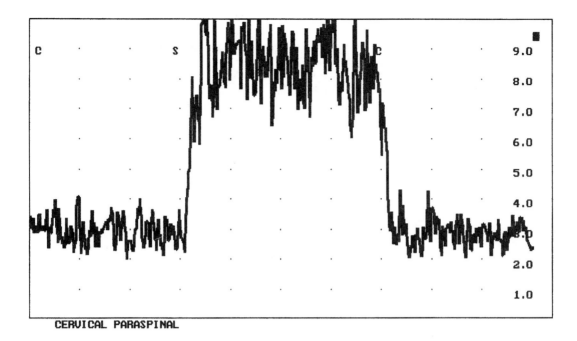

CERVICAL PARASPINAL

Figure 5–18 Postural training with use of SEMG feedback from cervical paraspinal muscles. A substantial difference in signal magnitude is associated with the patient's corrected postural alighnment (**C**) versus the spontaneous, forward head alignment (**S**) displayed before training.

bar paraspinal activity during the early portion of the lift, compared with use of a lumbar lordosis and anterior pelvic tilt.[70] It can be argued that because intradiscal pressure is likely to be higher with increased flexion angle, and because slack on posterior soft tissues is taken up with increased flexion angle, lifting in kyphosis is not a preferred maneuver. The increased muscle activity associated with lordosis might serve a protective role. Thus the effects on all components of the motion segment must be taken into account when body mechanics are considered. Muscle activity should be produced to achieve the movement goal in a way that efficiently controls load on joint structures. The therapist should seek a suitable joint alignment and then encourage the patient to find the minimal level of SEMG activity that supports that arrangement. Furthermore, SEMG activity should return to the resting baseline at the conclusion of the task.

14. Therapeutic Exercises with SEMG Feedback

SEMG feedback is combined with therapeutic exercises for two purposes: exercise selection and technique instruction. Use of SEMG to evaluate the efficacy of specific exercises and exercise equipment has been commonly reported.[71–75] Fundamentally, SEMG has been used to assess recruitment specificity and inferences made as to purported conditioning effects. After scrutiny with SEMG, some exercises have failed to produce the results that prevailing clinical opinion might have predicted.[76,77]

Wolf and colleagues[78] have also discussed the evaluation of individual patient programs with SEMG. Recording with SEMG helps therapists determine which exercise variants are most suitable for any particular patient. Monitoring with SEMG reduces the guesswork for therapists in grading the intensity and isolation ability of

---

Clinical Procedure—Body Mechanics Instruction with SEMG Feedback

1. Prepare several objects of light to moderate weight and minimal to moderate volume for practice—for example, a pencil, a book, a dish, a simulated bag of groceries, a small crate with variable weights, a cart, an old vacuum cleaner, a telephone, or items for personal grooming.

2. Set up a series of surfaces at table height, shoulder height, and eye level. If possible, set up a bin that approximates a standard car trunk and other bins that simulate a bathroom sink, a kitchen sink, and a dishwasher or low drawer.

3. Instruct the patient to practice lifting the light items from floor to table height. Also ask the patient to practice holding and carrying the items a short distance.

4. While suitable care is taken to avoid injury, observe effects at the SEMG display as an object is held close to the body axis compared with arm's length, or straight in front versus off to the side. Paraspinal SEMG activity is considerably reduced when the object is held close to the trunk. Asymmetries are produced with off-center maneuvers or lifts that involve trunk twisting (Figure 5–19).

5. Compare lifting with knees straight with knees bent. Demonstrate appropriate lifting technique, and by using anatomic charts, explain the effects of inefficient loading on spinal structures. Compare lifting with a lumbar lordosis and anterior pelvic tilt, a lumbar kyphosis and posterior pelvic tilt, and a neutral spine and pelvis.

6. Once the patient has been instructed in optimal techniques with a light object, repeat with heavier, larger objects and the higher lifts.

7. In the same manner, practice optimal techniques for routine personal care, household, and office tasks.

8. Document changes in peak SEMG amplitude, symmetry, or baseline recovery during practice with key maneuvers.

---

strengthening exercises. Activity is displayed during evaluation of potential stretching techniques to ensure that patients successfully relax target muscles. Thus individual differences are accounted for, and patients receive exercise programs that are tailored to their needs. SEMG feedback can then be used to practice the selected exercises. The feedback aids skill acquisition, motivates, and builds confidence in both patient and therapist that the program is being performed properly. Presumably, this process facilitates compliance and attention to technique when the patient practices independently at home. See the box "Clinical Procedure—Therapeutic Exercises with SEMG Feedback."

An example of the use of SEMG monitoring for exercise prescription is shown in Figure 5–20. This patient had unilateral neck pain, apparent upper trapezius hyperactivity and lower trapezius hypoactivity. The goal was to identify a home exercise to promote isolation and uptraining of the lower trapezius relative to the upper trapezius. Prone shoulder lateral rotation best achieved this objective and was chosen for home practice.

Figure 5–21 illustrates an example of the effects of SEMG feedback training during exercise instruction. SEMG activity was recorded while a subject prepared for intense strengthening exercise with a low precursor training load. The presentation of SEMG feedback assisted with neuromuscular recruitment strategies for an improved pattern of pacing, tonic amplitude, and peak activation.

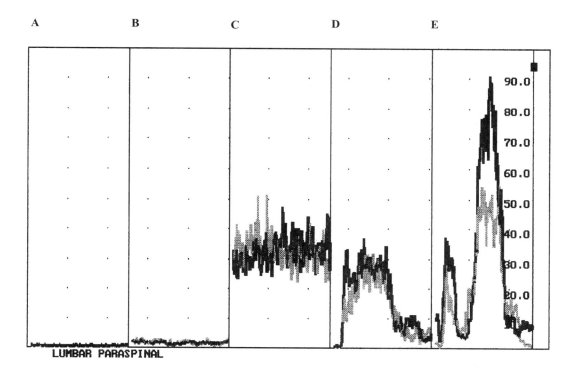

Figure 5–19 Body mechanics instruction with use of SEMG feedback from the left (black) and right (gray) lumbar paraspinal muscles. (**A**) Patient in standing position with neutral trunk alignment and arms relaxed at sides of the trunk. (**B**) Neutral standing with a 10 lb weight held close to the trunk. (**C**) Neutral standing with the same 10 lb weight held at arm's length. (**D**) Symmetric lifting of a 10 lb weight from floor to table height, bending the knees, maintaining an approximately neutral lumbar spine, and attempting to keep the weight as close to the trunk as possible. (**E**) Off-center asymmetric lifting of a 10 lb weight from floor to table height, twisting the trunk as the lift proceeds, beginning with knees straight and the lumbar spine flexed, with no attempt to keep the weight closely aligned to the trunk.

Figure 5–22 displays cervical paraspinal activity from a patient with chronic neck pain during an upper extremity pulley rowing exercise. The subject initially stabilized the head and neck with about 16 to 20 µV of peak activity during each repetition. Using feedback from the SEMG display, as well as from the therapist regarding exercise technique, the patient learned to produce satisfactory stabilization with a rhythmic increase to less than 10 µV. The tonic amplitude was also reduced. She learned that more activity was superfluous and came to realize that she was guarding her neck unnecessarily. This patient was engaged in a comprehensive work condi-tioning program, and Figure 5–23 shows cervical paraspinal activity during a strengthening exercise of the quadriceps. The task was performed with seated exercise apparatus, and the head and trunk were well supported. The patient learned how to decrease habitual but unnecessary cervical muscle activity. By the end of the session, she felt less apprehensive about her exercise program and could execute it with less neck pain and fatigue.

SEMG activity of the hamstring from a patient with persistent lower extremity pain, positive dural stretch signs, and extremely limited straight leg raising mobility is represented in

Clinical Procedure—Therapeutic Exercises with SEMG Feedback

Exercise prescription:

1. Monitor the desired muscle as standard exercises for that muscle are performed.
2. Consider using additional channels to record the activity of muscles that might act antagonistically to, or substitute for, the preferred muscle effect.
3. Experiment with known variations in positioning and adjunctive techniques while observing effects on the SEMG display.
4. Prescribe those strength-conditioning or neuromuscular re-education exercises that demonstrate the greatest isolated SEMG output. Select those stretching methods that are accompanied by the least SEMG activity.
5. Document average or peak SEMG amplitudes during each of the tested exercises.
6. Refer to Chapters 8 through 14 for specific clinical suggestions.

Technique instruction:

1. Instruct the patient to repeat the prescribed exercise while monitoring SEMG activity from the agonist muscle.
2. Consider using additional channels to record activity of muscles that might act antagonistically to, or substitute for, the preferred muscle effect.
3. For strengthening or neuromuscular re-education exercises, instruct the patient to maximize agonist SEMG activity while minimizing activity from the other channels. Consider setting a threshold marker to be exceeded for the agonist and another threshold for an antagonistic or substituting muscle. SEMG activity is to be maintained below the latter, perhaps linked to an audio function, so that excessive activity is signaled as an alarm. Alternatively, a rewarding audio tone may be yoked to a prescribed ratio of one channel's activity relative to the other.
4. Cue the patient to produce a microrest (see Clinical Procedure—Deactivation Training) between repetitions. Use the waxing and waning of the SEMG display to teach appropriate exercise rhythm across repetitions. Instruct the patient in a full macrorest between exercise sets if appropriate.
5. For stretching exercises, teach the subject to lengthen the muscle, elongating through the range for which minimal SEMG activity is preserved. Slightly decrease length and use prolonged holds, abdominal breathing, cognitive relaxation methods, or contract–relax cycles if SEMG activity rises.
6. For comprehensive gym programs, monitor the target muscle as each exercise is performed. Maximize activity during strengthening exercises designed to have an impact on the target muscle, and minimize activity during associated stretching exercises. With all other exercises, instruct the patient in the use of proper body alignment while controlling the level of stabilizing activity from the recorded muscle. Cue relaxation if the recorded muscle does not play a biomechanically relevant role. Maximize efficiency of the target muscle through the total program.

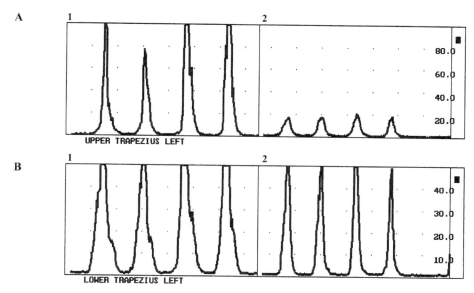

Figure 5–20 Exercise prescription with use of SEMG monitoring of the upper trapezius (**A**) and lower trapezius (**B**). The goal was to identify a home exercise that would isolate, uptrain, and condition the lower trapezius. (**A1, B1**) Straight arm lift from prone with the arm over the edge of a plinth, corresponding to lower trapezius manual muscle testing position. (**A2, B2**) Shoulder lateral rotation in prone with the arm supported in 90 degrees of abduction, forearm over the edge of a plinth. Isolation of the lower trapezius from the upper trapezius is superior with the lateral rotation maneuver.

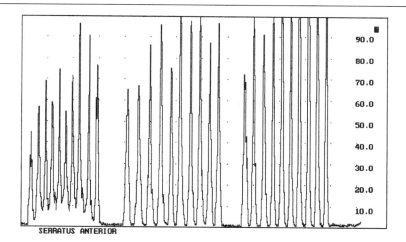

Figure 5–21 Exercise instruction with use of SEMG feedback from the lower serratus anterior during a seated upper extremity press–scapular protraction task with resistive gym equipment. Results of three sets of 10 repetitions each are shown. Resistance was constant across sets at approximately 10% of the patient's one-repetition maximum (insufficient to induce a subjective sense of fatigue). After the first few repetitions of the first set, the patient was cued to relax transiently and inhale between press/exhalation trials. The patient was subsequently cued to refine the exercise movement and maximally engage the serratus anterior. Combined with visual observation, it was judged that the patient learned to perform the exercise in a satisfactory manner by the conclusion of the third set. Additional exercise sets were then monitored as the load was increased to maximal capacity for high-level conditioning.

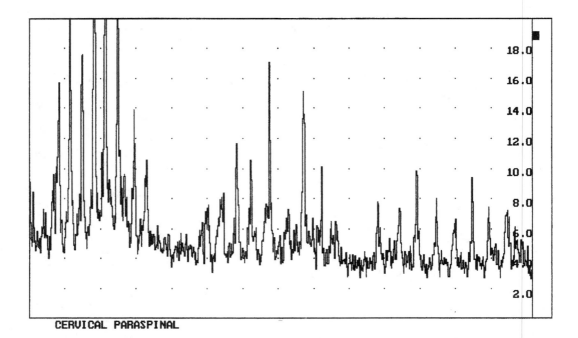

CERVICAL PARASPINAL

Figure 5–22 Exercise instruction with use of SEMG feedback from the cervical paraspinal muscles of a patient with chronic neck pain and elevated muscle tension. Results of three sets of eight repetitions each of an upper extremity pulley rowing exercise are shown. Low-level resistance and correct body alignment (continuously monitored by a therapist) were constant across the exercise sets. By the third set, the patient learned to pace transient muscle relaxation between repetitions and to stabilize the neck appropriately with far less cervical muscle activity.

Figure 5–24. This patient was being seen 8 weeks after undergoing laminectomy for a severe intervertebral disc herniation. There was no improvement following a course of manual mobilization and an independent stretching program. The figure shows the effects of different stretching methods. The first panel illustrates SEMG activity during a "bouncing stretch" maneuver that the patient performed prior to injury. The activity displayed in the third panel was generated during a prolonged, seemingly gentle hold with appropriate joint alignment. It was judged, however, that the level of muscle activity would not allow an optimal stretch. The amount of stretch was decreased until the SEMG amplitude dropped and a contract–relax cycle was performed, resulting in activity as shown in the fourth panel. With the patient in supine posi-

tion and the involved leg up along a door frame, an even lower activity level was produced, as displayed in the fifth panel. This latter method was repeated in a home program. The patient's pain decreased while mobility easily increased over the following weeks.

Synchronous recruitment of the lumbar paraspinal and abdominal muscles is shown in Figure 5–25. This patient complained of chronic low back pain and demonstrated segmental instability on radiographic study. A therapeutic exercise program was prescribed in which the patient maintained a neutral spinal position while performing extremity movements. This type of training is intended to teach the patient to program trunk muscles to stabilize the body core in a biomechanically satisfactory alignment.[79] Proximal musculature sets a foundation for dy-

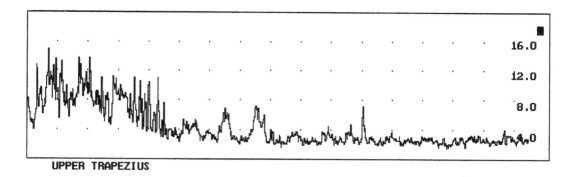

UPPER TRAPEZIUS

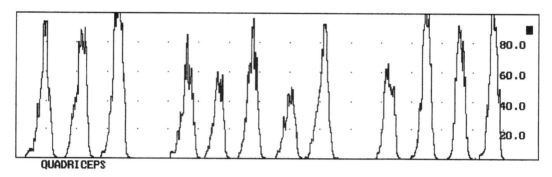

QUADRICEPS

Figure 5–23 Exercise instruction with use of SEMG feedback from cervical paraspinal muscles of the same patient as described in Figure 5–22. Repetitions of a quadriceps pulley strengthening exercise are shown with the patient's head and trunk supported by the exercise apparatus. Despite initial tendency to activate the cervical paraspinals, the patient quickly responded to cueing by a therapist and learned that the exercise could be performed safely without much cervical muscle activation.

namic extremity use. Patients are taken through an exercise progression and into functional tasks. SEMG feedback was used in this case to facilitate a neutral spine position during a contralateral upper extremity–lower extremity lift from a hands-and-knees position. Small sized electrodes were centered over the lower multifidus muscles and external obliques. The patient incorporated the feedback cues as he explored various motor strategies to maintain trunk alignment. Optimal positioning was associated with synchronous, higher amplitude recruitment of the oblique abdominals along with decreased lumbar paraspinal muscle activity.

Exercises that integrate well with SEMG feedback training are suggested for selected clinical syndromes in Chapters 8 through 14. These methods are, however, intended as starting points, and the reader is referred to texts of exercise prescription for sophisticated approaches that can be used with patients with musculoskeletal injury.[49,80–82]

15. Functional Activity Performance with SEMG Feedback

All training leads to this procedure. Motor control must be practiced under the real-life conditions that threaten it. Functional rehabilitation is a focal point for multidisciplinary chronic pain management programs[83] and SEMG training fits well with this framework.

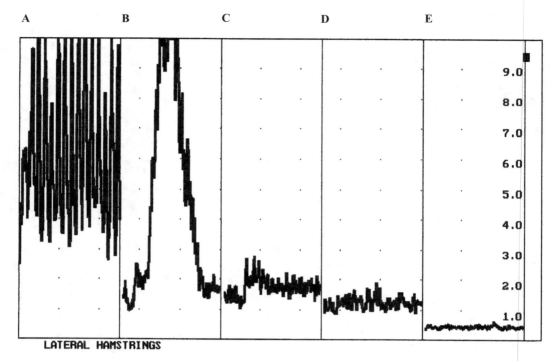

Figure 5–24 Exercise instruction with use of SEMG feedback from hamstrings during hamstring stretching. (**A**) Standing, heel up on chair, "bouncing." (**B**) Supine active knee extension. (**C**) Half long-sitting on a bench, the lower extremity to be stretched straight on the bench, the other lower extremity over the side of the bench, trunk upright; no feedback. (**D**) Same as **C** but with SEMG feedback. (**E**) Supine, lower extremity to be stretched up along a door frame.

Lessons learned from the other feedback training techniques are useless if they cannot be successfully applied to functional activities. The strategies discussed previously for deactivation, postural, and body mechanics training each incorporate some degree of functional tasking. That focus is expanded and tailored now. Functional activities are selected that were identified during evaluation as having exacerbated symptoms and being accompanied by aberrant SEMG patterns. Assignments may include routine activities of daily living or highly specialized work or sport movements. It is recommended that SEMG training be integrated with functional activities during every clinic session. This can be accomplished with activity simula-

tions in the clinic or with portable SEMG units at the actual activity sites.

Efficient movement is characterized by achievement of the task goal with an economy of effort. There are two aspects of treatment to be addressed with SEMG feedback. One is potential ergonomic modifications of the task equipment. The other involves the application of movement skill. Muscles with stabilizing or prime moving roles should be recruited in a coordinated way and only to the degree necessary to produce an appropriate movement pattern. When movement is terminated, the involved muscles should return promptly to baseline postural activity levels. SEMG feedback is used to demonstrate graphically to patients what is best

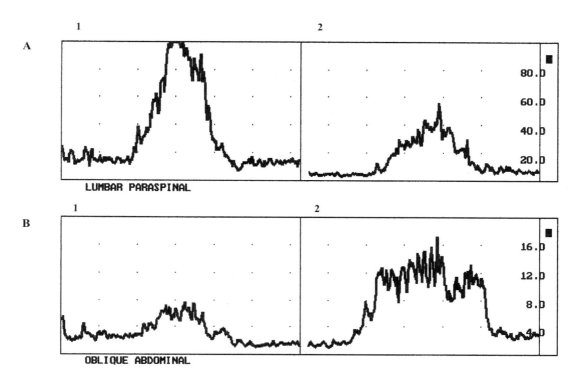

Figure 5–25 Exercise instruction with use of SEMG feedback, training synchronous recruitment of lumbar paraspinal muscles (**A**) and oblique abdominal muscles (**B**) to stabilize the trunk in neutral alignment. (**A1, B1**) Hands-and-knees position, contralateral upper extremity–lower extremity lift as spontaneously performed, accompanied by trunk extension and rotation. (**A2, B2**) Same exercise as in **A1, B1**, but with neutral lumbar spine alignment.

for them to do, and not do, in regulating their muscle activity. Patients become empowered to make constructive changes in their movement patterns and task environment. They learn behaviors to avoid dysfunction and associated symptoms and how best to respond if problems do occur. See the box "Clinical Procedure— Functional Activity Performance with SEMG Feedback."

The therapist and patient may come to the same ergonomic plan that they would have without the SEMG display, but with the SEMG signal, those interventions with the greatest likelihood for success can be identified more efficiently. For example, Figure 5–26 shows SEMG activity from a bicyclist with neck pain

and who planned to participate in an upcoming long distance race. The seat position and handlebars of her mountain bike were modified, which resulted in decreased cervical and trapezius SEMG activity. Figure 5–27 shows SEMG activity from the thoracic paraspinal muscles of another patient with upper back pain associated with work at an electronics repair job. This person's SEMG activity was reduced by incorporating a lumbar role at the work seat and raising and tilting the assembly surface by using a drafting table during simulation trials. Rather than field testing a wider range of interventions over a period of many weeks, the adjustments for these patients were identified in a single session and were followed by a resolution of com-

Clinical Procedure—Functional Activity Performance with SEMG Feedback

1. Set up a simulation, or ask the patient to perform problematic functional tasks.
2. If there are a large number of functional limitations, prioritize for those that will have the greatest impact on the patient's disability and be easiest to affect. Consider the patient's vocational, recreational, personal care, and familial roles.
3. Integrate movement strategies learned from the previous training procedures with activity performance.
4. Also consider potential equipment modifications, alterations in activity technique, sequencing, and pacing.
5. Consult with occupational therapists, physical therapists, vocational counselors, ergonomists, athletic trainers, exercise physiologists, or coaches if unfamiliar with the functional tasks.
6. Have the patient try one thing at a time, and observe the effects at the SEMG display.
7. Document the equipment and task site modifications that have a significant impact on SEMG activity. Document the movement control strategies that have a positive effect on muscle function.
8. Repeat favored maneuvers with a faded feedback schedule until the patient is able to reproduce them over multiple trials without any SEMG feedback.
9. Randomize performance of training tasks, add distractions, and introduce unpredictable variations, as relevant to real-life circumstances.

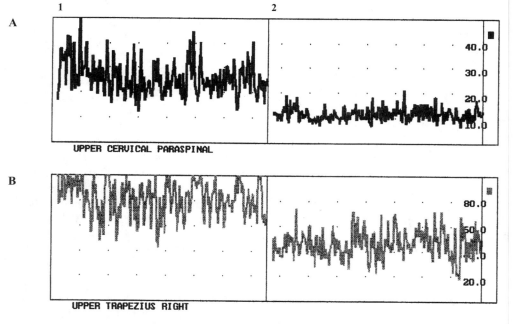

Figure 5–26 SEMG activity of left (black) and right (gray) (**A**) upper cervical paraspinal and (**B**) upper trapezius muscles. Activity was recorded from a mountain bicyclist with neck pain during stationary pedaling (**1**) before and (**2**) after modification of bike seat position and handlebars. The modifications were associated with decreased neck pain during subsequent rides in the field.

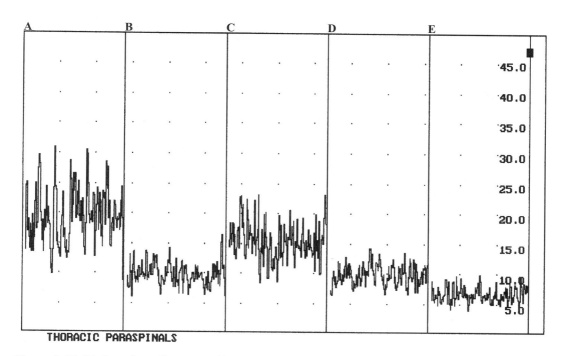

THORACIC PARASPINALS

Figure 5–27 Work station adjustment with use of SEMG monitoring of thoracic paraspinal muscles during simulated performance of an electronics repair job. (**A**) Sample tracing during the standard job task and original work station alignment. (**B**) Same as in **A** but with a lumbar roll. (**C**) Same as in **A** but with increased work table height. (**D**) Same as in **A** but with increased table height and tilt. (**E**) Same as in **A** but with a lumbar roll and increased table height and tilt.

plaints. Critical interventions were planned in a shorter time, with fewer return visits, thus reducing the total cost of care.

Figure 5–28 shows SEMG activity from the right upper trapezius of a patient who worked as a soda bottle loader. She experienced right cervical and suprascapular pain that progressed through each work shift and increased cumulatively over the workweek. Prior physical agents and manual therapies were only temporarily beneficial. Integration of neck stretches and job rotation principles were partially helpful. The patient then practiced the isolation and deactivation feedback procedures and tried to adapt those strategies to the bottle loading task. Note the deeper trough phase displayed in Figure 5–28 after functional retraining. This was accomplished within a session by the patient consciously dropping trapezius activity as the bottle was brought across the midline, with the use of

SEMG feedback as a guide. There was no lasting compromise of work speed or body mechanics alignment, or job safety. The patient successfully incorporated the trapezius microrest into her work day, and her symptoms resolved without further difficulty.

SEMG activity from a golfer with left shoulder subacromial pain is shown in Figure 5–29. Pain was sharply produced during the follow-through phase of each golf swing and cumulatively over each round. Prior use of anti-inflammatory medications and shoulder therapeutic exercises had little effect. After comprehensive evaluation, it was believed that the patient had poor dynamic scapular control. The patient next practiced isolating and uptraining the lower trapezius using SEMG feedback. He progressed in movement arc and speed while performing shoulder abduction and then integrated the skills with golf swings. The patient increased recruitment of the lower

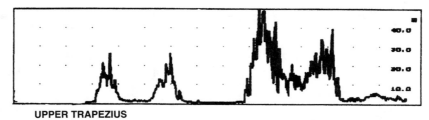

UPPER TRAPEZIUS

Figure 5–28 Work technique modification with SEMG feedback from the upper trapezius in a patient with chronic, work-related cervical and suprascapular pain. Activity was recorded during simulated performance of the patient's work as a soda bottle loader. The first two peaks show corrected performance. Note the decreased peak amplitude and production of a microrest between task phases. The second two peaks show spontaneous performance. A bottle is picked up during the first peak, brought across the body midline during the trough phase, and loaded into a tray during the second peak.

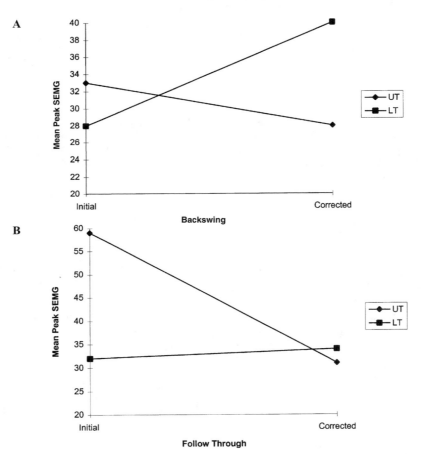

Figure 5–29 SEMG activity of the upper trapezius and lower trapezius recorded from a golfer with a chronic impingement syndrome of the nondominant shoulder. Peak microvolt scores during **(A)** backswing and **(B)** follow through were respectively averaged over multiple swings and are illustrated for the patient's initial and corrected swing styles, with intervening SEMG feedback training and expert coaching. Training was followed by decreased shoulder pain and improved golf scores.

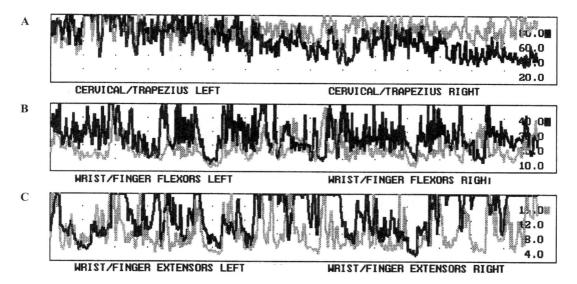

Figure 5–30 Monitoring of performing artist technique with use of SEMG feedback from (**A**) cervical paraspinal–upper trapezius muscles, (**B**) wrist and finger flexors, and (**C**) wrist and finger extensors from left (black) and right (gray) sides. Recordings were derived from an improvisational string bass player with chronic, bilateral occipital headache, neck and suprascapular pain, and forearm pain and parasthesias during performance. High level, tonic activity of neck muscles is apparent. Resting baseline activity from all muscles was less than 2 µV (not shown). The signals therefore indicate continuous muscle activity and little rest during performance.

trapezius and decreased activity of the upper trapezius during the follow-through and backswing phases, and expert opinion was used to alter other components of the swing. The patient could then swing the golf club without pain, and he actually lowered his golf score.

A final case is illustrated in Figure 5–30. Forearm and cervical SEMG activity is displayed from an improvisational jazz musician who had complaints of occipital headache, bilateral neck and suprascapular pain, and bilateral forearm pain and parasthesias. The symptoms progressively emerged during long sets while he played the string bass. A forward head, kyphotic thoracic posture was noted, along with abducted arms and an extremely aggressive fingering style. The patient was in the habit of sustaining high-level isometric contractions for prolonged periods. Decreased symptoms were associated with a more upright trunk posture and dropping of the elbows, as well as reductions in the tonic amplitude and peak levels of SEMG activity and increased production of microrests. His consid-

erable challenge was to generate these changes without compromising his artistic style.

THE BOTTOM LINE

Table 5–1 classifies the SEMG feedback techniques by uptraining, downtraining, and coordination of training objectives. The most basic recommendation, though, is for the operator to do whatever it is that he or she would normally do with the patient, but with the added benefit of the SEMG display. It is not necessary for the therapist to get caught up in fancy equipment or difficult protocols.

Continually evaluating the SEMG results, seeing whether they fit together with the practitioner's other observations, and facilitating the patient's learning are the important points. The SEMG machine need not be thought of as an entity unto itself. Rather, SEMG serves as an extension of the patient's and therapist's senses, helping to integrate the different aspects of treatment and enhancing any approach.

Table 5–1 Summary Selection of SEMG Feedback Training Techniques

	Assessment		
	Hypoactivity	Hyperactivity	Faulty Timing, Faulty Multimuscle Coordination
		Training Goal	
Training Technique	Uptraining	Downtraining	Coordination Training
Isolation of target muscle activity	X	X	X
Relaxation-based downtraining		X	
Threshold-based uptraining/downtraining	X	X	
Tension recognition threshold training		X	
Tension discrimination training	X	X	X
Deactivation training		X	X
Generalization to progressively dynamic movement	X	X	X
SEMG–triggered neuromuscular electrical stimulation	X		X
Left/right equilibration training	X	X	X
Motor copy training	X		X
Promotion of correct muscle synergies and related coordination patterns			X
Postural training with SEMG feedback		X	
Body mechanics instruction with SEMG feedback	X	X	X
Therapeutic exercises with SEMG feedback	X	X	X
Functional activity performance with SEMG feedback	X	X	X

REFERENCES

1. Kee WG, Middaugh SJ, Pawlick KL. Persistent pain in the older patient: evaluation and treatment. In: Gatchel RJ, Turk DC, eds. *Psychological Perspectives and Treatment Approaches.* New York: Guilford Press; 1996.

2. Buckelew SP, Parker JC, Keefe FJ, et al. Self-efficacy and pain behavior among subjects with fibromyalgia. *Pain.* 1994;59:377–384.

3. Jensen MP, Turner JA, Romano JM, Lawler BK. Relationship of pain-specific beliefs to chronic pain adjustment. *Pain.* 1994;57:301–309.

4. Morley S, Wilkinson L. The pain beliefs and perceptions inventory: a British replication. *Pain.* 1995; 61:427–433.

5. Williams DA, Robinson ME, Geisser ME. Pain beliefs: assessment and utility. *Pain.* 1994;59:71–78.

6. Duda JL, Smart AE, Tappe MK. Predictors of adherence in the rehabilitation of athletic injuries: an application of personal investment theory. *J Sport Exerc Psychol.* 1989;11:367–381.

7. Kaplan RM, Atkins CJ, Reinsch S. Specific efficacy expectations mediate exercise compliance in patients with COPD. *Health Psychol.* 1984;3:223–242.

8. Oldridge NB. Compliance with exercise in cardiac rehabilitation. In: Dishman RK, ed. *Exercise Adherence: Its Impact on Public Health.* Champaign, IL: Human Kinetics; 1988;283–304.

9. Bigos S, Bowyer O, Braen G, et al. *Acute Low Back Problems in Adults.* Rockville, MD: Agency for Health Care Policy and Research, Public Health Service, US Dept of Health and Human Services; 1994. Clinical Practice Guideline No. 14, AHCPR publication 95-0642.

10. Davis M, Eshelman ER, McKay M. *The Relaxation & Stress Reduction Workbook.* Oakland, CA: New Harbinger Publications; 1982.

11. McKay M, Davis M, Fanning P. *Thoughts and Feelings: The Art of Cognitive Stress Intervention.* Richmond, CA: New Harbinger Publications; 1981.

12. Peper E, Holt C. *Creating Wholeness: A Self-Healing Workbook Using Dynamic Relaxation, Images and Thoughts.* New York: Plenum Publishing; 1993.

13. Travis JW, Ryan RS. *The Wellness Workbook.* 2nd ed. Berkeley, CA: Ten Speed Press; 1988.

14. Hislop HG, Montgomery J. *Daniels and Worthingham's Muscle Testing: Techniques of Manual Examination.* 6th ed. Philadelphia: WB Saunders Co; 1995.

15. Kendall FP, McCreary EK, Provance PG. *Muscles, Testing and Function.* 4th ed. Baltimore: Williams & Wilkins; 1993.

16. Basmajian JV, ed. *Biofeedback: Principles and Practice for Clinicians.* 3rd ed. Baltimore: Williams & Wilkins; 1989.

17. Flor H, Birbaumer N. Comparison of the efficacy of electromyographic biofeedback, cognitive-behavioral therapy, and conservative medical interventions in the treatment of chronic musculoskeletal pain. *J Consult Clin Psychol.* 1993;61:653–658.

18. Gaarder KR, Montgomery PS. *Clinical Biofeedback: A Procedural Manual.* Baltimore: Williams & Wilkins; 1977.

19. Lehrer PM, Carr R, Sagunaraj D, Woolfolk RL. Stress management techniques: are they all equivalent, or do they have special effects? *Biofeedback Self Regul.* 1994;19:353–401.

20. Peper E, Ancoli S, Quinn M, eds. *Mind/Body Integration: Essential Readings in Biofeedback.* New York: Plenum Publishing; 1979.

21. Schwartz MS, ed. *Biofeedback: A Practitioner's Guide.* New York: Guilford Press; 1995.

22. White L, Tursky B, eds. *Clinical Biofeedback: Efficacy and Mechanisms.* New York: Guilford Press; 1982.

23. Cram JR, Kasman GS. *Introduction to Surface Electromyography.* Gaithersburg, MD: Aspen Publishers; 1997.

24. Schwartz MS. The use of audiotapes for patient education and relaxation. In: Schwartz MS, ed. *Biofeedback: A Practitioner's Guide.* New York: Guilford Press; 1995;301–312.

25. Davidson RJ, Schwartz GE. The psychobiology of relaxation and related states: a multiprocess theory. In: Motolsky D, ed. *Behavior Control and the Modification of Physiological Activity.* Englewood Cliffs, NJ: Prentice Hall; 1976;399–441.

26. Jacobsen E. *Modern Treatment of Tense Patients.* Springfield, IL: Charles C Thomas; 1970.

27. Barber TX. Changing "unchangeable" bodily processes by (hypnotic) suggestions: a new look at hypnosis, cognitions, imagining, and the mind-body problem. In: Sheikh AA, ed. *Imagery and Healing.* New York: Baywood Publishing; 1984.

28. Norris P. Clinical psychoneuroimmunology: strategies for self-regulation of immune system responding. In: Basmajian JV, ed. *Biofeedback: Principles and Practice for Clinicians.* 3rd ed. Baltimore: Williams & Wilkins; 1989;57–66.

29. Luthe W, ed. *Autogenic Therapy.* Vol 1–4. New York: Grune & Stratton; 1969.

30. Stoyva JM. Autogenic training and biofeedback combined: a reliable method for induction of general relaxation. In: Basmajian JV, ed. *Biofeedback: Principles and Practice for Clinicians.* 3rd ed. Baltimore: Williams & Wilkins; 1989;169–186.

31. Bacon M, Poppen R. A behavioral analysis of diaphragmatic breathing and its effects on peripheral temperature. *J Behav Ther Exp Psychiatry.* 1985;16:15–21.

32. Harris V, Katlick E, Lick J, Habberfield T. Paced respiration as a technique for modification of autonomic response to stress. *Psychophysiology.* 1976;13:386–391.

33. Peper E. Strategies to reduce the effort of breathing: electromyographic and incentive spirometry biofeedback. In: von Euler C, Katz-Salamon M, eds. *Respiratory Psychophysiology.* London, England: Macmillan Press; 1988;113–122.

34. Peper E, Crane-Gockley V. Towards effortless breathing. *Med Psychother.* 1990;3:135–140.

35. Schwartz MS. Breathing therapies. In: Schwartz MS, ed. *Biofeedback: A Practitioner's Guide.* New York: Guilford Press; 1995;248–287.

36. Goldfried MP. Reduction of generalized anxiety through a variant of systematic desensitization. In:

Goldfried MR, Merbaum M, eds. *Behavior Change Through Self Control.* New York: Holt, Rinehart and Winston; 1973;159–182.

37. Lazarus AA. *Behavior Therapy and Beyond.* New York: McGraw-Hill; 1971.

38. Meichenbaum D. *Cognitive Behavior Modification.* New York: Plenum Publishing; 1977.

39. Suinn RM, Richardson F. Anxiety management training: a non-specific behavior therapy program for anxiety control. *Behav Ther.* 1971;2:498–510.

40. Stoyva J, Budzynski T. Cultivated low arousal—an antistress response? In: Peper E, Ancoli S, Quinn M, eds. *Mind/Body Integration: Essential Readings in Biofeedback.* New York: Plenum Publishing; 1979; 7–46.

41. Wolpe J. *The Practice of Behavior Therapy.* 2nd ed. New York: Pergamon Press; 1973.

42. Green EE, Green AM. General and specific applications of thermal biofeedback. In: Basmajian JV, ed. *Biofeedback: Principles and Practice for Clinicians.* 3rd ed. Baltimore: Williams & Wilkins; 1989;209–221.

43. Peek CJ. A primer of biofeedback instrumentation. In: Schwartz MS, ed. *Biofeedback: A Practitioner's Guide.* New York: Guilford Press; 1995;45–95.

44. Brucker BS. Biofeedback in rehabilitation. In: Ince LP, ed. *Behavioral Psychology in Rehabilitation Medicine: Clinical Applications.* Baltimore: Williams & Wilkins; 1980;188–217.

45. Fogel ER. Biofeedback-assisted musculoskeletal therapy and neuromuscular re-education. In: Schwartz MS, ed. *Biofeedback: A Practitioner's Guide.* New York: Guilford Press; 1995;560–596.

46. Wolf SL, Binder-Macleod SA. Electromyographic biofeedback in the physical therapy clinic. In: Basmajian JV, ed. *Biofeedback: Principles and Practice for Clinicians.* 3rd ed. Baltimore: Williams & Wilkins; 1989; 91–104.

47. Alders SS, Beckers D, Buck M. *PNF in Practice.* Heidelberg, Germany: Springer-Verlag; 1993.

48. Knott M, Voss DE. *Proprioceptive Neuromuscular Facilitation.* 2nd ed. New York: Harper & Row; 1969.

49. Sullivan PE, Markos PD. *Clinical Procedures in Therapeutic Exercise.* 2nd ed. Stamford, CT: Appleton & Lange; 1996.

50. Bayles GH, Cleary PJ. The role of awareness in the control of frontalis muscle activity. *Biol Psychol.* 1986; 22:23–35.

51. Glaros AG, Hanson K. EMG biofeedback and discriminative muscle control. *Biofeedback Self Regul.* 1990; 15:135–143.

52. Pollard RQ Jr, Katkin ES. Placebo effects in biofeedback and self-perception of muscle tension. *Psychophysiology.* 1984;21:47–53.

53. Segreto J. The role of EMG awareness in EMG biofeedback learning. *Biofeedback Self Regul.* 1995;20:155–167.

54. Stilson DW, Matus I, Ball G. Relaxation and subjective estimates of muscle tension: implications for a central efferent theory of muscle control. *Biofeedback Self Regul.* 1980;5:19–36.

55. Flor H, Schugens MM, Birbaumer N. Discrimination of muscle tension in chronic pain patients and healthy controls. *Biofeedback Self Regul.* 1992;17:165–177.

56. Jonsson B. The static load component in muscle work. *Eur J Appl Physiol.* 1988;57:305–310.

57. Middaugh SJ. Upper trapezius overuse in chronic headache and correction with EMG biofeedback training. In: *Proceedings of the Association for Applied Psychophysiology and Biofeedback (AAPB) 26th Annual Meeting, Cincinnati, Ohio, March 1995.* Wheat Ridge, CO: AAPB; 1995;89–92.

58. Milerad E, Ericson MO, Nisell R, Kilbom A. An electromyographic study of dental work. *Ergonomics.* 1991;34:953–962.

59. Veiersted KB. Sustained muscle tension as a risk factor for trapezius myalgia. In: Nielsen R, Jorgensen K, eds. *Advances in Industrial Economics and Safety.* London: Taylor & Francis Publishers; 1993;V:15–19.

60. Veiersted KB, Westgaard RH. Development of trapezius myalgia among female workers performing light manual work. *Scand J Work Environ Health.* 1993;19:277–283.

61. Veiersted KB, Westgaard RH, Andersen P. Electromyographic evaluation of muscular work pattern as a predictor of trapezius myalgia. *Scand J Work Environ Health.* 1993;19:284–290.

62. Winkel J, Westgaard RH. Occupational and individual risk factors for shoulder-neck complaints, part II: The scientific basis (literature review) for the guide. *Int J Indust Ergon.* 1992;10:85–104.

63. Ettare DL, Ettare R. Muscle learning therapy—a treatment protocol. In: Cram JR, ed. *Clinical EMG for Surface Recordings.* Vol 2. Nevada City, CA: Clinical Resources; 1990;197–234.

64. Donaldson S, Donaldson M. Multichannel EMG assessment and treatment techniques. In: Cram JR, ed. *Clinical EMG for Surface Recordings.* Vol 2. Nevada City, CA: Clinical Resources; 1990;143–173.

65. Skubick DL, Clasby R, Donaldson CCS, Marshall WM. Carpal tunnel syndrome as an expression of muscular dysfunction of the neck. *J Occup Rehabil.* 1993;3:31–44.

66. Donaldson S, Romney D, Donaldson M, Skubick D. Randomized study of the application of single motor unit biofeedback training to chronic low back pain. *J Occup Rehabil.* 1994;4:23–37.

67. Wolf SL, LeCraw D, Barton L. Comparison of motor copy and targeted biofeedback training techniques for restitution of upper extremity function among patients with neurologic disorders. *Phys Ther.* 1989;69:719–735.

68. Travell JG, Simons DG. *Myofascial Pain and Dysfunction.* Baltimore: Williams & Wilkins; 1983.

69. Nachemson AL, Andersson GB, Schultz AB. Valsalva maneuver biomechanics: effects on lumbar trunk loads of elevated intraabdominal pressures. *Spine.* 1986; 11:476–479.

70. Vakos JP, Nitz AJ, Threlkeld AJ, Shapiro R, Horn T. Electromyographic activity of selected trunk and hip muscles during a squat lift. *Spine.* 1994;19:687–695.

71. Ballantyne BT, O'Hare SJ, et al. Electromyographic activity of selected shoulder muscles in commonly used therapeutic exercises. *Phys Ther.* 1993;73:668–682.

72. Cuddeford T, Williams AK, Medeiros JM. Electromyographic activity of the vastus medialis oblique and vastus lateralis muscles during selected exercises. *J Ortho Phys Ther.* 1996;4:10–15.

73. McCann PD, Wootten ME, Kadaba MP, Bigliani LU. A kinematic and electromyographic study of shoulder rehabilitation exercises. *Clin Orthop Rel Res.* 1993; 288:170–188.

74. Moseley JB, Jobe FW, Pink M, Perry J, Tibone J. EMG analysis of the scapular muscles during a shoulder rehabilitation program. *Am J Sports Med.* 1992;20:128–135.

75. Soderberg GL, Duesterhaus Minor S, Arnold K, et al. Electromyographic activity of selected leg musculature in subjects with normal and chronically sprained ankles performing on the BAPS board. *Phys Ther.* 1991; 71:514–522.

76. Fiebert I, Keller CD. Are "passive" extension exercises really passive. *J Orthop Sports Phys Ther.* 1994; 19:111–116.

77. Karst GM, Jewett PD. Electromyographic analysis of exercises proposed for differential activation of medial and lateral quadriceps femoris muscle components. *Phys Ther.* 1993;73:286–295.

78. Wolf SL, Edwards DI, Shutter LA. Concurrent assessment of muscle activity (CAMA): a procedural approach to assess treatment goals. *Phys Ther.* 1986; 66:218–224.

79. Lee WWM. Progressive muscle synergy and synchronization in movement patterns: an approach to the treatment of dynamic lumbar instability. *J Manual Manipulative Ther.* 1994;2:133–142.

80. Basmajian JV, Wolf SL, eds. *Therapeutic Exercise.* 5th ed. Baltimore: Williams & Wilkins; 1990.

81. Hall CM, Thein L, eds. *Therapeutic Exercise for the Musculoskeletal Patient.* Philadelphia: Lippincott-Raven Publishers. In press.

82. Kisner C, Colloy LA. *Therapeutic Exercise: Foundations and Techniques.* 3rd ed. Philadelphia: FA Davis; 1996.

83. Hazard RG. Spine update: functional restoration. *Spine.* 1995;20:2345–2348.

SEMG-Triggered Neuromuscular Electrical Stimulation

Surface electromyography (SEMG) feedback training has long been used as a therapeutic modality for rehabilitation. Neuromuscular electrical stimulation (NMES) has also been used to improve motor control after orthopaedic or neurologic insult. Combining the two techniques would seem to be a logical step for the clinician to take. Easy-to-use, affordable systems are available commercially in which delivery of NMES is triggered by the patient's SEMG activity. By bringing SEMG and NMES together, the inherent weaknesses of each technique are canceled, and the strengths of each are complemented.

In this chapter, the concept of, and physiologic rationale for, combined SEMG-triggered NMES (SEMG-NMES) will be discussed. Indications and basic applications, as well as contraindications and precautions, for the combined modalities will be highlighted. Commentary will also focus on clinical guidelines for the use of SEMG-NMES, as well as on special applications and home practice considerations. Finally, three cases with the use of SEMG-NMES will be presented.

CONCEPT

With NMES, muscles are activated indirectly through stimulation of peripheral motor nerves. The method is considered to be safe and effective in facilitating neuromuscular re-education, strength, and range of motion, as well as for spasticity management and functional orthosis in selected patients.[1–6] A maximum potential of motor units can be recruited with NMES, and this may support muscle contraction sufficient for therapeutic exercise and functional activity. The timing of target muscle contraction can be regulated and balanced to task requirements, as well as to the target muscle's synergists and antagonists. A limitation of the technique is that the muscle is activated by an extrinsic stimulus. The patient may be instructed to add his or her volitional attempt at contraction during the stimulation, but ultimately, the patient can remain passive during the process. If motor learning and integration are impaired, there is no guarantee that the patient's efforts will be directed into activation of the appropriate neuronal pathways. There is no practical way to ensure that the patient's central nervous system (CNS) will be actively engaged with the stimulation machine, working toward the same goal.

SEMG evaluation and feedback applications have been reviewed for use in neuromuscular re-education, coordination, strengthening, spastic motor control, gait disorders, and chronic pain management.[7–16] Surface electrodes record a representative sum of muscle action potentials that lead to generation of muscle tension. This bioelectric signal is differentially amplified; filtered; rectified (typically), integrated, or averaged in some fashion; and transduced to an auditory or visual microvoltage display. A clinician can discriminate a patient's ability to activate a target neuromuscular pathway by examining the outcome at the display screen. The magnitude of the response can be quantified, reflecting the total of spatial and temporal motor unit summation.[17] Recruitment and decruitment timing can be assessed by following the rise and fall of the voltage wave form. The display also gives the patient access to relatively instantaneous, performance-contingent muscle feedback. The patient uses this information to learn to relax overly tense muscles, as well as to activate weak muscles or coordinate activity among agonists, antagonists, and synergists more efficiently.

Although the objective in using SEMG feedback is to improve motor control over a course of training, the number and temporal pattern of recruited motor units initially will be suboptimum. For patients attempting to increase muscle output, recruitment levels may be insufficient to support functional activity or vigorous therapeutic exercises. Any proprioceptive feedback generated by the muscle contractions and subsequent structural loading will probably also be suboptimum.

In considering SEMG and NMES together, the strength of each technique is the weakness of the other (Exhibit 6–1). NMES can be used to generate large amounts of muscle tension; produce structural load, proprioceptive feedback, tissue conditioning, and force output; and support directly the performance of functional activities. It cannot, however, define the patient's inherent abilities of motor control, or ensure cognitive involvement during the training process. SEMG can be used to measure correct activation of a target neuromuscular pathway and provide feedback, but it cannot maximally recruit, or regulate, target muscles in a predictable manner. In the SEMG-NMES paradigm, SEMG and NMES are coupled together, so that an extrinsic electrical stimulus is delivered to a target muscle once a prescribed SEMG microvolt threshold is exceeded. Thus specifically desired, intrinsic neural activity re-

Exhibit 6–1 Comparative Advantages and Disadvantages of SEMG, NMES, and SEMG-NMES

	ADVANTAGES	*DISADVANTAGES*
SEMG	Enables discrimination and quantification of patient's intrinsic recruitment ability. Provides highly sensitive, performance-contingent muscle feedback.	No means of extrinsic, immediate regulation of motor control.
NMES	Enables immediate and precise regulation of motor recruitment amplitude and onset timing. With brisk contractions, generates robust proprioceptive feedback. Can produce muscle-conditioning effects when volitional control is limited.	No inherent means of discriminating intrinsic recruitment ability; no assurance of integration of NMES and volition. No patient feedback system.
SEMG-NMES	Provides all advantages of SEMG and NMES. Links volitional recruitment with enhanced intrinsic, somatotopic feedback.	

sults in motor unit recruitment that is augmented by artificially induced motor recruitment (Figure 6–1).

PHYSIOLOGIC RATIONALE

To identify the substrates of motor learning with SEMG-NMES, it is helpful to consider sensory and motor relationships in the CNS and the principle of somatotopy in particular.

Normal motor control requires peripheral somatic sensory input.[18] Sensory and motor systems are anatomically and physiologically linked at all levels of the neuraxis, in a plastic way, and with a level of integration that ranges from stereotyped, monosynaptic stretch reflexes to sophisticated neuronal ensembles.

Somatotopy is the concept that the body's somatic sensory fields are mapped out throughout the CNS, represented at the postcentral gyrus of the cerebral cortex by the well-known homunculus.[19] At the cortical homunculus, a neuron that responds to mechanical stimulation of the hand, for example, is located close to neurons with receptive fields at the wrist. A corresponding map is found over the motor strip at the precentral gyrus, and these sensory and motor maps are anatomically connected.[20–22] Cortical motor neurons that generate activity for a specific muscle receive sensory input from that muscle and related body surfaces[23,24] (Figure 6–2).

The maps are regular but disproportionate to body surfaces in that larger amounts of neural tissue are devoted to body areas with greater

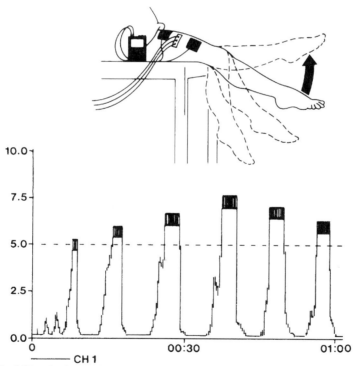

Figure 6–1 Standard SEMG-triggered NMES setup. EMG electrodes detect a voltage sum derived from muscle action potentials. The EMG signal is processed in a routine manner, and when the display magnitude exceeds a predetermined value, a relay causes a neuromuscular electrical stimulator to deliver current to the same muscle. The EMG display is nullified during electrical stimulation because the device would record voltage associated with injection of artificial current, masking the small muscle action potential signal. Courtesy of Verimed International, Inc., Coral Springs, Florida.

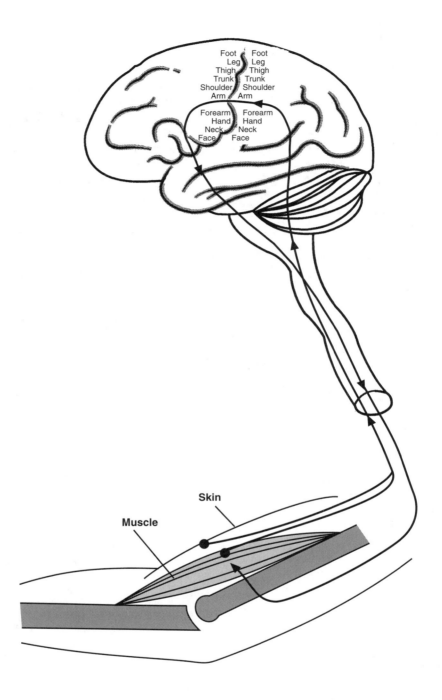

Figure 6–2 Anatomically correspondent areas on the sensory and motor strips of the cerebral cortex are linked. Cortical neurons involved in programming a particular muscle receive sensory input from that muscle and the overlying skin.

somatic or motor sensibility.[25] Cortical reorganization has been demonstrated in humans after limb amputation.[26,27] In the cortical somatic sensory homunculus of monkeys, the proportionate size representation for a body area has been shown to vary with the level of ongoing peripheral stimulation.[28–31] Thus high levels of peripheral sensory activity from a given muscle and its related body surfaces may bring about plastic changes in central sensorimotor integration, influencing efferent drive to that same muscle. Somatotopic afferent–efferent relationships also exist subcortically throughout the brainstem reticular formation, cerebellum, and spinal cord.[32] Motor learning influences these relationships,[33,34] even at the spinal reflex level.[35–37] The notion that motor neurons are affected by sensory stimulation from their target innervated muscle and the covering skin has also been a basis for manually facilitated exercise techniques.[38]

The muscle contractions and biomechanical loads that are augmented by NMES increase the output of sensory receptors in the muscle–tendon–joint complex. These generate proprioceptive feedback to the CNS. The CNS receives additional input through electrical activation of cutaneous sensory fibers that overlie the stimulated muscle. In a SEMG–contingent NMES system, the SEMG component detects when the patient correctly activates the target neuromuscular pathway and immediately triggers NMES to enhance cutaneous sensation and proprioception. The feedback to the CNS is somatotopically linked and time locked to the volitional muscle contraction. Presumably, the process acts to reinforce the CNS motor program that produced the initial, desired peripheral response (Figure 6–3). SEMG-NMES may be used in a clinical setting with a muscle contraction that can be initiated but not sustained over time or through a range of motion arc. Augmented contractions may give the patient more time to integrate feedback cues and can make the difference in the patient's ability to use a motor response in a functional context.

Feedback with SEMG-NMES differs uniquely from other forms of biologic feedback in that the information is somatosensory based. Thus direct somesthetic-motor coupling becomes an advantage. Traditional audio and visual SEMG feedback cues are probably processed through more complex pathways in sensory association cortex. Because the SEMG-NMES system uses a traditional SEMG feedback display, all types of feedback loops are facilitated. Heterosensory feedback accesses multiple sensorimotor systems and levels of the CNS, maximizing the synaptic volume of opportunities for integration, plasticity, and learning.

Use of SEMG as a control signal for clinical electrical stimulation has been described in the literature.[39–45] These SEMG-contingent electrical stimulation devices have been designed for patients with proprioceptive neglect and paresis after stroke, spinal cord paraplegia, and other neurologic and orthopaedic impairments. In terms of patient outcomes, there have been a number of anecdotal comments[12,41,46,47] and studies, the latter of which relate to pediatric cerebral palsy[48] and stroke in adults.[42,49,50] The investigators have documented positive results with SEMG-NMES in facilitating wrist extension and hand functional ability, as well as ankle dorsiflexion and functional gait, in patients with chronic deficits refractory to conventional therapies. Treatment sessions ranged from 30 to 60 minutes, three times per week, over 8 to 12 weeks.

Although SEMG-NMES has been compared with conventional therapies, there have been no direct comparisons of SEMG-NMES versus the singular use of either modality. However, methods that approach the point were used in two studies. Kraft and colleagues[50] demonstrated significantly greater gains in functional motor control of the hand with SEMG-NMES, compared with a manually facilitated clinic exercise program or no treatment, with a poststroke population. They also included a group treated with submotor electrical stimulation combined with voluntary movement and found lower but

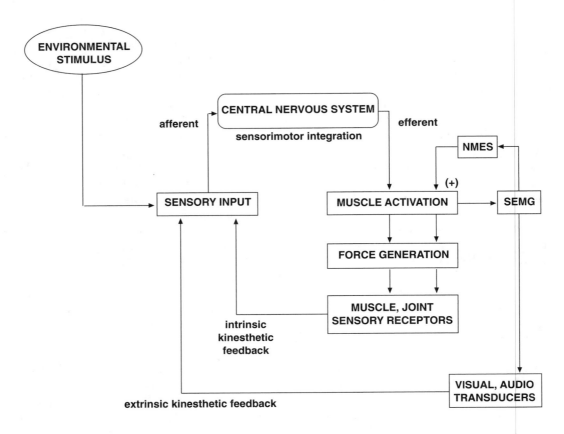

Figure 6–3 Schematic illustration of SEMG-triggered NMES paradigm. Some environmental stimulus, abstracted and evaluated in the central nervous system, creates a need for a motor outcome. A voluntary set of motor commands is programmed in response, followed by muscle activation and force generation. Sensory receptors detect changes in mechanical events. This intrinsic feedback is conducted to the central nervous system, where it is integrated to evaluate the success of the motor program relative to the movement goal. Coincidentally, SEMG electrodes detect a voltage sum associated with muscle action potentials, and a representative electrical signal is transmitted and processed for visual and auditory display. This artificial extrinsic feedback is integrated with intrinsic feedback in the subject's central nervous system. If the processed SEMG signal satisfies the training goal criteria, a neuromuscular electrical stimulator augments activation of the target muscle. The augmented contraction reinforces intrinsic feedback and sensorimotor integration.

nonsignificant gains in this group, compared with findings in the group treated with SEMG-NMES. Subject number, however, was limited and duration and frequency of treatment were not equivalent across groups.

Cozean and associates[51] also studied a poststroke population, in this case measuring several gait parameters. All subjects received

30-minute treatment sessions, three times per week, for 6 weeks. Participants were provided with gait training and one of four other therapies: (1) conventional exercise therapy, (2) SEMG feedback for ankle dorsiflexor facilitation and possibly plantarflexor relaxation, (3) ankle dorsiflexor NMES, or (4) SEMG feedback and NMES. The group working with the fourth therapy option did so in blocked trials; there was no SEMG-NMES contingency or combined use within trials. Nevertheless, the group treated with SEMG feedback and NMES demonstrated the greatest improvements.

Gains noted for hemiplegic patients who were treated with SEMG-NMES[50] and motion-triggered NMES[52] have been maintained for 9- to 12-month follow-up periods. Motion-triggered NMES incorporates a strategy close to that used in SEMG-NMES in that NMES is triggered once a subject volitionally moves and meets a preset goniometric criterion. Results of one study showed significant improvements in isometric wrist extension torque and volitional wrist extension range of motion compared with a manually facilitated clinic exercise program conducted over a 4-week period.[52] Findings in another investigation showed significant improvements in knee extension torque and range of motion, compared with a conventional treatment regimen.[53] The idea of a therapist manually triggering NMES, using an external switch, as a patient performs volitional movement sequences has similarly been discussed.[1]

INDICATIONS AND BASIC APPLICATIONS

SEMG-NMES is indicated for neuromuscular facilitation and re-education. Essentially, SEMG-NMES may be considered any time NMES or SEMG feedback would be used individually to increase motor output. Situations include uptraining a poorly recruited agonist in generating peak power or attempting to retrain the timing and relative recruitment magnitude of the muscular components of a complex force couple. SEMG-triggered NMES can be helpful in overcoming a patient's postsurgical inhibition (eg, after undergoing total knee replacement or shoulder repair), as well as for neuromuscular re-education after tendon transplantation. The treatment may also be used with chronic musculoskeletal dysfunction involving

- shoulder girdle dysfunction and suspected insufficiency of the lower trapezius, serratus anterior, and infraspinatus
- low back and hip syndromes with gluteus maximus or medius hypoactivity
- patellofemoral dysfunction with vastus medialis oblique insufficiency
- neuromuscular inhibition due to reflex sympathetic dystrophy or learned disuse

Neuromuscular electrical stimulation requires an intact peripheral nerve conduction system. Illustrative cases for musculoskeletal rehabilitation are reviewed later in this chapter.

CONTRAINDICATIONS AND PRECAUTIONS

There are few precautions for the use of SEMG. Indeed, this is one of the primary advantages of SEMG procedures. There are, however, a number of concerns regarding the application of electrical currents.[3,54,55]

1. NMES is contraindicated for patients with demand type pacemakers.
2. NMES is contraindicated where active muscle contraction or active range of motion is contraindicated, eg, recent fusions, fractures, tissue repairs, infection, or malignancies.
3. NMES is contraindicated over the carotid sinus, laryngeal or pharyngeal muscles, eyes, or over superficial metal implants. Transcranial, transpectoral, and transthoracic applications are contraindicated.
4. SEMG and NMES electrodes should be applied only to intact skin.
5. NMES should not be used in patients with history of cardiac disease or brain seizure disorder unless appropriately screened by a physician.
6. Use of NMES during pregnancy is not recommended.
7. NMES should be used with caution in patients with perceptual or cognitive deficits.

8. SEMG-NMES should be attempted only with equipment specifically designed with a compatible interface system and approved for use by appropriate regulatory agencies.

CLINICAL GUIDELINES

The SEMG component of the SEMG-NMES system is a standard SEMG device with a few additional hardware and software features. An external relay connects via a cable to the accessory port of an independent, standard NMES unit. The accessory port is more commonly used to drive stimulation from either a heel switch placed in the patient's shoe or a hand switch controlled by the therapist. Those switches are traditionally used to match stimulation timing to a naturally occurring functional movement sequence. The SEMG and NMES components can alternatively be housed together, eliminating the need for separate devices and connecting cables. In any case, the clinician programs the SEMG device to display a threshold goal level based on the patient's recruitment ability. If the threshold is exceeded (possibly with a mandatory prescribed hold time), the stimulator is triggered to deliver current (see Figure 6–1). The clinician watches the SEMG display to observe the success of the patient's volitional recruitment strategy, and the patient also watches, or listens to an audio tone, for conventional feedback. During delivery of electrical stimulation, the patient's bioelectric SEMG signal is masked by the stimulator voltage, and the SEMG display is nullified. Once a prescribed stimulation period elapses, the stimulator current is terminated, and the system reverts back to SEMG recording. Some systems allow for a mandatory rest period before stimulation can be retriggered.

All routine guidelines for application of SEMG feedback training and NMES are pertinent for SEMG-NMES. Elaboration of these methods is beyond the scope of this discussion, and the reader is referred to other chapters in this book, as well as to the companion publication to this book[56] and other materials on SEMG recording.[7,9,12,16,17,57] Several resources for NMES are also recommended.[54,58–61] Application of NMES is legally restricted in many localities. The potential for harm with NMES is significant. Therefore NMES should be performed by a licensed therapist or physician with specific training in stimulation safety and methods, or by assistants or aides who are appropriately certified and supervised. Because initial equipment setup and software operation for SEMG-NMES can be more complicated than with either SEMG or NMES alone, and because each modality is itself technique sensitive, clinicians who use SEMG-NMES should first become practiced with SEMG recording and NMES as independent entities. For properly trained individuals, SEMG-NMES methods are mastered without difficulty, and setup becomes relatively facile.

There are a few issues unique to SEMG-NMES that require consideration. When separate SEMG and NMES devices are coupled together, the on:off timing functions of the stimulator are usually controlled by the SEMG unit's program. However, stimulator intensity and any rise:fall ramping of that intensity remain a control feature of the NMES device. Some SEMG-NMES units can record and stimulate through the same set of electrodes. It is recommended that separate electrodes be used for all applications other than those involving small muscles. Electrodes designed for NMES generally do not have good recording characteristics; they should not be used to detect SEMG signals. SEMG electrodes, on the other hand, are acceptable for electrical stimulation as well as recording. However, the surface area of SEMG electrodes is typically too small to allow for a comfortable and effective dissipation of electrical current density for NMES of medium to large muscles. SEMG electrodes, therefore, may be used for electrical stimulation over the hand and forearm, but separate recording and stimulating electrodes are preferred elsewhere.

When separate stimulating and recording electrodes are used over a medium-sized muscle, physically fitting all the electrodes at their optimum locations may be difficult. Placement preference is granted to the stimulating electrodes in these cases. The NMES system should be set up first because to achieve efficient activation of the target muscle, the stimulating electrodes may have to be picked up and moved over several trials of current delivery. SEMG electrodes are then positioned in the best possible way for recording. The therapist should ensure that stimulating and recording electrodes do not touch each other as this contact could confound recording. Sample electrode placements for medium-sized muscles are illustrated in Figures 6–4 through 6–6.

The microvolt threshold level of the SEMG unit used to trigger NMES may be variably set. The triggering threshold is initially set at a level that can be successfully reached about 80% of attempts. The threshold may be increased as the patient's intrinsic recruitment ability improves. This process allows the patient to do as much as possible on his or her own. To the extent that the stimulation is viewed as a contingent reward for activation of the target neuromuscular pathway, the therapist can advance the threshold to enhance patient motivation and shape progressively stronger responses. In some situations, however, it is more helpful to leave the threshold at a relatively low value. This is the case when

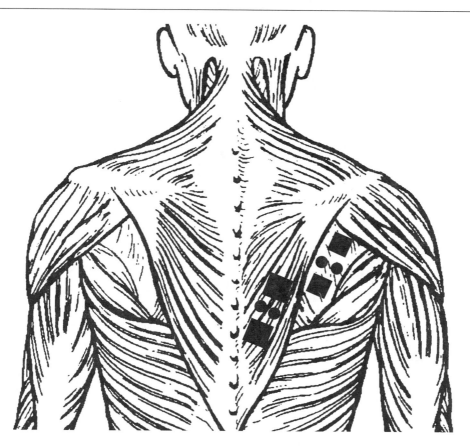

Figure 6–4 Sample electrode placements for the infraspinatus and lower trapezius with bipolar neuromuscular electrical stimulation (squares) and SEMG (active electrodes; circles).

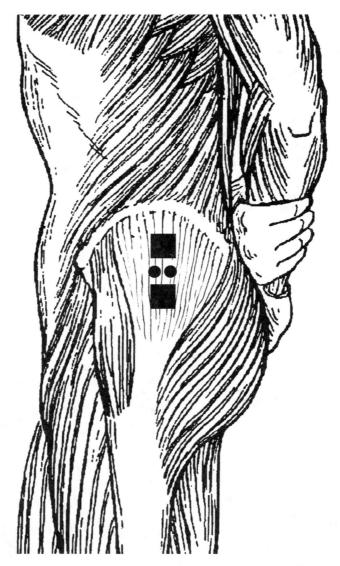

Figure 6–5 Sample electrode placements for the gluteus medius with bipolar neuromuscular electrical stimulation (squares) and SEMG (active electrodes; circles).

SEMG-NMES is used during a functional activity, and stimulation is required to bring the task to meaningful completion with a smooth, fluid movement quality. The patient's SEMG activity might be sufficient to reach a higher threshold, but only with an effort that produces substitution patterns and untoward compensation at adjacent joint segments.

The threshold can also be left at a lower value if the goal is to facilitate earlier recruitment of a target muscle during movement. One component of a muscle synergy may be seen to activate strongly under some circumstances, but recruit late, weakly, or both relative to an antagonist or a synergist during a functional movement arc. This phenomenon might be seen, for example, in

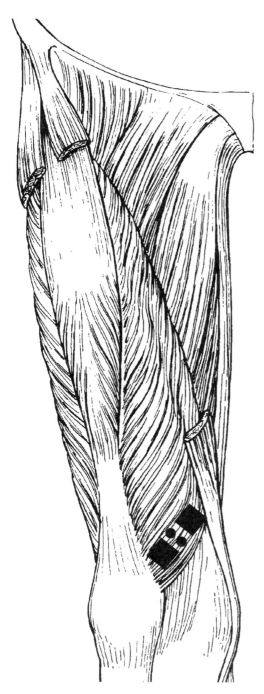

Figure 6–6 Sample electrode placements for the vastus medialis oblique with bipolar neuromuscular electrical stimulation (squares) and SEMG (active electrodes; circles).

some cases of patellofemoral dysfunction during a partial squat maneuver or in faulty relationships between the upper and lower portions of the trapezius during shoulder abduction. In the first example, the vastus medialis oblique is thought to provide medial stabilization of the patella as it dynamically tracks in the femoral trochlear groove, opposing a laterally directed moment created by the vastus lateralis, passive restraints, and other biomechanical factors.[62,63] With the second example, the upper trapezius, lower trapezius, and lower fibers of the serratus anterior synergistically contract, each with a specific timing, to rotate the scapula cephalad.[64] In both cases, the threshold would be set to a low value so that the target muscle (ie, vastus medialis oblique or lower trapezius) triggers a facilitory NMES response early in the movement sequence, before an antagonist or a synergist dominates inappropriately. If the triggering threshold were linked to a high value, the NMES unit would fire too late to be of benefit. An inefficient muscular force couple would persist throughout most of the movement.

The therapist usually has to take a trial-and-error approach in setting the trigger value. He or she should instruct the patient to perform several repetitions of the desired task at a consistently moderate speed. The therapist observes both the patient and the SEMG-NMES device, noting the point in the range of motion arc at which stimulation is initiated. A judgment that the NMES is being triggered too far into the movement arc is followed by a decrease in the threshold value. The NMES will then be activated earlier for most functional movements. If the NMES is triggered too soon, the threshold is increased. The sequence is repeated until the most natural timing for muscle facilitation is obtained. Consider, for example, a patient with a shoulder impingement syndrome, faulty scapular control, and apparent lower trapezius hypoactivity. It would be undesirable to deliver strong NMES to the lower trapezius at the very start of shoulder flexion. This would cause the lower trapezius to generate too much tension too early in the motion and result in gross overcorrection of the original problem. Scapular mechanics would be disturbed in a different direction. Instead, the threshold would be adjusted until the NMES is triggered at about 30 to 40 degrees of flexion, perhaps with a 0.25- to 0.5-second NMES intensity ramp, so that recruitment increases as the motion continues.

SPECIAL APPLICATIONS

A number of special approaches are possible with SEMG-NMES, depending on patient and equipment particulars. The most salient of these applications will be considered next.

Orthotic Substitution during Gait: Ankle Dorsiflexion Assist

NMES has been used as a functional orthosis for ankle dorsiflexion during gait when regulated by the patient with a heel-pressure switch or therapist with a hand switch.[65,66] There is, however, no fixed contingency between the trigger for stimulation and a patient's volitional attempt at dorsiflexion. The protocol may be adapted for use with SEMG-NMES. With careful selection of stimulation ramping and on:off cycles, the SEMG-NMES system is timed to match the gait cycle. If, for example, the patient ambulates at a slow cadence, the use of a low triggering threshold, a 0.8 second stimulation on time with instant rise and fall times, and a 1.2-second mandatory off time can be effective. The use of miniaturized system components clipped onto the patient's belt allows for freedom from extraneous leads and reduction of movement artifact.

SEMG-Triggered Submotor Electrical Stimulation

Situations may arise in which submotor electrical stimulation is contingently tied to SEMG recording. The system operates as discussed above for SEMG-NMES, but with electrical stimulation at a lower intensity. Electrical stimulation is used to excite superficial afferent sensory fibers. The obvious application is when patients do not tolerate a stimulation intensity sufficient for muscle activation. Discomfort may be an issue during the initial stages of training, with patient apprehension, high electrical impedance of the skin, peripheral neuropathic dysesthesias, or reflex sympathetic dystrophy. Use of SEMG contingent submotor electrical stimulation has also been proposed for dystonic, spasmodic torticollis[67] and nocturnal bruxism.[68] In these latter cases, stimulation is delivered over a body surface nonanatomically related to the recording muscle (eg, a forearm) as a means of cueing inappropriate muscle activation that might otherwise go unrecognized.

Muscle Flaccidity

When the muscle for which activation is desired is flaccid or nearly so, there will be insufficient SEMG voltage to act as a control signal for NMES. A reasonable option is to derive the control SEMG signal from the contralateral homologous muscle and use bilateral symmetric movements. Alternatively, NMES of a flaccid target muscle may be triggered by a SEMG signal from a lesser involved synergist on the same side. For example, a scapular motor control may be impaired in patients with selected peripheral nerve injuries, and a shoulder impingement syndrome may develop. If serratus anterior muscle function is insufficient, the anterior deltoid could be used to generate a control signal for stimulation over the lower fibers of the serratus anterior during reaching movements. The recording electrodes would then be moved to the serratus anterior as soon as an adequate SEMG signal is produced.

Dual Channel Stimulation

Sometimes it is appropriate to record from one muscle and stimulate that muscle and another muscle simultaneously. Many of the standard NMES units that are coupled with SEMG devices have dual channel capability. One scenario applies to mechanically synergistic muscles. For example, maximal elbow flexion can be produced by recording from and stimulating a poorly recruited biceps, and using a second stimulation channel to activate the brachioradialis simultaneously. Another example would be to record and stimulate the gluteus maximus and additionally stimulate the hamstrings for hip extension during sit-to-stand or stair-stepping maneuvers.

Another instance for use of dual channel NMES involves functional synergists; that is, muscles with different but complementary joint actions for functional movements. The gluteus maximus and quadriceps, or the quadriceps and triceps surae, could be used in this manner to facilitate stance control and prevent collapse of the lower extremity kinetic chain into flexion. The quadriceps might also be used with the gluteus medius to promote knee stability and lateral pelvic control, respectively, with weight acceptance onto that limb. At the upper extremity, components of proprioceptive neuromuscular facilitation[69] diagonal patterns could be dually facilitated.

Finally, joint antagonists can be stimulated simultaneously to support co-contraction around an unstable joint. The quadriceps and hamstrings could be jointly facilitated to generate stance control in the presence of give-way weakness and recurvatum that is due to quadriceps weakness. The quadriceps would be used as the recording and primary stimulation site, and the hamstrings would act as an accessory stimulation site. Before applying this method, the therapist should evaluate the patient's trunk, hip, and ankle function and correct any problems as much as possible. The technique would be inappropriate, for example, in attempting control of knee recurvatum that occurs in compensation for restricted ankle mobility. Independent stimulation timing for each channel is helpful to achieve precise control of the joint during weight bearing. The quadriceps would be timed to contract immediately on weight acceptance to prevent collapse of the lower extremity into flexion, and the hamstrings timed to contract 0.2 to 0.5 second later to stabilize the joint and prevent knee

hyperextension. This could be accomplished by using either a slower ramping function for the hamstring channel intensity or a function that delays hamstring stimulation onset from the external trigger.

SUGGESTIONS FOR HOME UNITS

SEMG-NMES systems are available both as clinical units and portable home trainers. The patient's physical impairments, cognitive limitations, and tolerance of gadgets should be considered in assessing his or her ability to manage a home system. A friend or family member can be trained to operate the system if the patient is unable to do so. As with NMES, SEMG-NMES should not be used as an orthotic substitute for stance support unless a qualified therapist is present to protect the patient from a fall. It may be helpful first to send the patient home with NMES alone. Once competence is demonstrated and the whole SEMG-NMES setup has been practiced in the clinic, the SEMG component can be added for home practice. Written instructions for all phases of the setup should be provided to the patient. A videotape of a supervised practice session is best, or a descriptive audiotape may help. Although rental fees will be incurred, it may be far more cost effective to dispense a home unit and reduce the frequency of clinic visits. A home unit will also enable patients to practice on a daily basis and with multiple sessions per day.

CASE HISTORIES

Three case histories have been included to describe application of SEMG-NMES with patients.

Case 1: Quadriceps Weakness after Total Knee Replacement

Figure 6–7A shows the SEMG activity recorded during a maximal effort, isometric quadriceps contraction from a 67-year-old man 6 days after total knee replacement for osteoarthri-

A
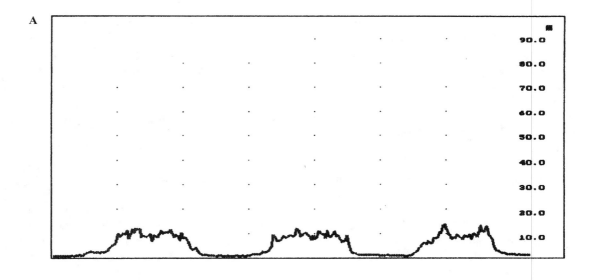

B
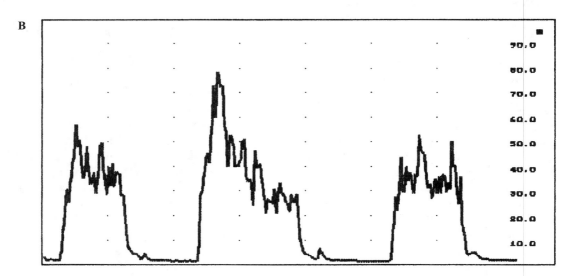

Figure 6–7 SEMG activity of the quadriceps recorded from a patient after total knee replacement. (**A**) Activity before SEMG-triggered NMES. (**B**) Activity after SEMG-triggered NMES.

tis. SEMG activity at this time was judged as inadequate on the basis of conversion of the peak value to a percentage of maximal effort before surgery and comparison of the normalized score with expected values for this clinical pathway (G S Kasman and colleagues, unpublished data, 1991). This corresponded to an inability to perform an independent terminal knee extension or straight leg raise, as well as to slow progress with transfers and ambulation. The previous morning the patient had met with little success by training with SEMG feedback alone. Application of NMES on the previous afternoon helped facilitate independent recruitment to some extent, but the effect did not carry over to the next day. Figure 6–7B shows peak recruitment effort after 15 minutes of SEMG-NMES (after NMES was discontinued). The effect was significant in enhancing independent movement control during terminal knee extension. Results carried over and were extended the following 2 days. The patient was then ready for discharge on postoperative day 8, eliminating the need for an anticipated transfer to a rehabilitation unit and a longer hospital stay.

Case 2: Reflex Sympathetic Dystrophy

Figure 6–8 shows SEMG activity from the anterior and posterior compartments of the leg during volitional ankle dorsiflexion in a supine position. Activity from a 13-year-old female with bilateral, severe dysesthetic foot pain, 6 months after onset is shown (Figure 6–8A1) versus a normal subject (Figure 6–8A2) for comparison. Note the elevated activity from the posterior compartment and minimal anterior compartment recruitment in the patient. Dorsiflexion in the patient had been graded at 0/5 by manual muscle test. Her pain began after running a half-marathon, progressed in intensity, and became accompanied by skin that was discolored, hyperhydrotic, and poorly thermoregulated. She had ambulated for most of the previous 6 months up on the balls of her feet to minimize pain. As a consequence, profoundly reduced myofascial extensibility and passive length had developed in the posterior compartment and Achilles tendon, with secondary compensations throughout the lower extremities and trunk. Moreover, there was marked family discord and behavioral dysfunction. No progress was made with superficial heat, ultrasound, manual soft tissue mobilization, stretching, or SEMG feedback for relaxation or facilitated ankle dorsiflexion. Electrical stimulation was then applied over the anterior compartment, gradually building in intensity over the course of two sessions until motor threshold was reached. Dual channel SEMG feedback was next coupled to the NMES. The anterior compartment signal

was visually observed by the patient and used as the signal for NMES, while the posterior compartment channel triggered an audio tone if activity significantly increased above baseline. Figure 6–9B shows the results after 12 sessions of 30 minutes each, spaced over a 4-week period. Manual muscle testing for ankle dorsiflexion then scored 5/5, and SEMG-NMES was discontinued in favor of periodic assisted stretching, a self-directed home exercise program, behavioral counseling, and progressive resumption of normal functional activities.

Case 3: Patellofemoral Dysfunction and Pain

The final case involves a 43-year-old female with chronic right anterior knee pain who was employed as a taxicab driver. The patient began each day without pain but progressively experienced pain and swelling during the course of her work shift. Moving from the accelerator to the brake pedal was definitively exacerbating, as was going up and down stairs or squat maneuvers. Physical examination findings were consistent with a patellofemoral cause. Asymmetric tightness of the right rectus femoris and iliotibial band was also noted. A previously prescribed general stretching and quadriceps strengthening program had been ineffective at reducing symptoms. Pain was now causing time loss from work.

SEMG activity recorded from the vastus medialis oblique (VMO) was depressed on the involved side whereas that of the vastus lateralis (VL) was symmetric. Activity for each recording site was also normalized as a percentage of maximal effort, isometric SEMG value, and then expressed as a VMO:VL ratio. The VMO:VL ratio on the right consistently ranged between 0.91 and 1.19 during submaximal contractions in non–weight-bearing positions, values well within expected limits (see Chapter 13) and similar to those from the left side. However, the VMO:VL ratio on the right decreased to 0.69 to 0.84 during squat and stair activities. When pressing down with moderate force on a brake pedal after moving from an accelerator was

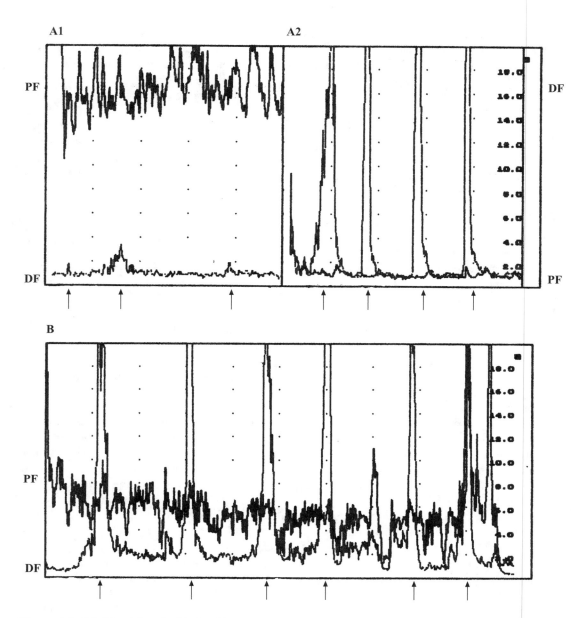

Figure 6–8 SEMG activity of ankle dorsiflexors (**DF**) and plantar flexors (**PF**). (**A1**) Activity from a patient with reflex sympathetic dystrophy during attempted ankle dorsiflexion (**arrows**). (**A2**) Activity from a normal subject during ankle dorsiflexion for comparison. (**B**) Activity from the patient (in **A1**) after treatment program with use of SEMG-triggered NMES.

simulated, the VMO:VL ratio initially averaged 0.64 and then increased as the movement range was completed. SEMG-NMES was then per-formed over the VMO for 20 minutes. Trials were started with the patient in a sitting position and quickly progressed into weight-bearing and simulated driving movements. Next, NMES was withdrawn, and SEMG was retested with all activities showing a VMO:VL ratio greater than 0.94. A home program was designed combining SEMG-NMES, patellofemoral taping,[70] and stretching to be performed daily for 7 days. With follow-up testing, the patient demonstrated independent carry-over of VMO:VL SEMG ratios greater than 0.85 for all activities and was nearly pain free and able to return to driving a full shift. SEMG-NMES was discontinued, whereas taping and exercise were continued at home, tapering over a 5-week period. SEMG feedback was also used to help make changes in seat position and motor habit that decreased recruitment of the tensor fascia latae and rectus femoris during simulated driving.

CONCLUSION

SEMG-NMES is an elegant means of eliminating disadvantages of SEMG training and NMES that occur when each modality is used alone. The SEMG display is used by the clinician to assess the success of the patient's volitional recruitment strategy and by the patient to obtain traditional feedback cues. NMES facilitates motor contraction and sensory stimulation beyond the patient's inherent capabilities and generates performance-contingent, somatotopic, time-ordered feedback. It is proposed that this process enhances sensorimotor integration, leading to neuromuscular re-education and improved functional motor control. Competencies in SEMG recording and display methods, NMES techniques, and combined SEMG-NMES strategies are required. Manufacturers are sensitive to the need to minimize setup complexity. Significant advances in hardware and software will likely come to commercial markets over the next few years. Although SEMG feedback and NMES have each been studied extensively, reports that conclusively establish outcome values and cost efficiencies for combined SEMG-NMES methods will be of principal importance. In all cases, SEMG-NMES should be regarded as one component of a comprehensive treatment program that addresses underlying pathologies and advances patients toward functional independence.

REFERENCES

1. Baker LL. Clinical uses of neuromuscular electrical stimulation. In: Nelson RP, Currier DP, eds. *Clinical Electrotherapy*. 2nd ed. Norwalk, CT: Appleton & Lange; 1991;143–170.

2. Currier DP. Neuromuscular stimulation for improving muscular strength and blood flow and influencing changes. In: Nelson RP, Currier DP, eds. *Clinical Electrotherapy*. 2nd ed. Norwalk, CT: Appleton & Lange; 1991;171–200.

3. DeVahl J. Neuromuscular electrical stimulation (NMES) in rehabilitation. In: Gersh MR, ed. *Electrotherapy in Rehabilitation*. Philadelphia: FA Davis; 1992;218–268.

4. Morrissey MC. Neuromuscular electrical stimulation in the rehabilitation of orthopedic injury. *Phys Ther Pract*. 1992;1:20–29.

5. Packman-Braun R. Electrotherapeutic applications for the neurologically impaired patient. In: Gersh MR, ed. *Electrotherapy in Rehabilitation*. Philadelphia: FA Davis; 1992;362–397.

6. Stralka SW. Application of therapeutic electrical currents in the management of the orthopedic patient. In: Gersh MR, ed. *Electrotherapy in Rehabilitation*. Philadelphia: FA Davis; 1992;345–361.

7. Basmajian JV, ed. *Biofeedback: Principles and Practice for Clinicians*. 3rd ed. Baltimore: Williams & Wilkins; 1989.

8. Binder-Macleod SA. Biofeedback in stroke rehabilitation. In: Basmajian JV, ed. *Biofeedback: Principles and Practice for Clinicians*. 2nd ed. Baltimore: Williams & Wilkins; 1983;73–89.

9. Cram JR. *Clinical EMG for Surface Recordings*. Vol 2. Nevada City, CA: Clinical Resources; 1990.

10. Fogel ER. Biofeedback-assisted musculoskeletal therapy and neuromuscular re-education. In: Schwartz

MS, ed. *Biofeedback: A Practitioner's Guide*. 2nd ed. New York: Guilford Press; 1995;560–596.

11. Krebs DE. Biofeedback in neuromuscular re-education and gait training. In: Schwartz MS, ed. *Biofeedback: A Practitioner's Guide*. 2nd ed. New York: Guilford Press; 1995;525–559.

12. LeCraw DE, Wolf SL. Electromyographic biofeedback (EMGBF) for neuromuscular relaxation and re-education. In: Gersh MR, ed. *Electrotherapy in Rehabilitation*. Philadelphia: FA Davis; 1992;291–327.

13. Moreland J, Thomson MA. Efficacy of electromyographic biofeedback compared with conventional physical therapy for upper-extremity function in patients following stroke: a research overview and meta-analysis. *Phys Ther*. 1994;74:534–544.

14. Schleenbaker RE, Mainous AG. Electromyographic biofeedback for neuromuscular reeducation in the hemiplegic stroke patient: a meta-analysis. *Arch Phys Med Rehabil*. 1993;74:1301–1304.

15. Tries J. EMG biofeedback for the treatment of upper extremity dysfunction: can it be effective? *Biofeedback Self Regul*. 1989;14:21–53.

16. Wolf SL. Electromyographic biofeedback: an overview. In: Nelson RP, Currier DP, eds. *Clinical Electrotherapy*. 2nd ed. Norwalk, CT: Appleton & Lange; 1991;361–384.

17. Basmajian JV, De Luca CJ. *Muscles Alive: Their Functions Revealed by Electromyography*. 5th ed. Baltimore: Williams & Wilkins; 1985.

18. Carew TJ. Descending control of spinal circuits. In: Kandel ER, Schwartz JH, eds. *Principles of Neural Science*. New York: Elsevier; 1983:312–322.

19. Penfield W, Rasmussen T. *The Cerebral Cortex of Man*. New York: Macmillan; 1950.

20. Eccles JC. *The Understanding of the Brain*. 2nd ed. New York: McGraw-Hill; 1977.

21. Jones EG, Powell TPS. Connexions of the somatic sensory cortex of the rhesus monkey, I. ipsilateral cortical connexions. *Brain*. 1969;92:477–502.

22. Woolsey CN. Organization of the somatic sensory and motor areas of the cerebral cortex. In: Harlow HF, Woolsey CN, eds. *Biological and Biochemical Bases of Behavior*. Madison: University of Wisconsin Press; 1958;63–81.

23. Asanuma H. Cerebral cortical control of voluntary movement. *Physiologist*. 1973;16:143–166.

24. Powell TPS, Mountcastle VB. Some aspects of the functional organization of the cortex of the postcentral gyrus of the monkey: a correlation of findings obtained in single unit analysis with cytoarchitecture. *Bull Johns Hopkins Hosp*. 1959;105:133–162.

25. Kandel ER. Somatic sensory system, III: central representations of touch. In: Kandel ER, Schwartz JH, eds.

Principles of Neural Science. New York: Elsevier; 1983;184–198.

26. Elbert T, Flor H, Birbaumer N, et al. Extensive reorganization of the somatosensory cortex in adult humans after nervous system injury. *Neuroreport*. 1994;5:2593–2597.

27. Flor H, Elbert T, Knecht S, et al. Phantom-limb pain as a perceptual correlate of cortical reorganization following arm amputation. *Nature*. 1995;375:482–484.

28. Jenkins WM, Merzenich MM, Ochs MT, Allard T, Guic Robes E. Functional reorganization of primary somatosensory cortex in adult owl monkeys after behaviorally controlled tactile stimulation. *J Neurophysiol*. 1990;63:82–104.

29. Merzenich MM, Kaas JH, Wall MJ, Nelson JR, Felleman DJ. Progression of change following median nerve section in the cortical representation of the hand in areas of 3b and I in adult owl and squirrel monkeys. *Neuroscience*. 1983;20:639–665.

30. Merzenick MM, Nelson JR, Stryker MP, Cynader MS, Scoppmann A, Zook JM. Somatosensory cortical map changes following digit amputation in adult monkeys. *J Comp Neurol*. 1986;224:591–605.

31. Pons TP. Massive cortical reorganization after sensory deafferentiation in adult macaques. *Science*. 1991; 13:1857–1860.

32. Carpenter MR. *Core Textbook of Neuroanatomy*. 2nd ed. Baltimore: Williams & Wilkins; 1978.

33. Horak FB. Assumptions underlying motor control for neurologic rehabilitation. In: *Contemporary Management of Motor Control Problems: Proceedings of the II STEP Conference*. Alexandria, VA: Foundation for Physical Therapy; 1991;11–27.

34. Schmidt RA. Motor learning principles for physical therapy. In: *Contemporary Management of Motor Control Problems: Proceedings of the II STEP Conference*. Alexandria, VA: Foundation for Physical Therapy; 1991;49–63.

35. Segal RL, Wolf SL. Variability of human biceps brachii spinal stretch reflexes: control conditions. *J Electromyogr Kinesiol*. 1993;3:24–32.

36. Wolf SL, Segal RL, Heter ND. Contralateral and long latency effects of human biceps brachii stretch reflex conditioning. *Exp Brain Res*. 1995;107:96–102.

37. Wolf SL, Segal RL. Conditioning of the spinal stretch reflex. *Phys Ther*. 1990;70:652–656.

38. Sullivan PE, Markos PD, Minor MA. *An Integrated Approach to Therapeutic Exercise*. Reston, VA: Reston Publishing Co; 1982.

39. Campbell JA, Tallis R. Contingency transcutaneous stimulator for patients with unilateral tactile and proprioceptive neglect. *Med Biol Eng Comput*. 1985;23:90–92.

40. Graupe D. EMG pattern analysis for patient-responsive control of FES in paraplegics for walker supported walking. *IEEE Trans Biomed Eng.* 1989;711–719.

41. Graupe D, Kohn KH. A critical review of EMG-controlled electrical stimulation. *Crit Rev Biomed Eng.* 1987;15:187–210.

42. Hansen GVO. EMG-controlled functional electrical stimulation of the paretic hand. *Scand J Rehabil.* 1979;11:189–193.

43. Hefftner G, Jaros GG. The electromyogram (EMG) as a control signal for functional neuromuscular stimulation, Part II: practical demonstration of the EMG signature discrimination system. *IEEE Trans Biomed Eng.* 1988;35:238–311.

44. Hefftner G, Zucchini W, Jaros GG. The electromyogram (EMG) as a control signal for functional electrical stimulation, Part I: autoregressive modeling as a means of EMG signature discrimination. *IEEE Trans Biomed Eng.* 1988;35:230–237.

45. Vodovnik L, Rebersek S. Information content of myocontrol signals for orthotic and prosthetic systems. *Arch Phys Med Rehabil.* 1974;55:52–56.

46. Kasman GS. Use of integrated electromyography for the assessment and treatment of musculoskeletal pain: guidelines for physical medicine practitioners. In: Cram JR, ed. *Clinical EMG for Surface Recordings.* Vol 2. Nevada City, CA: Clinical Resources; 1990;255–302.

47. Kraft DE. EMG-triggered muscle stimulation. *Arch Phys Med Rehabil.* 1988;73:220–227.

48. Atwater SW, Tatarka ME, Kathrein JE, Shapiro S. Electromyography-triggered electrical muscle stimulation for children with cerebral palsy: a pilot study. *Pediatr Phys Ther.* 1991;3:190–199.

49. Fields RW. Electromyographically triggered electrical muscle stimulation for chronic hemiplegia. *Arch Phys Med Rehabil.* 1987;68:407–414.

50. Kraft GH, Fitts SS, Hammond MC. Techniques to improve function of the arm and hand in chronic hemiplegia. *Arch Phys Med Rehabil.* 1992;73:220–227.

51. Cozean CD, Pease WS, Hubbell SL. Biofeedback and functional electrical stimulation in stroke rehabilitation. *Arch Phys Med Rehabil.* 1988;69:401–405.

52. Bowman BR, Baker LL, Waters RL. Positional feedback and electrical stimulation: an automatic treatment for the hemiplegic wrist. *Arch Phys Med Rehabil.* 1979;60:497–502.

53. Winchester P, Montgomery J, Bowman H, Hislop H. Effects of feedback stimulation and cyclical electrical stimulation on knee extension in hemiplegic patients. *Phys Ther.* 1983;63:1096–1111.

54. Benton LA, Baker LL, Bowman BR, Waters RL. *Functional Electrical Stimulation—A Practical Guide.* Downey, CA: Rancho Los Amigos Rehabilitation Engineering Center; 1980.

55. Mannheimer JS, Lampe GN. *Clinical Transcutaneous Electrical Nerve Stimulation.* Philadelphia: FA Davis; 1984.

56. Cram JR, Kasman GS. *Introduction to Surface Electromyography.* Gaithersburg, MD: Aspen Publishers; 1997.

57. Schwartz MS. ed. *Biofeedback: A Practitioner's Guide.* 2nd ed. New York: Guilford Press; 1995.

58. American Physical Therapy Association, Section of Clinical Electrophysiology. *Electrotherapeutic Terminology in Physical Therapy.* Alexandria, VA: American Physical Therapy Association; 1990.

59. Gersh MR, ed. *Electrotherapy in Rehabilitation.* Philadelphia: FA Davis; 1992.

60. Nelson RP, Currier DP. *Clinical Electrotherapy.* 2nd ed. Norwalk, CT: Appleton & Lange; 1991.

61. Robinson AJ, Synder-Mackler L. *Clinical Electrophysiology.* Baltimore: Williams & Wilkins; 1995.

62. Lieb FJ, Perry J. Quadriceps function: an anatomical and mechanical study using amputated limbs. *J Bone Joint Surg Am.* 1968;50:1535–1548.

63. Shelton GL, Thigpen LK. Rehabilitation of patellofemoral dysfunction: a review of the literature. *J Orthop Sports Phys Ther.* 1991;14:243–249.

64. Bagg SD, Forrest WJ. Electromyographic study of the scapular rotators during arm abduction in the scapular plane. *Am J Phys Med.* 1986;65:111–124.

65. Cranston B, Larrson LE, Prevec TF. Improvement of gait following functional electrical stimulation: investigations on changes in voluntary strength and proprioceptive reflexes. *Scand J Rehabil Med.* 1977;9:7–13.

66. Packman RA, Ewaski B. *Gait Training Protocol.* Minneapolis, MN: Medtronic, Inc; 1983.

67. Cleeland CS. Behavioral techniques in the modification of spasmodic torticollis. *Neurology.* 1973;23:1241–1247.

68. Hudzinski LG, Zebrick LA. *Use of portable electromyographs and faradic shock in determining and treating chronic nocturnal bruxism.* Abstracts of papers presented at 24th annual meeting, Association for Applied Psychophysiology and Biofeedback. Wheat Ridge, CO; 1993.

69. Alders SS, Beckers D, Buck M. *PNF in Practice.* Heidelberg, Germany: Springer-Verlag; 1993.

70. McConnell JS. Management of patellofemoral problems. *Manual Ther.* 1996;1:60–66.

CHAPTER 7

SEMG and Muscle Dysfunction: Impairment Syndromes

In Chapter 2, a three-tiered surface electromyography (SEMG) assessment process was introduced. Level 1 assessment is used to determine candidacy for SEMG intervention and to identify a clinical path for SEMG procedures. Specific SEMG tests are conducted and interpreted during the level 2 assessment. SEMG profiles are constructed from a menu of possible options. Finally, level 3 assessment consists in part of assigning an impairment syndrome to the SEMG results. Designation of a syndrome category helps the therapist sort complex findings into meaningful clusters. The level 3 assessment then can be used to drive treatment planning.

The same SEMG pattern may be produced for different reasons. Figure 7–1 illustrates a hypothetical finding of elevated baseline activity of the upper trapezius. Six patients are represented, all with neck pain after a motor vehicle accident. The root cause of the muscle hyperactivity, however, is different in each case. It is important that the underlying problem be differentiated because each patient is best treated in a different way. No simple neck pain protocol would suffice across the board. A complex protocol that takes in all patient types would be time consuming, expensive, and contain elements that are unnecessary for specific patient subtypes. Greater clinical value can be obtained by linking assessment with treatment through the impairment syndromes (Figure 7–2). The model applies to any region of the body.

Use of SEMG impairment syndromes simplifies the therapist's selection of intervention procedures. Treatment is planned in a rational way for any patient. The syndrome scheme provides a structure for clinical reasoning without imposing rigid protocols on multivariate problems. Fundamentally, the therapist treats what is found, adapting the procedures to meet the unique needs of each patient.

Eight impairment syndromes involving aberrant motor activity are proposed (Exhibit 7–1). The syndromes are not mutually exclusive, nor is the scope exhaustive. Patients may exhibit some of or all the qualities of one of or all the syndromes. The reader is referred to Chapter 1 for a detailed discussion of the pathologic mechanisms subserving each syndrome, Chapter 2 for particulars on the evaluation profiles, and Chapters 5 and 6 for specifics regarding feedback training procedures.

IMPAIRMENT SYNDROMES

Psychophysiologic, Stress-Related Hyperactivity

Recognition of this syndrome emerged from early studies of relaxation training.[1–4] Relaxation with physiologic feedback modalities was, and continues to be, used to address psychologic stress-based disorders. The focus is on establishing voluntary control of autonomic function. An underlying construct is that certain cognitions

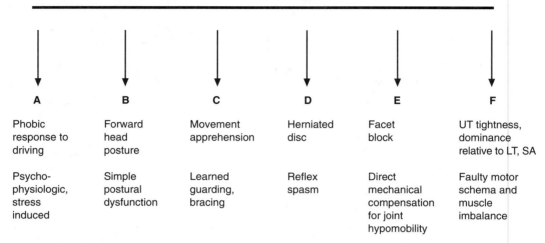

Figure 7–1 Potential causes of elevated upper trapezius (UT) electromyographic activity in six patients (A–F) after motor vehicle accident. Lower trapezius (LT); serratus anterior (SA).

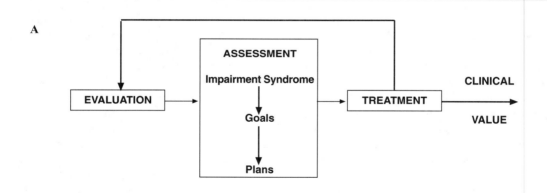

Figure 7–2 (**A**) Relationships among evaluation, assessment, treatment, and clinical value. (**B**) Clinical value equation.

and affective states lead to autonomic arousal and increased muscle tone (Figure 7–3). Stress-relaxation models are incorporated as fundamental concepts in physiologic feedback training programs as well as in books on the topic.[5–10] Musculoskeletal dysfunction may coexist, but behavioral/cognitive intervention of some sort is warranted. The ideas continue to receive a great deal of experimental attention, and it has been suggested recently that effects of the sympathetic nervous system may be mediated through the muscle spindle apparatus.[11–15]

Exhibit 7–1 SEMG-Related Impairment Syndromes

- psychophysiologic, stress-related hyperactivity
- postural dysfunction
- weakness/deconditioning
- reflex spasm/inhibition
- learned guarding/bracing
- learned inhibition
- chronic compensation for joint hypermobility/hypomobility
- faulty motor schema and muscle imbalance

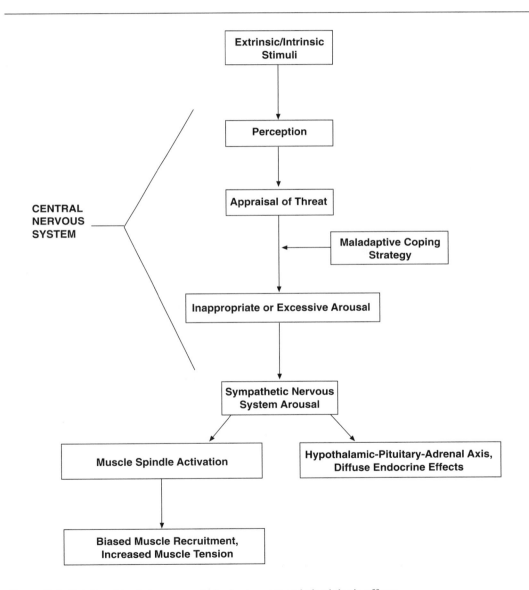

Figure 7–3 Relationships between psychologic stressors and physiologic effects.

Psychophysiologic, Stress-Related Hyperactivity

Identification
- SEMG activity shows discrete, diffuse, or global hyperactivity.*
- Hyperactivity
  1. varies with emotional arousal
  2. precedes onset or exacerbation of pain
- Psychophysiologic stress profile shows positive findings.
- Examination findings are otherwise relatively unremarkable.

Treatment Goals
- Decouple muscle tension responses from cognitions.
- Resolve or mediate key psychologic issues.
- Facilitate self-efficacy and an internal health locus of control.
- Resolve functional limitations and social role disabilities.

General Plans
- behavioral/cognitive psychotherapy
- wellness counseling (as indicated):
  1. exercise
  2. nutrition
  3. posture
  4. body mechanics
  5. activity pacing
  6. stress management.
- SEMG feedback training
  1. general muscle relaxation–based downtraining
  2. specific muscle isolation training
  3. specific muscle threshold–based downtraining
  4. tension recognition threshold training
  5. tension discrimination training
  6. deactivation training
  7. generalization methods for functional situations, for example:
     –systematic desensitization
     –mental rehearsal
     –rational/affirmative self-talk
     –relaxation trigger words, images, hand positions

Case Example
   A 44-year-old female presents for evaluation 4 months after sustaining a cervical whiplash injury in a rear-end motor vehicle accident. She no longer has pain with routine activities, with the exception of driving. Physical examination findings are benign. She volunteers that she feels anxious while driving and notes feelings of tension about the neck and shoulders. These sensations progress to stiffness and pain. Symptoms abate over a period of several hours once driving is concluded. Baseline SEMG activity recorded from cervical and suprascapular regions is unremarkable. Activity remains uneventful during performance of pressured mental arithmetic but markedly increases while the patient generates imagery related to driving. Counseling is provided for a rational cognitive interpretation of events associated with driving. SEMG feedback is combined with relaxation training, tension recognition, and systematic desensitization techniques. Over the following weeks, she learns to decouple muscle tension from stressors, and her phobic response resolves.

---

   *Discrete refers to a particular muscle or muscle group; diffuse, to several adjacent muscles within a particular topographic region; and global, to multiple muscles across topographic regions of the body.

Postural Dysfunction

With this syndrome, aberrant motor activity varies as a function of posture. The syndrome may occur in conjunction with other syndromes, but in its pure form, there is nothing else wrong. Pain probably results from untoward loading of articular structures and chronic ligament stretch. McKenzie[16] likens this to the discomfort caused by bending back one's finger for a long period. Over time, though, the involved joint segments become subject to degenerative mechanical disease and muscle imbalances.[17–22] Muscle length–tension relationships become inefficient with poor posture. Also, load moments are increased by lengthening the lever arm through which gravity acts on kinetic segments. Normal force couples are disrupted as some muscles recruit at an increased level while the antagonists are relieved of their normal contribution. Movement that proceeds from a poor postural foundation is bound to be inefficient. For example, increased cervical paraspinal activity is readily noted from patients in forward head postures (Figure 7–4). Postural effects on SEMG activity have been reported for patients with headache, cervical and upper quadrant dysfunction, and low back problems.[6,23–27]

Weakness, Deconditioning

Muscle function problems may result from radiculopathies, plexopathies, neuropathies, myopathies, and central neuromotor diseases. This syndrome, however, involves individuals without neurologic or myopathic disease who have become impaired because of simple muscle disuse. This disuse may be related to immobilization after injury or surgery or the cumulative effect of poor motor habits and decreased general activity. The situation involves atrophic loss of muscle cross-sectional area, inefficient vascularization, and compromised biochemical and physiologic function.[28–32] There are also changes

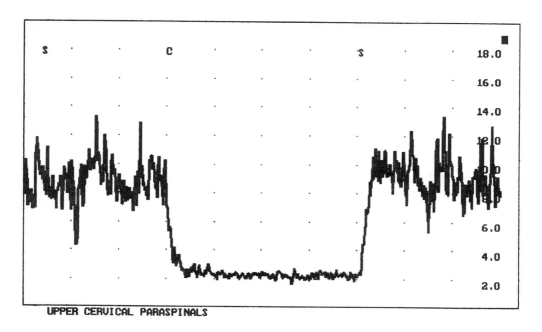

UPPER CERVICAL PARASPINALS

Figure 7–4 SEMG activity of the upper cervical paraspinal muscles recorded during a patient's spontaneous forward head posture (**S**) and corrected postural alignment (**C**).

Postural Dysfunction

Identification

- Intake is notable for apparent poor posture, ergonomic setup, and activity pacing.
- SEMG activity shows discrete or diffuse hyperactivity (less often, discrete hypoactivity—eg, passively suspended on ligaments with an accentuated thoracic kyphosis).*
- Aberrant SEMG activity varies with posture.
- Stereotyped responses occur on posture repetition.
- Other than above, SEMG activity is uneventful.

Treatment Goals

- Improve posture and associated joint, soft tissue dysfunction.
- Resolve functional limitations and social role disabilities.

General Plans

- postural training with SEMG feedback as an adjunct
- generalization cues, ergonomics assist, activity pacing
- correction of associated myofascial, joint mobility imbalances as required
- reassessment with SEMG

Case Example

A 44-year-old female physician complains of headaches and low back pain that start in the afternoon and build through the remainder of the work day. Symptoms tend to be worse on days during which she stands for long periods. Static posture shows diminished lumbar lordosis, increased thoracic kyphosis, and protracted head and shoulder girdles. SEMG activity is markedly elevated at cervical and lumbar paraspinal sites (Figure 7–5). After the therapist instructs her to raise the sternum, SEMG amplitudes fall dramatically. She is instructed to monitor and correct her posture throughout the day. Her symptoms rapidly decrease over the following weeks. The single visit is the only therapy-related expense.

It is worth noting that the therapist would instruct the patient in postural correction even without recording SEMG activity. The difference is that with SEMG recording the therapist develops a high degree of confidence that posture is a contributory factor and that correction likely will be an important issue. Using SEMG feedback, the patient also sees this relationship and becomes motivated to comply with the instruction.

---

*Discrete refers to a particular muscle or muscle group, whereas diffuse refers to several adjacent muscles within a particular topographic region.

in neural drive that accompany muscle-conditioning levels.[33,34] In all likelihood, both central and peripheral factors contribute to the decreased SEMG activity seen during maximal effort contractions. Other impairments include weakness on manual muscle testing, decrements in peak torque, power deficits (inabilities to sustain force through range of motion arcs), and lowered endurance. Muscular endurance can be assessed by analyzing the frequency content of SEMG signals. Frequency spectral decrements have been implicated in chronic neck[35] and low back pain.[36,37]

Reflex Spasm/Inhibition

Spasm is involuntary hypertonicity induced by reflex systems.[38–42] Muscle tone is increased through central mechanisms that respond to noxious mechanical and chemical stimulation in the periphery.[43–48] Inhibition is a neurologic suppression of muscle activity. Reflexive inhibition occurs because of pain and joint effusion.[49–57] An active inflammatory response is implied with either reflexive inhibition or spasm. Active trigger points have also been proposed as a causative factor of hypertonicity or hypotonicity, depend-

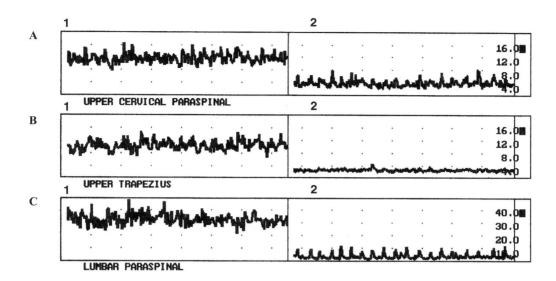

Figure 7–5 SEMG activity of the upper cervical paraspinals, upper trapezius, and lumbar paraspinals from a patient with chronic headaches and low back pain. (**A1, B1, C1**) Activity of respective muscles with patient in spontaneous standing posture. (**A2, B2, C2**) Activity of respective muscles with correction of patient's posture by gentle elevation of sternum.

Weakness, Deconditioning

Identification

- Weakness is seen on manual muscle testing, and decrements in peak torque, power, and endurance are observed on isokinetic and functional tests.
- Atrophy and decreased limb girth may be observed.
- Peak SEMG amplitude is decreased during maximal volitional isometric contraction.
- During submaximal contractions, SEMG activity shows
  1. hypoactivity
  2. symmetry
  3. hyperactivity
     variable, depending on severity, chronicity, and contraction type and intensity. Hypoactivity can exist with maximal volitional contractions; symmetry, with light tasks; and hyperactivity, with activities requiring moderate effort.
- Roughly symmetric muscle recruitment and decruitment timing occurs during light to moderate contraction tasks.
- Compared with the noninvolved homologue, the involved side shows a greater decrease in the plot of SEMG median frequency versus time during sustained, high-intensity contraction.

Treatment Goals

- Restore normal strength, power, endurance.
- Integrate gains with purposeful movements.
- Resolve functional limitations and social role disabilities.

General Plans
- treatment of associated musculoskeletal dysfunction
- exercise prescription
- SEMG feedback training
  1. muscle isolation training
  2. threshold-based uptraining—isometric and during range of motion
  3. generalization to progressively dynamic movement
  4. motor copy training
  5. SEMG-triggered neuromuscular electrical stimulation
  6. integration with functional activities

Case Example

A 62-year-old female is seen following 6 weeks of knee immobilization and restricted weight bearing after sustaining a leg fracture. There is decreased limb girth due to quadriceps atrophy, as well as restricted range of motion, decreased strength on manual muscle testing, and impaired functional mobility. Maximal effort isometric SEMG activity is decreased on the involved side. However, submaximal dynamic contractions are associated with increased activity, presumably reflecting decreased neuromuscular efficiency (Figure 7–6). SEMG feedback is used during the initial stages of exercise prescription and training. Objectives include maximizing neural drive and teaching appropriate exercise technique. The patient makes rapid gains in strength assessed with manual muscle tests, and SEMG feedback is discontinued. She continues with a home exercise program and functional activity progression.

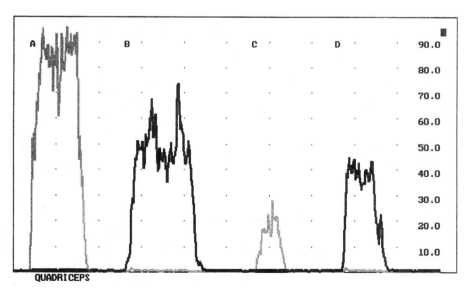

Figure 7–6 SEMG activity from the left (black) and right (gray) quadriceps recorded from a patient with muscle impairments after fracture and immobilization of the left lower extremity. (**A**) Maximal effort, right isometric quadriceps set. (**B**) Maximal effort, left isometric quadriceps set. (**C**) Right terminal knee extension from hooklying with a bolster under the distal thighs and 7-lb cuff weight affixed to the ankle. (**D**) Left terminal knee extension from hooklying with a bolster under the distal thighs and a 7-lb cuff weight affixed to the ankle. Maximal effort activity is asymmetrically decreased on the left, but asymmetrically increased on the left for the equivalent submaximal task.

ing on the involved muscle.[58,59] Reflex changes may be produced with acute injuries or chronic cumulative strain and recurrent trauma.

Learned Guarding/Bracing

Guarding or bracing is heightened muscle activity that is a learned response to pain occurring on movement or postural loading. Responses are performed in an attempt to avoid pain and perceived potential further injury. Muscle hyperactivity is used to stiffen joints against possible displacement into a painful range. Protective guarding has long been discussed as a dysfunctional response to injury[60] and has been a core

---

Reflex Spasm/Inhibition

Identification

- SEMG activity shows discrete or diffuse hyperactivity, discrete hypoactivity.*
- SEMG baseline activity may show exceptional magnitude and variance if hyperactive.
- SEMG frequency spectrum may be unusually broad if hyperactive.
- Stereotyped aberrant responses occur with
    1. all activating movements.
    2. passive stretch
    3. (potentially) non–weight-bearing rest.
- Syndrome
    1. is associated with
        –clear signs of trauma
        –decreased range of motion or increased range or motion/instability
        –joint accessory motion dysfunction
    2. may be associated with active trigger points
- Findings on SEMG are well correlated with patient's subjective reports of symptom exacerbation.

Treatment Goals

- Restore normal tonus.
- Resolve acute injury or effects of cumulative trauma.
- Resolve functional limitations and social role disabilities.

General Plans

- adjunctive therapies:
    1. rest/therapeutic exercise prescription
    2. orthosis
    3. physical agents
    4. manual therapies
    5. medications
- reassessment with SEMG
- preventative long-term counseling (as indicated):
    1. exercise
    2. nutrition
    3. posture
    4. body mechanics
    5. ergonomics
    6. activity pacing
    7. workplace domestic, recreational/athletic safety

Case Examples

1:

A 32-year-old male presents with severe low back pain and history of a weight-bearing trunk flexion injury. Static posture is flexed and laterally shifted, with visibly and palpably elevated lumbar paraspinal tone and poor sitting tolerance. Presence of a severely herniated disc is confirmed by radiographic findings. SEMG activity appears markedly elevated and asymmetric, higher on the side opposite to the shift (Figure 7–7). It is believed that SEMG feedback training for tone reduction is pointless; therefore, it is not attempted. The patient does respond to manipulation, positioning, and lumbar extension exercises, which are presumed to help reduce the disk herniation.

2:

A 27-year-old female reports knee pain and swelling after catching an edge on rough ice and falling while skiing. Physical examination reveals knee effusion and severe anterior cruciate ligament laxity. SEMG activity from the quadriceps on the involved side is depressed relative to the contralateral side during a partial squat task (Figure 7–8). Surgical intervention is chosen to repair the anterior cruciate ligament, followed by a rehabilitation program.

3:

A 55-year-old male complains of exacerbated right scapular and arm pain 10 weeks after aggressively increasing push-up repetitions during his exercise routine. Sleep and functional activities are significantly disrupted. Symptoms are reproduced by palpation of trigger points along the right medial scapular border. SEMG activity over the right mid-trapezius/rhomboid region is increased relative to that from the left side during shoulder elevation or push-up tasks (Figure 7–9). Pain is reduced, and SEMG responses approach symmetry after treatment with transcutaneus electrical nerve stimulation, manual soft tissue mobilization, and stretching. He is then counseled for gradual exercise progression. Stretching and other strengthening exercises are prescribed for balanced muscle training.

---

*Discrete refers to a particular muscle or muscle group, whereas diffuse refers to several adjacent muscles within a particular topographic region.

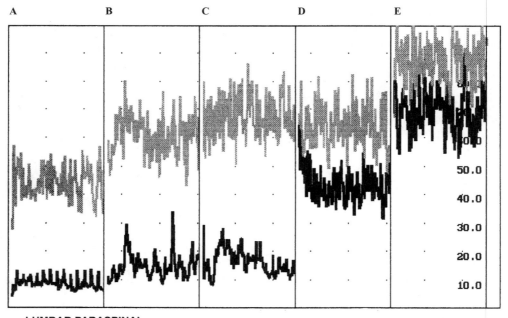

LUMBAR PARASPINAL

Figure 7–7 SEMG activity from the left (black) and right (gray) lumbar paraspinal muscles recorded from a patient with a herniated disc; severe right low back and lower extremity pain; and flexed, left lateral postural shift. (**A**) Supine with hips and knees comfortably bent and lower extremities supported on pillows. (**B**) Supine with lower extremities straight. (**C**) Prone. (**D**) Sitting in chair with lumbar support. (**E**) Standing. Lumbar hyperactivity and asymmetry change in magnitude but persist in all positions.

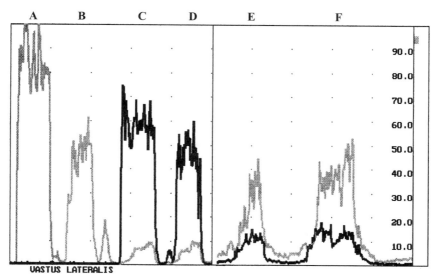

Figure 7–8 SEMG activity of the left (black) and right (gray) vastus lateralis recorded from a patient with an injured left anterior cruciate ligament. (**A**) Non–weight-bearing, straight knee, maximal effort isometric quadriceps set right. (**B**) Non–weight-bearing, bent knee, maximal effort isometric quadriceps set right. (**C**) Non–weight-bearing, straight knee, maximal effort isometric quadriceps set left. (**D**) Non–weight-bearing, bent knee, maximal effort isometric quadriceps set left. (**E**) and (**F**) Bilateral partial squat, equal lower extremity weight-bearing monitored with a scale under each of the patient's feet. Activity from left side appears inhibited relative to that seen on the right in weight-bearing, as well as in non–weight-bearing with an extended knee.

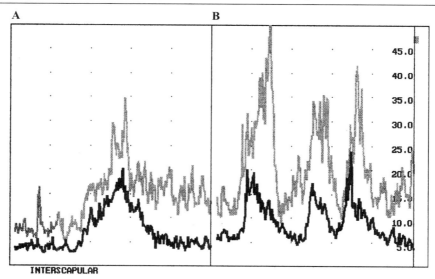

Figure 7–9 SEMG activity of left (black) and right (gray) interscapular muscles recorded from a patient with right periscapular and arm pain. (**A**) Bilateral simultaneous symmetric arm abduction. (**B**) Three repetitions of standard floor push-ups; each left/right set of peaks corresponds to one repetition. Muscle activity on the right side is consistently elevated above that on the left side during all movements. Also note the failure to recover to baseline amplitude after abduction on the right (**A**) and altered timing pattern on the right during push-ups (**B**).

underpinning for diagnostic models used by practitioners who work with SEMG feedback.[23,61,62] In some cases involving complex behavioral dysfunction, guarding responses may be performed to declare pain and disability. Abnormal posturing becomes a pain behavior, a vehicle for communicating distress.[63] Diffuse, compensatory, or seemingly illogical SEMG patterns can result.

This syndrome may be closely related to the psychophysiologic, stress-related hyperactivity syndrome discussed earlier. The key distinction is that stress-related hyperactivity leads to muscle hyperactivity, which in turn causes the discomfort. With guarding, fear occurs in response to potentially painful movement, and muscle hyperactivity is a learned compensation.

Learned Inhibition

In rare cases, individuals learn to inhibit motor activity to avoid pain, a concept similar but opposite in direction to guarding/bracing. These individuals perceive that muscle activation results in pain, and pain implies tissue damage. This belief induces patients to avoid muscle activation. Patients then alter patterns of functional activity to evade contraction. The learn-

---

Learned Guarding/Bracing

Identification

- SEMG activity shows diffuse or global hyperactivity, potentially marked magnitude and erratic variance.*
- With unilateral involvement, SEMG hyperactivity may be ipsilateral to the painful side or bilateral.
- Marked agonist/antagonist co-contraction tends to be displayed.
- Syndrome is
  1. associated with decreased range of motion and a non-fluid, potentially "ratchety" movement quality
  2. accompanied by verbal and nonverbal pain behaviors
- SEMG baseline activity increases with anticipated movement.
- Hyperactivity
  1. persists from weight-bearing to non–weight-bearing movement, active range of motion or passive stretch; sharp increase in SEMG amplitude and co-contraction occurs with increased velocity
  2. varies with emotional arousal
- Movement repetition elicits nonstereotyped SEMG responses.
- Aberrant SEMG patterns are ameliorated by cognitive, behavioral attempts for relaxation and improved fluidity.

Treatment Goals

- Restore normal tonus.
- Resolve anticipatory movement anxiety, facilitate movement confidence and an internal health locus of control.
- Restore normal range, fluid movement.
- Resolve functional limitations and social role disabilities.

General Plans

- treatment of underlying musculoskeletal, psychologic issues
- exercise prescription, movement re-education, exercise and functional activity quotas
- SEMG feedback training
  1. general relaxation-based training
  2. specific muscle isolation and relaxation
  3. tension discrimination training
  4. deactivation training

5. threshold-based downtraining during
   –passive static stretch
   –passive range of motion
   –active range of motion
6. generalization to progressive dynamic tasks
7. integration with functional activities

In extreme cases, SEMG feedback work may reinforce guarding and other pain behaviors and should be deferred until later in the treatment course.

Case Example

A 42-year-old male presents with chronic right cervical, suprascapular, and interscapular pain after sustaining a work injury while lifting heavy piping for overhead installation. Resting SEMG activity appears diffusely elevated over all recording sites (Figure 7–10A). Activity increases further while the therapist gives instructions for movement testing, but before any actual movement takes place. Test results for range of motion show decreased excursion, impaired quality, and marked co-contraction around the shoulder complex. Activity patterns improve after the patient is educated regarding healing processes, breathing and feedback relaxation techniques, and gentle progressive movement. In Figure 7–10B, improvement is demonstrated by lowered baseline activity and decreased left/right co-activation during movement. Amplitudes of the right side muscles are increased because the excursion of motion is greater.

---

*Diffuse refers to several adjacent muscles within a particular topographic region, whereas global refers to multiple muscles across topographic regions of the body.

A

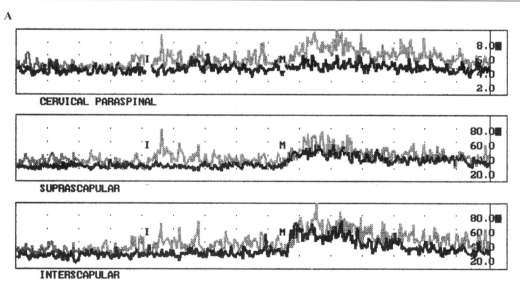

continues

Figure 7–10 SEMG activity from left (black) and right (gray) cervical paraspinal, suprascapular, and interscapular sites recorded from a patient with chronic right cervical, suprascapular, and interscapular pain. (**A**) At (**I**), the patient is told that he will be asked to abduct the right arm, and the abduction motion is demonstrated by a therapist. The patient initiates abduction movement at (**M**). Note the increase in right side activity during the instruction period, before any movement begins, as well as left side coactivation during right side movement. (**B**) Three repetitions of right arm abduction at a later date. Baseline activity is reduced, muscle activation and deactivation are promptly coupled to actual movement, and right side coactivation is nearly eliminated. Overall, the signals are smoother and look less erratic.

Figure 7–10 continued

B

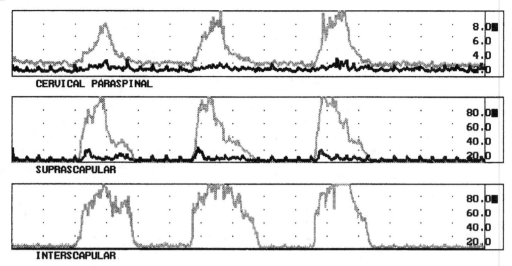

ing process seems to proceed subconsciously in some persons. Over time, they believe that the muscle "just doesn't work." Continuation of the syndrome results in atrophy and increased vulnerability of myofascial tissue to repeated injury. Exacerbation of pain reinforces the dysfunctional perception–belief–behavior–injury cycle. In very rare instances, individuals present with hysterical weakness as a manifestation of serious psychopathology. Hysterical weakness is a different and much more difficult problem.

Chronic Compensation for Joint Hypermobility/Hypomobility

In this syndrome, dysfunctional SEMG activity occurs as a consequence of chronic joint hypermobility or hypomobility. The neuromuscular system compensates by attempting to stabilize lax joint structures, effecting movement against joint stiffness, or subserving linked compensatory movements over kinetic chains.[64–68] Although SEMG activity is aberrant, the pri-

---

Learned Inhibition

Identification

- SEMG activity shows discrete or diffuse hypoactivity.*
- Marked muscle weakness can be seen.
- No current, identifiable anatomic or physiologic lesion can be identified through physical examination, radiographic testing, or medical electrodiagnostic testing to explain the observed weakness.
- Hypoactivity persists across all test procedures involving volitional muscle activation.
- Nonstereotypic responses occur during volitional muscle activation as compared to reflexive activation (eg, induced by unanticipated postural perturbation).
- Patients with hysterical weakness may additionally show
  1. inconsistent responses during formal testing, compared with informal observation
  2. nonanatomic aberrant responses
  3. grossly inappropriate affect, thought, and judgment
  4. positive hysterical profiles on psychometric testing

Treatment Goals
- Restore normal muscle recruitment and movement.
- Resolve movement anxiety, facilitate movement confidence and an internal health locus of control.
- Address psychologic dysfunction.
- Resolve functional limitations and social role disabilities.

General Plans
- treatment of any associated musculoskeletal dysfunction
- cognitive, behavioral support
- exercise prescription, movement re-education, exercise and functional activity quotas
- SEMG feedback training:
  1. muscle isolation training
  2. threshold-based uptraining—isometric and during active range of motion
  3. tension discrimination training
  4. motor copy training
  5. SEMG-triggered neuromuscular electrical stimulation
  6. generalization to progressively dynamic movement
  7. integration with functional activities

Case Example

An otherwise healthy 31-year-old male aeronautical engineer sustains recurrent strain of the right hip adductor muscles while playing racquetball. The pain becomes severe whenever the adductor muscles contract during functional activities. He learns how to get in and out of his bed or car with less adductor activity, modify the way he turns away from a urinal, and get up from the floor and engage in play with his children differently. His movement deviations are subtle and tend not to be recognized by others. There is no time loss from work, although recreational athletics are curtailed. His problem proves refractory to multiple therapeutic interventions, and there is no ready explanation from clinical examination, extensive radiologic studies, or intramuscular EMG evaluation. He scores in a relatively unremarkable fashion on somatization and hysteria psychometric scales. Adductor SEMG amplitude from the involved side appears decreased while he walks and markedly so during sustained unilateral stance or lunging. Right side SEMG activity is depressed with right adductor manual muscle testing, whereas left side activity is well preserved with left side testing (Figure 7–11). However, SEMG activity is bilaterally decreased when left and right adductor groups are simultaneously resisted. The effect is quite reproducible and persists despite coaching to recruit the right side. Pain is present but subjectively reported as mild. Anatomically, the problem must represent a centrally mediated reflex or learned phenomenon. The adductors are next seen to recruit to a level that exceeds voluntary activation when the patient's balance is suddenly disrupted. Thus the muscles are recruited with postural reactions to help prevent a fall. Inconsistent activation patterns are also observed with novel exercise equipment and cross-over stepping sequences, especially if there are simultaneous cognitive distractions. After reassurance, education, and 2 weeks of home SEMG-triggered neuromuscular electrical stimulation, he produces symmetric and robust adductor SEMG activity during all the same tasks. Symptoms gradually resolve with exercise and functional activity progression over the next few months.

---

*Discrete refers to a particular muscle or muscle group, whereas diffuse refers to several adjacent muscles within a particular topographic region.

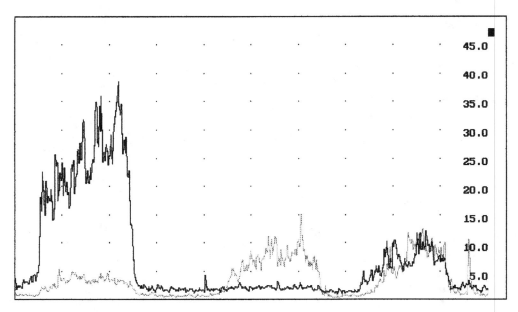

Figure 7–11 SEMG activity of the left (black) and right (gray) hip adductor muscles recorded from a patient with chronic right adductor strain and groin pain. Resisted left hip adduction (first peak) produces a robust signal response. Resisted right side hip adduction (second peak) produces a weak signal response. Simultaneous, bilaterally resisted hip adduction (third set of peaks) produces a bilaterally weak signal response.

mary problem is a biomechanical articular fault. The articular dysfunction causes a compensatory motor control pattern, which may spontaneously resolve on improvement in joint mechanics. In these cases, SEMG training is not the first choice of treatment. The joint dysfunction should be addressed first, followed by reassessment of SEMG activity.

Faulty Motor Schema and Muscle Imbalance

This eighth and final syndrome takes in all seven other syndromes. It results from their perpetuation and amalgamation over time. Muscle imbalance occurs when the relative stiffness of two or more muscles that participate in a con-

---

Chronic Compensation for Joint Hypermobility/Hypomobility

Identification
- SEMG activity
  1. shows discrete hyperactivity, inappropriate timing patterns*
  2. persists despite all cognitive, behavioral attempts to decrease it
  3. does not vary directly with emotional arousal, movement anticipation
- Stereotyped aberrant responses occur on movement repetition.
- Syndrome is associated with
  1. decreased joint range of motion or increased range of motion/instability
  2. specific joint accessory motion dysfunction

- Onset and duration of aberrant SEMG activity occur coincidentally with provocative range of motion arc but are not necessarily correlated with primary pain distribution.
- Aberrant SEMG activity varies as a function of
  1. weight bearing
  2. extrinsic joint load
  3. closed versus open kinetic chain function
  4. active versus passive range of motion
  5. movement velocity

  That is, aberrant activity changes with conditions that vary joint load and position.
- Volitional muscle control and tension awareness are unremarkable when joint load is minimized (eg, with low-intensity isometric contractions in a stable, pain-free joint position). SEMG activity associated with maximal effort isometric contractions also may be symmetric and otherwise unremarkable if they are generated in a stable, pain-free joint position.
- Aberrant SEMG patterns are ameliorated by specific joint mobilization or stabilization procedures.

Treatment Goals
- Restore normal arthokinematics (small accessory motions at the joint surfaces), osteokinematics (displacement of bones about joints), and muscle synergies.
- Resolve functional limitations and social role disabilities.

General Plans
- stretching or stabilizing of joint segment, as indicated, through
  1. manual therapies
  2. therapeutic exercise
  3. preparatory physical agents
  4. orthosis
- instruction in
  1. joint protection principles
  2. postures
  3. body mechanics
  4. ergonomics
  5. activity pacing
  6. nutrition
  7. workplace/athletic technique
- reassessment of SEMG activity

Case Example

A 52-year-old female with chronic left jaw pain displays hypomobility at the left temporomandibular joint (TMJ). The midpoint of the mandible deviates to the left during opening and closing, and there is a palpable difference between the arthrokinematic motions of left and right mandibular condyles. As opening is initiated, both condyles are felt to spin in place. The left condyle is then felt to translate a shorter anterior distance (relative to the right) as opening continues. Protrusion and manual distraction of the joint are also limited and painful on the left. SEMG activity shows greater recruitment of the right masseter compared to the left masseter during jaw opening/closing range of motion (Figure 7–12). The right mandibular condyle translates a greater distance than the left along the articular surface of the zygomatic process. Thus it is speculated that the right masseter is recruited to a larger degree than the left to subserve the greater range of motion. The fundamental problem, however, is not one of right greater than left masseter SEMG activity, but of left less than right joint mobility. SEMG activity becomes symmetric once the left TMJ is mobilized with manual techniques and exercise.

---

*Discrete refers to a particular muscle or muscle group.

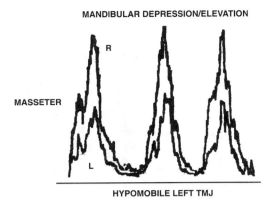

Figure 7–12 SEMG activity of the left (L) and right (R) masseter muscles recorded from a patient with chronic left TMJ pain during three repetitions of jaw opening/closing. Decreased left side muscle activity was associated with hypomobility of the left joint appreciated by manual examination.

certed way to execute a specific movement are inappropriately coordinated. Inefficient patterns of muscle stiffness arise from both passive and active tensile factors. These include passive myofascial length, active force-generating ability related to length–tension relationships and intrinsic muscle factors, psychologic variables, and faulty central nervous system motor programming. This last issue becomes the focus for this syndrome. Schmidt's motor schema theory[69–72] was discussed in Chapter 3, and its tenets play into this syndrome. According to this view, the elements of motor programs that specify phasing relationships between muscles, as well as their proportionate contraction intensities, are fixed for particular movements. Movement velocity and amplitude may vary, but the relationships between the muscles are preserved. Prototypic programming rules for phasing and proportionate intensity become subverted in this syndrome. Clinically, the normal magnitude and timing among agonists, antagonists, and synergists are disturbed. Each muscle

generates too much or too little force at particular portions of the range of motion arc. As a result, muscles co-contract when they should not, fail to fire in a synchronous manner when they should, or otherwise function disproportionately out of phase. Inefficient motor plans are put into place, and they continue as a matter of course even after the original insult is resolved (Figure 7–13). There are now lasting problems with motor response selection and programming, regardless of the starting point. With the other seven impairment syndromes, the expression of a motor control problem is secondary to a distinct peripheral factor. In this syndrome, central processing becomes a primary problem in its own right. Treatment focuses on neuromuscular re-education, along with therapies for coincident joint segment and soft tissue dysfunction as well as cognitive/behavioral issues.

GUIDELINES FOR USE OF IMPAIRMENT SYNDROMES

The classification system outlined in this chapter is intended as a starting point for treatment. Syndrome schemes should be integrated with "best practice" care standards as defined by each clinician's scope of practice. A team approach among care providers is required to implement the more involved plans. Some of the syndromes may seem to blend together and be indistinguishable in certain persons. In those situations, the treatment plans suggested for each of the involved syndromes may be combined. Use of any one of the suggested treatment plans does not countermand the others. Application sequences may need to be prioritized differently to reflect the idiosyncrasies of each case. Table 7–1 summarizes hallmarks for syndrome identification. Treatment approaches for each syndrome are outlined in Table 7–2. Directed programs for specific body regions and clinical problems are provided in Chapters 8–13.

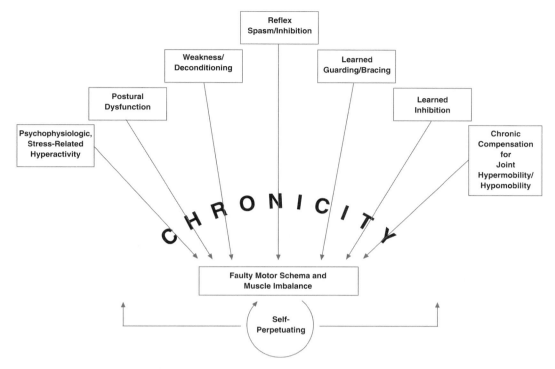

Figure 7–13 Factors contributing to the development of faulty motor schema and muscle imbalance.

Faulty Motor Schema and Muscle Imbalance

Identification
- SEMG activity
  1. shows discrete hyperactivity or discrete hypoactivity, inappropriate timing*
  2. shows premature termination or incomplete or delayed recovery to baseline during rest periods
  3. is quiescent during passive stretch until end range is approached
- Agonist–antagonist co-contraction, synergist imbalance manifests as faulty SEMG magnitude and timing patterns across recording channels.
- Aberrant SEMG activity
  1. is correlated to specific patterns of
     - muscle shortness (SEMG hyperactivity with shortened muscles)
     - muscle weakness (SEMG hypoactivity with weakened maximal effort contractions; variable hyperactivity, hypoactivity, symmetry with submaximal effort contractions)
     - inappropriate muscle dominance patterns (SEMG hyperactivity with muscles that appear to produce inappropriate muscle substitution patterns and faulty kinematics)
  2. may be associated with
     - decreased range of motion
     - increased range of motion/instability
     - joint accessory play dysfunction
     - active trigger points

3. may vary with emotional arousal as well as mechanical variables, such as
   –posture
   –load
   –velocity
   –open versus closed kinetic chain function
   –contraction as a prime mover, phasic stabilizer, or tonic postural stabilizer
4. is ameliorated by therapies that address
   –cognitive/behavioral variables
   –motor control
   –joint mobilization
   –joint stabilization

- Stereotyped aberrant responses occur on movement repetition.
- Motor control and tension awareness tend to be faulty during functional movements performed with both submaximal contractions and maximal effort.

Treatment Goals

- Restore normal agonist recruitment/decruitment timing, magnitude, endurance relative to antagonists and synergists (ie, restore normal muscle force couple relationships).
- Restore passive muscle length and myofascial balance.
- Resolve other musculoskeletal, psychologic issues.
- Resolve functional limitations and social role disabilities.

General Plans

- correction of postural faults
- instruction (as indicated) in appropriate
  1. body mechanics
  2. ergonomics
  3. nutrition
  4. activity pacing
  5. stress management
- addressing of joint and soft tissue passive mobility problems with
  1. stretching
  2. manual therapies
  3. adjunctive physical agents
  4. temporary orthosis
- active exercise, movement re-education
- SEMG feedback training:
  1. muscle isolation training
  2. tension recognition training/tension discrimination training
  3. threshold-based uptraining/downtraining
  4. deactivation training
  5. left/right equilibration training
  6. motor copy training
  7. SEMG-triggered neuromuscular electrical stimulation
  8. generalization from static training to progressively dynamic movement with appropriate agonist, antagonist, synergist relationships
  9. postural training, body mechanics instruction, and exercise instruction with SEMG feedback
  10. functional activity modification with SEMG feedback

Case Example

A 35-year-old male is seen with chronic unilateral headaches, neck pain, and shoulder pain of insidious onset. Symptoms are exacerbated by lifting activities at work and playing basketball. He has no pain with a single repetition of any task. Discomfort cumulatively arises over many trials and then limits performance. During bilateral symmetric shoulder flexion, the peak SEMG amplitude of the symptomatic right side upper trapezius is increased, whereas activity of the right lower serratus anterior is decreased, each respectively to its homologous mate (Figure 7–14). The serratus anterior is also slower to increase activity on the involved side through an equivalent left/right range of motion arc. These findings are associated with passive tightness of the upper trapezius and weakness of the serratus anterior on manual muscle testing. Upper trapezius levator scapulae, and rhomboid bulk seem hypertrophied on the symptomatic side. Total shoulder range of motion is roughly symmetric. With close visual inspection, however, differences in the pattern of scapular displacement between the two sides are observed. The scapula on the symptomatic side appears to elevate more and abduct and rotate cephalad less. Accessory joint play testing is without provocation through the shoulder girdle, cervical and thoracic spine, and ribs. Emotional stressors increase symptoms if they are already flared but are otherwise without effect. The patient shows poor abilities to recognize muscle tension and isolate SEMG signals on the involved side. Using feedback, he learns to isolate the SEMG activity of the serratus anterior from the other scapular muscles. Exercises are identified that selectively facilitate the serratus anterior, and those movements are incorporated into a home exercise program. The patient also practices stretching the upper trapezius while minimizing SEMG activity. Recruitment of the serratus anterior is increased during overhead lifting simulations for work and sports. The patient corrects ergonomic alignment at work, learns to recognize and ameliorate the effects of emotional stressors, and trains with a coach to improve basketball shooting skills. Symptoms resolve, and there are no further recurrences during ad libitum performance of functional activities.

*Discrete refers to a particular muscle or muscle group.

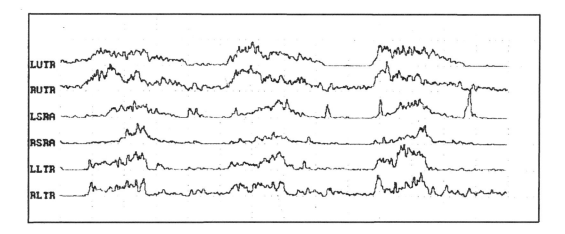

Figure 7–14 SEMG activity from the left (**L**) and right (**R**) upper trapezius (UTR), lower serratus anterior (SRA), and lower trapezius (LTR), recorded from a patient with right side headaches, neck pain, and shoulder pain during three repetitions of bilateral symmetric shoulder flexion. During the concentric portion of the motion, corresponding to leading half of each set of peaks, there is a tendency for increased right upper trapezius activity and decreased/delayed serratus anterior activity.

Table 7-1 Summary of Hallmarks in SEMG Impairment Syndromes

SEMG Impairment Syndromes	Variations with Emotional Arousal	Variations with Movement	Stereotyped	Diffuse Hyperactivity	Discrete Hyperactivity	Discrete/Diffuse Hypoactivity	Frank Joint Restriction/Instability	Variations in Active Range of Motion vs Passive Range of Motion Weight Bearing vs Non–Weight Bearing	Asymmetric Maximal Effort Isometric Activity	Other
Psychophysiologic, Stress-Related Hyperactivity	×			×	×					Positive findings on psychophysiologic stress profile; Apparent life stressors on examination
Postural Dysfunction		×	×	×	×	×		×		Apparent poor posture, ergonomic setup, activity pacing
Weakness/Deconditioning		×	×		×	×			×	History of deconditioning; Decreased strength, bulk; Increased frequency spectral changes

	Reflexive Spasm/Inhibition	Learned Guarding/Bracing	Learned Inhibition	Chronic Compensation for Joint Hypermobility/Hypomobility	Faulty Motor Schema and Muscle Imbalance
Associated with clear signs and history of acute or cumulatively acute trauma	×	×	×		×
Nonfluid movement quality	×			×	×
Marked agonist/antagonist co-contraction, often bilaterally	×	×		×	×
Increased activity with movement anticipation	×		×		×
Nonstereotypic responses—volitional vs reflexive activation or postural perturbation	×			×	×
No current identifiable anatomic lesion or physiologic dysfunction that explains symptoms		×		×	×
Good tension recognition and control when joint load is minimized	×			×	×
Resolution with joint mobilization/stabilization	×	×	×	×	×
Emphasis on faulty agonist/antagonist/synergist relationships	×	×	×		×
Chronic consequence of any other syndrome or independent result of pain/myofascial dysfunction		×	×		×

Table 7-2 Summary of Treatment Techniques for SEMG Impairment Syndromes

SEMG Impairment Syndromes	SEMG Feedback Training Techniques*												Other**
	Isolation of Target Muscle Activity	Relaxation-Based Downtraining	Threshold-Based Uptraining/Downtraining	Tension Recognition Threshold Training	Tension Discrimination Training	Deactivation Training	Generalization to Progressively Dynamic Movement	SEMG-Triggered Neuromuscular Electrical Stimulation	Left/Right Equilibration Training	Motor Copy Training	Promotion of Correct Muscle Synergies and Related Coordination Patterns	Therapeutic Exercises with SEMG Feedback	
Psychophysiologic, Stress-Related Hyperactivity	X	X	X	X	X	X							Provide behavioral/cognitive therapy; Transfer relaxation skills to functional contexts, provide generalization cues
Postural Dysfunction							X	X		X	X		Emphasize postural correction with feedback, generalization cues, activity pacing, ergonomics
Weakness/Deconditioning	X		X					X		X	X	X	Address any underlying dysfunction; Prescribe therapeutic exercises

Dysfunction	Treatment**
Reflexive Spasm/Inhibition	Treat with rest/therapeutic exercise, manual therapies, physical agents, orthosis, medications. Reassess SEMG activity if needed
Learned Guarding/Bracing	Address underlying issues. Prescribe therapeutic exercise quotas, movement re-education
Learned Inhibition	Address any underlying dysfunction. Provide behavioral support. Prescribe therapeutic exercises, quotas, movement re-education
Chronic Compensation for Joint Hypermobility/Hypomobility	Mobilize/stabilize joint. Consider manual therapies, orthosis, exercise. Instruct in work, athletics, activities of daily living technique/ergonomics
Faulty Motor Schema and Muscle Imbalance	Treat with manual therapies, physical agents, temporary orthosis. Prescribe therapeutic exercises, quotas, movement re-education. Provide behavioral support

*See Chapter 5 for details regarding SEMG feedback training techniques.
**In general, consider SEMG feedback with postural training, body mechanics instruction, functional activity modification, stress management, activity pacing, nutrition, exercise, wellness.

REFERENCES

1. Budzynski TH, Stoyva SM. An instrument for producing deep muscle relaxation by means of analog information feedback. *J Appl Behav Anal*. 1969;2:231–237.

2. Budzynski TH, Stoyva SM, Adler CS, Mullaney DJ. EMG biofeedback and tension headache: a controlled outcome study. *Psychosom Med*. 1973;35:484–496.

3. Lader MH, Matthews AH. Electromyographic studies of tension. *J Psychosom Res*. 1971;15:479–486.

4. Matthews AM, Gelder MG. Psychophysiological investigations of brief relaxation training. *Psychosom Res*. 1969;13:1–12.

5. Basmajian JV, ed. *Biofeedback: Principles and Practice for Clinicians*. 3rd ed. Baltimore: Williams & Wilkins; 1989.

6. Cram JR, ed. *Clinical EMG for Surface Recordings*. Vol 2. Nevada City, CA: Clinical Resources; 1990.

7. Gaarder KR, Montgomery PS. *Clinical Biofeedback: A Procedural Manual*. Baltimore: Williams & Wilkins; 1977.

8. Peper E, Ancoli S, Quinn M, eds. *Mind/Body Integration: Essential Readings in Biofeedback*. New York: Plenum Publishing; 1979.

9. Schwartz MS, ed. *Biofeedback: A Practitioner's Guide*. 2nd ed. New York: Guilford Press; 1995.

10. White L, Tursky B, eds. *Clinical Biofeedback: Efficacy and Mechanisms*. New York: Guilford Press; 1982.

11. Hubbard D, Berkoff G. Myofascial trigger points show spontaneous EMG activity. *Spine*. 1993;18:1803–1807.

12. Lewis C, Gervitz R, Hubbard D, Berkoff G. Needle trigger point and surface frontal EMG measurements of psychophysiological responses in tension-type headache patients. *Biofeedback Self Regul*. 1994;19:274–275.

13. McNulty W, Gervitz R, Berkoff G, Hubbard D. Needle electromyographic evaluation of trigger point response to a psychological stressor. *Psychophysiology*. 1994;31:313–316.

14. Johansson H, Sojka P. Pathophysiological mechanisms involved in genesis and spread of muscular tension in occupational muscle pain and in chronic musculoskeletal pain syndromes: a hypothesis. *Med Hypotheses*. 1991;35:196–203.

15. Selkowitz DM. The sympathetic nervous system in neuromotor function and dysfunction and pain: a brief review and discussion. *Funct Neurol*. 1992;7:89–95.

16. McKenzie RA. *The Lumbar Spine: Mechanical Diagnosis and Therapy*. Waikanae, New Zealand: Spinal Publications Limited; 1981.

17. Darnell MW. A proposed chronology of events for forward head posture. *Phys Ther*. 1983;1:50–54.

18. Greigel-Morris P, Larson K, Mueller-Klaus K, Oatis CA. Incidence of common postural abnormalities in the cervical, shoulder, and thoracic regions and their association with pain in two age groups of healthy subjects. *Phys Ther*. 1992;72:26–32.

19. Harrison AL, Barry-Greb T, Wojtowicz G. Clinical measurements of head and shoulder posture variables. *J Orthop Sports Phys Ther*. 1996;23:353–361.

20. Kendall FP, McCreary EK, Provance PG. *Muscles, Testing and Function*. Baltimore: Williams &Wilkins; 1993.

21. Rocabado M, Iglarsh ZA. *Musculoskeletal Approach to Maxillofacial Pain*. Philadelphia: JB Lippincott Co; 1991.

22. Sahrmann S. Adult posturing. In: Kraus S, ed. *TMJ Disorders: Management of the Craniomandibular Complex*. New York: Churchill Livingstone; 1988;295–310.

23. Cram JR. EMG muscle scanning and diagnostic manual for surface recordings. In: Cram J, ed. *Clinical EMG for Surface Recordings*. Vol 2. Nevada City, CA: Clinical Resources; 1990;1–142.

24. Cram JR, Engstrom D. Patterns of neuromuscular activity in pain and nonpain patients. *Clin Biofeedback Health*. 1986;9:106–115.

25. Cram JR, Steger JC. EMG scanning in the diagnosis of chronic pain. *Biofeedback Self Regul*. 1983;8:229–241.

26. Middaugh SJ, Kee WG, Nicholson JA. Muscle overuse and posture as factors in the development and maintenance of chronic musculoskeletal pain. In: Grzesiak RC, Ciccone DS, eds. *Psychological Vulnerability to Chronic Pain*. New York: Springer Publishing Co; 1994;55–89.

27. Schuldt K, Ekholm J, Harms-Ringdahl K, Nemeth G, Arborelius UP. Effects of changes in sitting work posture on static neck and shoulder muscle activity. *Ergonomics*. 1986;29:1525–1537.

28. Davies CTM, Sargeant AJ. Effects of exercise therapy on total and component tissue leg volumes of patients undergoing rehabilitation from lower limb injury. *Ann Hum Biol*. 1975;2:327–335.

29. Eriksson E. Rehabilitation of muscle function after sport injury: major problems in sports medicine. *Int J Sports Med*. 1981;2:1–6.

30. Haggmark T, Jansson E, Eriksson E. Fiber type area and metabolic potential of the thigh muscle in man after knee injury and immobilization. *Int J Sports Med*. 1981;2:12–17.

31. Komi PV. *Strength and Power in Sport*. Oxford, England: Blackwell Scientific Publications; 1992.

32. Stanish WD, Valiant GA, Bonen A, Belcastro AN. The effects of immobilization and electrical stimulation on

muscle glycogen and myofibrillar ATPase. *Can J Appl Sport Sci.* 1982;7:267–271.

33. Sale D. Neural adaptation to strength training. In: Komi PV, ed. *Strength and Power in Sport.* Oxford, England: Blackwell Scientific Publications; 1992;249–265.

34. Sale DG. Neural adaptation to resistance training. *Med Sci Sports Exerc.* 1988;20:S135–S145.

35. Gogia P, Sabbahi M. Median frequency of the myoelectric signal in cervical paraspinal muscles. *Arch Phys Med Rehabil.* 1990;71:408–414.

36. Klein AB, Snyder-Mackler L, Roy SH, De Luca CJ. Comparison of spinal mobility and isometric trunk extensor forces with electromyographic spectral analysis in identifying low back pain. *Phys Ther.* 1991;71:445–454.

37. Roy SH, De Luca CJ, Emley M, Buijs RJC. Spectral electromyographic assessment of back muscles in patients with low back pain undergoing rehabilitation. *Spine.* 1995;20:38–48.

38. Grieve GP. *Common Vertebral Joint Problems.* Edinburgh, Scotland: Churchill Livingstone; 1981.

39. Korr IM. Proprioceptors and somatic dysfunction. *J Am Osteopath Assoc.* 1975;74:638–650.

40. Kraus H. Muscle spasm. In: Kraus H, ed. *Diagnosis and Treatment of Muscle Pain.* Chicago: Quintessence Publishing Co; 1988;11–20.

41. Livingston WK. *Pain Mechanisms.* New York: Macmillan; 1943.

42. Patterson MM. A model mechanism for spinal segmental facilitation. *J Am Osteopath Assoc.* 1976;76:121–131.

43. Dahl JB, Erichsen CJ, Fugslang-fredriksen A, Kehlet H. Pain sensation and nociceptive reflex excitability in surgical patients and human volunteers. *Br J Anaesth.* 1992;69:117–121.

44. Hu JW, Yu X-M, Vernon H, Sessle BJ. Excitatory effects on neck and jaw muscle activity of inflammatory irritant applied to cervical paraspinal tissues. *Pain.* 1993;55:243–250.

45. Wall PD, Woolf CJ. Muscle but not cutaneous C-afferent input produces prolonged increases in the excitability of the flexion reflex in the rat. *J Physiol (Lond).* 1984;356:443–458.

46. Woolf CJ. Long term alterations in the excitability of the flexion reflex produced by peripheral tissue injury in the chronic decerebrate rat. *Pain.* 1984;18:325–343.

47. Woolf CJ, McMahon SB. Injury-induced plasticity of the flexor reflex in chronic decerebrate rats. *Neuroscience.* 1985;16:395–404.

48. Woolf CJ, Wall PD. Relative effectiveness of C primary afferent fibers of different origins in evoking a prolonged facilitation of the flexion reflex in the rat. *J Neurosci.* 1986;6:1433–1442.

49. Blockey NJ. An observation concerning the flexor muscles during recovery of function after dislocation of the elbow. *J Bone Joint Surg Am.* 1954;36:S33–S40.

50. deAndrade JR, Grant C, Dixon A. Joint distension and reflex muscle inhibition in the knee. *J Bone Joint Surg Am.* 1965;47:313–322.

51. Fahrer H, Rentsch HU, Gerber NJ, Beyeler C, Hess C, Grunig B. Knee effusion and reflex inhibition of the quadriceps. *J Bone Joint Surg Br.* 1988;70:635–638.

52. Shakespeare DT, Stokes M, Sherman KP, Young A. Reflex inhibition of the quadriceps after meniscectomy: lack of association with pain. *Clin Physiol.* 1985;5:137–144.

53. Spencer JD, Hayes KC, Alexander J. Knee joint effusion and quadriceps reflex inhibition in man. *Arch Phys Med Rehabil.* 1984;65:171–177.

54. Stokes M, Young A. The contribution of reflex inhibition to arthrogenous muscle weakness. *Clin Sci.* 1984;67:7–14.

55. Stratford P. Electromyography of the quadriceps femoris muscles in subjects with normal knees and acutely effused knees. *Phys Ther.* 1981;62:279–283.

56. Swearingen RL, Dehne E. A study of pathological muscle function following injury to a joint. *J Bone Joint Surg Am.* 1964;46:1364.

57. Wood L, Ferrell WR, Baxendale RH. Pressures in normal and acutely distended human knee joints and effects on quadriceps maximal voluntary contractions. *Q J Exp Physiol.* 1988;73:305–314.

58. Headley BJ. Evaluation and treatment of myofascial pain syndrome utilizing biofeedback. In: Cram J, ed. *Clinical EMG for Surface Recordings.* Vol 2. Nevada City, CA: Clinical Resources; 1990;235–244.

59. Taylor W. Dynamic EMG biofeedback in assessment and treatment using a neuromuscular reeducation model. In: Cram J, ed. *Clinical EMG for Surface Recordings.* Vol 2. Nevada City, CA: Clinical Resources; 1990;175–196.

60. Price JP, Clare MH, Ewehardt RH. Studies in low backache with persistent muscle spasm. *Arch Phys Med Rehabil.* 1948;29:703–709.

61. Whatmore G, Ellis R. Some neurophysiologic aspects of the depressed state. *Arch Gen Psychiatry.* 1959;1:70–80.

62. Whatmore G, Kohli D. *The Physiopathology and Treatment of Functional Disorders.* New York: Grune & Stratton; 1974.

63. Fordyce WE. *Behavioral Methods for Chronic Pain and Illness.* St. Louis, MO: CV Mosby; 1976.

64. Cerny K. Pathomechanics of stance: clinical concepts for analysis. *Phys Ther.* 1984;64:1851–1859.

65. Fish DJ, Nielsen JP. Clinical assessment of human gait. *J Prosthet Orthotics.* 1993;5:39–48.

66. Hertling D, Kessler RM. *Management of Common Musculoskeletal Disorders*. 2nd ed. Philadelphia: JB Lippincott Co; 1990.

67. Kamkar A, Irrgang JJ, Whitney SL. Nonoperative management of secondary shoulder impingement syndrome. *J Orthop Sports Phys Ther*. 1993;17:212–224.

68. Solomnow M, Barata RB, D'Ambrosia R. EMG-force relations of a single skeletal muscle acting across a joint: dependence on joint angle. *J Electromyogr Kinesiol*. 1991;1:58–67.

69. Schmidt RA. *Motor Learning and Performance: From Principles to Practice*. Champaign, IL: Human Kinetics; 1991.

70. Schmidt RA. Motor learning principles for physical therapy. In: Lister MJ, ed. *Contemporary Management of Motor Control Problems*. Alexandria, VA: Foundation for Physical Therapy; 1991;49–63.

71. Schmidt RA. *Motor Control and Learning: A Behavioral Emphasis*. Champaign, IL: Human Kinetics; 1988.

72. Schmidt RA. A schema theory of discrete motor learning. *Psychol Rev*. 1975;82:225–260.

CHAPTER 8

Tension-Type Headache

CLASSIFICATION AND DEFINITION

Headache is perhaps one of the most common medical maladies known; despite that, its primary cause probably is not of an organic nature. Silberstein and Silberstein[1] note that in any one year, 70% of the population will sustain at least one headache, and 5% will seek medical assistance. Headache can be classified into nine categories:[2]

1. migraine
2. tension-type headache
3. cluster headache and chronic paroxysmal hemicrania
4. miscellaneous headaches not associated with structural lesion
5. headache associated with head trauma
6. headache associated with vascular disorders
7. headache associated with nonvascular intracranial disorder
8. headache associated with substances, or with withdrawal related to discontinuing of their use
9. headache associated with noncephalic infection

Implicit in this categorization is the notion that headaches may have one or several origins and can be influenced by a variety of substances or circumstances, as well as with genetic disposition.

The tension-type headache may be defined as a constant tight or pressing sensation, often bilateral in nature; initially episodic; related to stress; but occurring almost daily without necessary association with obvious psychologic factors.[3] Thus it is distinct from migraine and may have several causes.[4] This reality may account for the discrepancy in the literature regarding a definitive treatment plan or the presentation of conclusive evidence favoring one particular, or a multifactorial, treatment approach. Tension-type headache may be further divided into episodic and chronic types with subsequent subclassification based on the presence of excessive jaw or scalp muscle contractions. The term chronic usually accompanies the term headache when an individual experiences more than 15 headaches each month.

SPECULATION ON CAUSE

For more than 30 years clinicians have attributed tension-type headaches to one of four causes:

1. muscle contractions
2. constriction of scalp arteries or small vessels, including those supplying the conjunctiva
3. prolonged maintenance of facial expressions
4. temporomandibular joint (TMJ) pain

The difficulty is that there is no clear evidence that any one agent is the most causally related, because treatment for one problem does not necessarily relieve the symptoms, even in two patients presenting with similar histories. Only recently has attention been drawn to the prospects that cervical musculature or structural pathology might contribute to headaches of this type. In reviewing multiple causes for tension-type headache, Sjaastad[5] notes that awkward neck movements, sustained stiffness, or trigger points in the upper quadrant musculature are often associated with headache onset and perpetuation. These observations require further exploration and certainly provide a rich exploratory ground for clinicians wishing to examine multiple muscle sites for aberrant or asymmetric surface electromyography (SEMG) activity.

SEMG has been used for many years as a feedback technique to treat various classifications of headache. The notion underlying these feedback applications is that by providing visual or auditory cues about muscle activity, typically, but not always, from facial or frontal muscles, patients could lower their muscle tension responses. General physiologic arousal contributing to the headache would thereby be diminished or eradicated. In an extensive review of this subject, Chapman[6] concluded that most controlled clinical trials to that point (ie, mid-1980s) yielded equivocal results. Specifically, although some data suggested that frontalis SEMG might contribute to muscle contraction headaches, this finding invariably did not apply to all patients with this diagnosis. Young patients who had not demonstrated any habituation to drug intake tended to respond better to feedback training. More specific observations in controlled trials comparing relaxation and feedback training (involving the frontalis or trapezius) indicated no decisive differences between those approaches.[7–11]

More recently, work from Arena and colleagues[12] has demonstrated that elderly individuals with tension-type headaches can lower frontal SEMG activity, and this decrease is associated with reduced overall headache activity in more than 90% of subjects. Moreover, by targeting the upper trapezius on SEMG training, greater clinical improvements were seen at 3-

month follow-up than with either frontal feedback training or relaxation therapy.[13] Although these results would seem to encourage the use of trapezius SEMG as a training vehicle, work by Peterson and associates[14] failed to correlate SEMG levels measured from five muscle sites with patient ratings of muscle tension or pain. These findings suggest that a site-specific relationship among chronic headache pain, subjective muscle tension reports, and quantified SEMG remains unclear.

Some discrepancies in these findings might be clarified from work reported by Jensen and coworkers,[15] who examined SEMG characteristics of right frontal and bilateral temporalis sites in 547 adults. Individuals with chronic headache had higher amplitude signals from their temporalis muscles at rest than those of migraineurs or subjects with episodic tension-type headaches. In patients actually experiencing headache, SEMG amplitudes were increased in frontal muscles at rest, suggesting heightened muscle tension. Among these subjects, amplitudes were decreased in all muscles monitored during maximal voluntary contractions, which leads to the possibility that these efforts were submaximal because of fatigue, morphologic changes, or metabolic differences. These factors typically have not been considered in evaluating variances in SEMG findings among patients with tension-type headache, and results of this study by Jensen and colleagues form the basis for worthwhile research and clinical investigations.

The need to examine more variables under specific circumstances is also emphasized by the findings of Sandrini and coworkers,[16] who observed that algometric and frontal muscle SEMG measures were more impaired among patients with episodic tension-type headache than among control subjects, or patients with migraine, when all were subjected to mental arithmetic stressors. Thus there may be a need to consider the impact of a headache on independent variable measures at the time of testing. Mathematical type stressors may induce differences in physiologic responses among people with different headache classes. This observation is supported by a report on 100 patients with headache by Jordy.[17] He found that without the use of stressors in the evaluation recommended by the Committee of the International Headache Society, a 24% to 32% diagnostic error can occur. He suggested that electromyography with stress be used as part of the diagnostic criteria for tension headache.

Added to the spectrum of variables the clinician needs to consider when using SEMG to evaluate or treat tension-type headache are behavioral trait characteristics of patients. Ficek and Wittrock[18] found that compared with headache-free control subjects, patients who experience recurrent tension-type headaches have higher levels of depression and trait anxiety. Although these two groups did not differ greatly in the use of coping skills, patients with headache perceived themselves as experiencing more stressful events than their headache-free counterparts. These observations indicate that personality profiles may be an essential element to include when developing a treatment strategy or when assessing the relative success of one. On the other hand, in working with 28 women who experienced frequent headaches, Lacroix and Corbett[19] were unable to find any relationship between targeting SEMG activity toward a defined level and expectation of a headache or discomfort. Finally, and perhaps most germane to practitioners who use SEMG in the treatment of contraction headaches are the observations offered by Hudzinski and Lawrence.[20] They suggest that clinicians should strongly consider the role of electrode placement specificity as a precursor to successful training. Recognition of muscle location and isolation may be critical in shaping patient responses and affecting overall physiologic arousal. For example, use of typical, broad-based frontal placements may be inappropriate if the levels are low at baseline and extraneous physiologic movements, such as jaw closure or excessive upper chest respiration, have been controlled. Some patients may display other postural abnormalities associated with headache, including unilaterally or bilater-

ally elevated activity of the upper trapezius. It would be relevant for the clinician to target this muscle in headache treatment. The clinician's task is to identify whether elevated SEMG activity is seen unilaterally or bilaterally, as well as whether this abnormality can be captured with narrow or wide electrode placement in the absence of contributing artifact, such as heartbeat or carotid pulse waves.

Two more noteworthy considerations involve electrical stimulation and pharmacologic management in the treatment of tension-type headaches. These issues are gaining more importance as electrophysiologic interventions are used to reveal pathologic responses in the central nervous system, and as drug interventions to "cure" headache receive increased recognition. Wang and Schoenen[21] have shown that electrical stimulation of the lip or finger region can lead to suppression of temporalis muscle activity, the "ES2" response. This suppression is most noted in patients with tension-type headache and may indicate an exceptional hyperexcitability of the reticular nuclei, which in turn might inhibit medullary interneurons mediating the ES2. Although ES2 duration tended to decrease with increasing duration of headache, Zwart and Sand[22] were unable to discern clear differences in the ES2 durations between control subjects and patients with cervicogenic headache, migraine, or chronic tension-type headache.

For pharmacologic management, many agents have been examined. Gobel and colleagues[23] found in a blind study that amitriptyline reduced tension-type headache by the third week of administration. Sensitivity to suprathreshold experimental pain was suppressed in the group receiving the drug, and reductions in daily headache duration were also reported. However, SEMG changes were not noted during relaxation or volitional muscle contraction. Collectively, results from this study introduce the intriguing paradox of decreased headache duration with a favorable drug but without concomitant changes in SEMG recordings in temporalis muscle.

CONCLUSION

Although SEMG has achieved more recognition in the treatment of tension-type headache than in migraine headache, its use still has some inherent difficulties. SEMG has been used successfully to discriminate among patients with headache under certain circumstances and has produced positive treatment outcomes in tension-type groups. However, environmental and behavioral factors are recognized as triggers of tension-type headache, and there is a need to continue to investigate the role of psychologic intervention. The effects of soft tissue and cra-

nial-cervical articular dysfunction also have yet to be clearly understood. Furthermore, some concerns exist about the appropriate target muscle(s) to train with SEMG feedback, as well as with the extent to which SEMG training can serve in lieu of pharmacologic management in particular patient subpopulations. A single best treatment approach cannot be defined at present. Regardless of these dilemmas, it is undeniable that the success of SEMG treatment must be based on the degree to which patients can abort or eliminate headache occurrences through application of training strategies in real-life contexts.

REFERENCES

1. Silberstein SD, Silberstein MM. New concepts in the pathogenesis of migraine headache. *Pain Management.* 1990;3:297–302.

2. Dalessio DJ, Silberstein SD. Diagnosis and classification of headache. In: Dalessio DJ, Silberstein SD, eds. *Wolff's Headache and Other Head Pain.* 6th ed. New York: Oxford University Press; 1993;1–18.

3. Lance JW. Tension-type headache. In: Lance JW, ed. *Mechanism and Management of Headache.* 5th ed. London: Butterworth-Heinemann; 1993;144–162.

4. Headache Classification Committee of the International Headache Society. Classification and diagnosis criteria for headache disorders, cranial neuralgias and facial pain. *Cephalalgia.* 1988;8(suppl 7):1–96.

5. Sjaastad O. Cervicogenic headache. In: Dalessio DJ, Silberstein SD, eds. *Wolff's Headache and Other Head Pain.* 6th ed. New York: Oxford University Press; 1993;203–208.

6. Chapman SL. A review and clinical perspective on the use of EMG and thermal biofeedback for chronic headaches. *Pain.* 1986;27:1–43.

7. Cott A, Golman JA, Pavloski RP, Kirschberg GJ, Fabich M. The long-term therapeutic significance of the addition of electromyographic feedback to relaxation training in the treatment of tension headache. *Behav Ther.* 1981;12:556–559.

8. Daly EJ, Donn PA, Galliher MJ, Zimmerman JS. Biofeedback applications to migraine and tension headaches: a double-blind outcome study. *Biofeedback Self Regul.* 1983;3:135–152.

9. Haynes SN, Griffin D, Mooney D, Parise M. Electromyographic biofeedback and relaxation instructions in the treatment of muscle contraction headaches. *Behav Ther.* 1975;6:672–681.

10. Janssen K. Differential effectiveness of EMG-feedback versus combined EMG-feedback and relaxation instructions in the treatment of tension headache. *J Psychsom Res.* 1983;27:243–253.

11. Schlutter LC, Golden CJ, Blume HG. A comparison of treatments for prefrontal muscle-contraction headaches. *Br J Med Psychol.* 1980;53:47–52.

12. Arena JG, Hannah SL, Bruno GM, Meador KJ. Electromyographic biofeedback training for tension headache in the elderly: a prospective study. *Biofeedback Self Regul.* 1991;16:379–390.

13. Arena JG, Bruno GM, Hannah SL, Meador KJ. A comparison of frontal electromyographic biofeedback training, trapezius electromyographic biofeedback training, and progressive muscle relaxation therapy in the treatment of tension headache. *Headache.* 1995;35:411–419.

14. Peterson AL, Talcott GW, Kelleher GW, Haddock CK. Site specificity of pain and tension in tension-type headache. *Headache.* 1995;35:89–92.

15. Jensen R, Fuglsang-Fredriksen A, Olsen J. Quantitative surface EMG of pericranial muscles I headache: a population study. *Electroencephalogr Clin Neurophysiol.* 1994;93:335–344.

16. Sandrini G, Antonaci F, Pucci E, Bono G, Nappi G. Comparative study with EMG, pressure algometry, and manual palpation in tension-type headache and migraine. *Cephalalgia.* 1994;14:451–457.

17. Jordy CF. Surface electromyography during experimental stress as a tool in the diagnosis of tension headache: results in 100 cases. *Arq Neuropsiquiatr.* 1995;53:437–440.

18. Ficek SK, Wittrock DA. Subjective stress coping in recurrent tension-type headache. *Headache.* 1995;35:455–460.

19. Lacroix JM, Corbett L. An experimental test of the muscle tension hypotheses of tension-type headache. *Int J Psychophysiol.* 1990;10:47–51.

20. Hudzinski LG, Lawrence GS. Significance of EMG surface electrode placement models and headache findings. *Headache.* 1988;28:30–35.

21. Wang W, Schoenen J. Reduction of temporalis exteroceptive suppression by peripheral electrical stimulation in migraine and tension-type headaches. Pain. 1994; 59:327–334.

22. Zwart JA, Sand T. Exteroceptive suppression of temporalis muscle activity: a blind study of tension-type headache, migraine, and cervicogenic headache. *Headache.* 1995;35:338–343.

23. Gobel H, Hamouz V, Hansen C, et al. Chronic tension-type headache: amitriptyline reduces clinical headache-duration and experimental pain sensitivity but does not alter pericranial muscle activity readings. *Pain.* 1994; 59:241–249.

SEMG Program for Tension-Type Headache

Refer to the discussion in Chapter 8 for a review of intervention approaches. The suggestions that follow are derived from those resources. Descriptions and operational definitions are provided to clarify optional practice patterns.

CANDIDATES

Implement for patients
- with chronic tension-type headache or mixed headache syndromes in whom muscle dysfunction is suspected.
- who have been diagnosed with an alternative headache category but in whom a muscular contribution is suspected. This includes patients
  1. with known history of cervical dysfunction, or clenching or bruxism of the teeth
  2. who report related tension sensations about the head, neck, and proximal area of the shoulder girdle
     Physical examination may show palpable hypertonicity, trigger points, or imbalances in muscle flexibility and strength.

EVALUATION OBJECTIVES

- Identify elevated or imbalanced muscle activity that potentially results in headache, myalgia, or secondary joint dysfunction.
- Assess effects of posture and dynamic movement on muscle activity.
- Assess effects of psychophysiologic factors on muscle activity.

FEEDBACK TRAINING OBJECTIVES

- Reduce excessive or imbalanced muscle tension.
- Resolve or reduce underlying cervical or TMJ mechanical dysfunction; improve postural function and ergonomic alignment.
- Decouple psychologic stressors and muscle tension responses.
- Retain and generalize improved motor control to functional contexts.
- Resolve or reduce functional limitations and disability.

RECORDING SITES

- Judge the utility of each recording site on the basis of history and physical examination results.
- Include muscles that
  1. underlie the pain distribution
  2. potentially refer symptoms to the patient's area of complaint
  3. reproduce the patient's symptoms when stretched, resisted, or palpated
- Consider use of an SEMG static scan procedure (see Chapters 5 and 6 in the companion book, *Introduction to Surface Electromyography*) to qualify sites for detailed postural and psychophysiologic assessments.

- Consult Chapter 14 in the companion book for specific electrode placement considerations.
- Confirm optimal sites from the following list by observation and palpation during isometric contraction:
  1. frontalis
  2. temporalis
  3. masseter
  4. sternomastoid
  5. cervical paraspinal groups (trapezius, splenius, semispinalis, erector spinae, suboccipitals, levator scapulae, rhomboids)
  6. upper trapezius, potentially in conjunction with the lower interscapular region (lower trapezius) or serratus anterior
  7. proximal interscapular region (trapezius, levator scapulae, rhomboids)
  8. lateral cervical region (levator scapulae, scalene)

EVALUATION PROCEDURES

- Select procedures that correspond to exacerbating and alleviating factors revealed by history and clinical examination.
- Refer to Chapter 2 for detailed discussion of evaluation methods.
- Perform at least five repetitions of each movement task to assess response consistency (consider discarding the results of the first one to two repetitions and averaging the results of the remaining repetitions). Many more repetitions may be needed to assess SEMG responses with reproduction of symptoms.
- Select relevant procedures from the following:
  1. psychophysiologic stress profile
  2. postural analysis
  3. active range of motion (AROM) for target recording muscles, as appropriate (observe for consistent excursion and velocity across test repetitions):
     –mandibular depression, elevation

     –cervical flexion, extension, side-bending, rotation, retraction, protraction
     –shoulder girdle elevation, depression, protraction, retraction; shoulder flexion, abduction, scaption (elevation in the scapular plane, between flexion and abduction)
  4. isometric contractions:
     –maximal
     –submaximal, progressively graded
  5. tension recognition thresholds
  6. analysis of muscle synergy patterns and reciprocal activity (eg, cervical paraspinals and sternomastoid, upper and lower portions of trapezius and serratus anterior)
  7. functional activity analysis:
     –job
     –home
     –recreation

ASSESSMENT

- Refer to Chapter 2 for detailed discussion of SEMG assessment.
- Refer to Chapter 14 in the companion book for representative SEMG tracings of normal function, as well as for benchmark baseline values for each site.
- Select SEMG assessment parameters from the following:
  1. Amplitude and variance of each channel during baseline. Activity during baseline should be stable and relatively quiescent. Mean amplitude values from nonpostural muscles should be close to internal noise levels of the recording device. Postural muscles may show low-level activity with the patient in weight-bearing positions (typically, about 2–6 μV RMS).
  2. Peak or average amplitude of each channel during activation. Activity can appear to be unremarkable, grossly excessive, or markedly depressed. For comparisons across nonhomologous muscles, magnitudes can be expressed as

–percentage of maximal volitional iso-metric contraction (%MVIC) ampli-tude with the use of standard manual muscle tests (test activity amplitude/MVIC × 100)

–percentage of some submaximal con-traction amplitude obtained with a standardized force intensity, joint angle, and body posture

3. Return to baseline amplitude after muscle activation. Qualitatively, recov-ery can be stated as prompt and com-plete versus elevated and delayed. Satisfactory baseline recovery is quanti-tatively defined (with a smoothing time constant of 0.1 second or less) as a re-turn to an SEMG amplitude within two standard deviations of the original baseline mean, within 3 seconds of movement cessation, and maintenance within that amplitude range for at least 30 seconds or until the next movement is initiated. Recovery can be characterized by the latency to achieve this criterion. More simply, the amplitude (expressed as percentage of baseline) observed 1 to 3 seconds after movement termination can be reported.

4. Quiescence of cervical paraspinal activ-ity in full flexion, the flexion–relaxation response.

5. Left/right peak amplitude symmetry for sagittal plane movements of the spine or bilateral symmetric movements of the extremities (eg, cervical flexion–exten-sion and bilateral shoulder flexion, re-spectively). Satisfactory symmetry is operationally defined as left/right scores within 35% as calculated [(higher val-ue – lower value)/higher value] × 100. Symmetry assessment assumes an equivalent left/right AROM excursion and velocity.

6. Left/right timing symmetry for sagittal plane movements of the spine or bilat-eral symmetric movements of the ex-tremities (eg, coincident recruitment,

peak, and decruitment patterns; sym-metric duration). When comparing the timing symmetry of synergist action, observe for changes in the recruitment order of muscles from one side to the other. For most clinical purposes, timing issues can be observed with rectified line tracings with a smoothing time con-stant of 0.1 second or less, SEMG sam-pling at 100 Hz or faster, frequency bandwidth filter low cutoff of 25 Hz or less, and a high resolution display with variable sweep speed. A graphic print-out is useful for documentation of subtle timing differences. Documentation can be quantified with calculations of aver-age slope, time to peak activity, or time to some percentage of MVIC activity that is clinically meaningful. Onset time can be reported simply as the latency to achieve a μV value equivalent to two standard deviations above the baseline mean. Duration may be noted as the amount of time between onset and baseline recovery as defined above.

7. Normal pattern of asymmetry for unilat-eral plane movements (eg, cervical rota-tion and unilateral shoulder flexion). Reciprocal symmetry of the patterns should be observed for reciprocal left/right tasks. Reciprocal asymmetry greater than 35% (assuming equal AROM excursion and velocity) is op-erationally an aberrant finding. Within a single side unilateral movement, similar levels of left/right co-activation are an aberrant finding.

8. Symmetrically proportionate left/right cervical paraspinal, lateral cervical, and sternomastoid amplitude patterns during evaluation procedures.

9. Symmetrically proportionate left/right upper trapezius, lower trapezius, and serratus anterior amplitude patterns dur-ing evaluation procedures.

10. Change in activity levels for a particular muscle and task across treatment ses-

sions. A normalization procedure is recommended when feasible. A reliable maximal manual muscle test effort or a standardized submaximal contraction is required. The average amplitude during the test task is divided by that day's reference contraction amplitude, and the quotient is multiplied by 100.

COMMON PATIENT PRESENTATIONS

Headache in General

Headache is due to a spectrum of associated and discrete causes. SEMG evaluation and feedback training may be of limited utility for true migraine. The techniques can be useful for mixed tension-type/migraine headaches. However, clinicians who practice regularly in this area also may consider use of thermal, photoplethysmographic, and other physiologic monitoring modalities. Before receiving SEMG intervention, patients with chronic headache should consult with a primary care physician to rule out occult disease or medication issues. Referral to a neurologist or other specialist may be warranted to address potentially serious medical problems.

Tension-Type Headache

Tension-related myalgia from pericranial muscles has been considered historically as the cause of tension-type headache (Figure 8–A–1). The role of pericranial muscle contraction is now regarded as controversial. The community of clinicians who use SEMG has broadened its focus to include referred trigger point pain, muscle hyperactivity, and imbalance from cervical and proximal shoulder girdle groups. Thus the sternomastoids, middle and lower cervical paraspinal, lateral cervical, and trapezius muscles may be considered for recording. To progress to SEMG feedback training, evaluation should demonstrate a relationship among specific examination maneuvers, symptom modification, and aberrant SEMG activity. Some patients show tonic muscle hyperactivity.

SEMG activity in other patients is quiescent until they are challenged with psychologic stressors.

Activity in patients of another subset appears unremarkable in static positions but becomes aberrant with movement. These patients demonstrate SEMG asymmetries during movement or failure to recover to postural baseline after movement. They may incur local or referred headache pain because of muscle overuse patterns and associated articular dysfunction. Detailed discussion of cervical and scapular muscle imbalances follows in Application Guides 10–A and 11–A, respectively.

TRAINING PROGRESSION

- Refer to Chapters 3 and 4 for detailed discussion of SEMG display setups and feedback structure.
- Refer to Chapters 5 and 6 for detailed discussion of SEMG feedback training techniques.
- As skill develops, generally
  1. Shape desired responses up or down.
  2. Add distractions.
  3. Randomize training activities.
  4. Withdraw continuous audio/visual feedback.
- Select relevant SEMG feedback training tasks from the following:
  1. isolation of target muscle activity
  2. postural training with SEMG feedback; training commonly requires cervical retraction or a sternal "lift." Monitor for inappropriate muscle bracing from upper trapezius; correct thoracic and lumbar postural faults
  3. relaxation-based downtraining
  4. threshold-based downtraining
  5. deactivation training
  6. tension recognition threshold training
  7. tension discrimination training
  8. left/right equilibration training. Emphasize isometric uptraining of the low amplitude side.
  9. therapeutic exercises with SEMG feed-

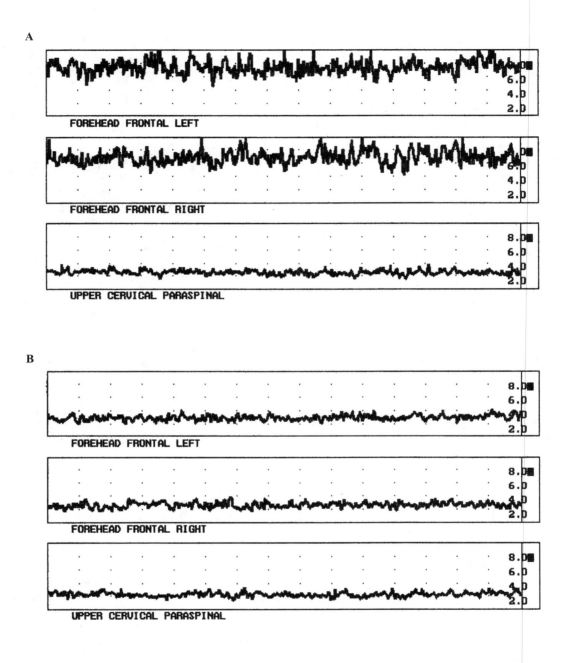

Figure 8–A–1 SEMG activity from left and right forehead frontal sites and bilateral upper cervical paraspinal muscles recorded from a patient with bifrontal tension-type headache. (**A**) Initial recording with headache subjectively rated at "6 out of 10" (the number 10 representing worst possible pain). (**B**) Recording after SEMG feedback downtraining and frontal muscle relaxation. Headache is now subjectively rated at "2 out of 10."

back. Assist relaxation during stretch, as indicated:

-suboccipitals

-sternocleidomastoid

-scalenes

-upper trapezius

-levator scapulae

-pectoralis group

10. promotion of correct muscle synergies and related coordination patterns between sternomastoid and cervical paraspinals or upper and lower portions of the trapezius and serratus anterior as indicated

11. functional activity performance with SEMG feedback

• Integrate SEMG feedback training into a comprehensive approach to patient management:

1. Refer patient to a mental health practitioner if psychologic stressors seem to be contributory.

2. Counsel patient for wellness. Include concepts relating to

-relaxation

-modification of stressful cognitive appraisals

-maintenance of appropriate postures and ergonomic setups

-sensible pacing of activities

3. Provide instruction in

-nutritional balance

-aerobic fitness

-general conditioning

-body weight management

4. Encourage moderation with intake of caffeine, nicotine, and alcohol, as well as with use of other psychoactive agents.

5. Monitor the patient closely for signs of medication abuse or rebound headaches associated with prescribed drugs.

• Promote transfer of relaxation skills to functional environments:

1. Instruct the patient in other related therapies, such as

-systematic desensitization

-stress inoculation

-positive self-talk

-relaxation trigger words

-hand positions

(Refer to Chapter 5.)

2. Have the patient practice an abbreviated relaxation technique in work, home, and recreational settings.

3. Instruct the patient in postural self-checks to use throughout the day.

4. Combine tactics in the three recommendations above with

-abdominal breathing

-cervical stretching

-adaptation of muscle deactivation and tension discrimination training procedures

5. Once basic competence is demonstrated with tension discrimination training in the clinic, have the patient practice at home without SEMG feedback, simply by estimating SEMG scores from the target muscles as if he or she were connected to the feedback machine.

• Prescribe frequent, brief practice sessions and adjunctive therapies for the patient with muscle asymmetries and dynamic imbalances.

1. Emphasize repetition of muscle equilibration procedures and recruitment of an underused antagonist or synergist.

2. Develop a careful plan to implement indicated changes in ergonomic setups and functional motor habits.

3. Consult other Application Guides in this book on TMJ, cervical, and shoulder girdle dysfunction for associated problems.

4. Consider consultation with a therapist or physician for

-adjunctive manual treatments

-exercise prescription

-physical agents

-functional activity modification

SUGGESTED READINGS

Arena JG, Bruno GM, Hannah SL, Meador KJ. A comparison of frontal electromyographic biofeedback training, trapezius electromyographic biofeedback training, and progressive muscle relaxation therapy in the treatment of tension headache. *Headache*. 1995;35:411–419.

Budzynski TH. Biofeedback strategies in headache treatment. In: Basmajian JV, ed. *Biofeedback: Principles and Practice for Clinicians*. 3rd ed. Baltimore: Williams & Wilkins; 1989;197–208.

Hudzinski LG, Lawrence GS. Significance of EMG surface electrode placement models and headache findings. *Headache*. 1988;28:30–35.

Jensen R, Fuglsang-Frederiksen A, Olsen J. Quantitative surface EMG of pericranial muscles: reproducibility and variability. *Electroencephalogr Clin Neurophysiol*. 1993;89:1–9.

Middaugh SJ, Kee WG, Nicholson JA. Muscle overuse and posture as factors in the development and maintenance of chronic musculoskeletal pain. In: Grzesiak RC, Ciccone DS, eds. *Psychological Vulnerability to Chronic Pain*. New York: Springer Publishing Co; 1994;55–89.

Sandrini G, Antonaci F, Pucci E, Bono G, Nappi G. Comparative study with EMG, pressure algometry, and manual palpation in tension-type headache and migraine. *Cephalalgia*. 1994;14:451–457.

Schwartz MS. Headache: selected issues and considerations in evaluation and treatment, part A: evaluation. In: Schwartz MS, ed. *Biofeedback: A Practitioner's Guide*. 2nd ed. New York: Guilford Press; 1995;313–353.

Schwartz MS. Headache: selected issues and considerations in evaluation and treatment, part B: treatment. In: Schwartz MS, ed. *Biofeedback: A Practitioner's Guide*. 2nd ed. New York: Guilford Press; 1995;354–410.

CHAPTER 9

Temporomandibular Joint Dysfunction and Myofacial Pain

The temporomandibular joint (TMJ) is a combined hinge and gliding joint. It is formed by the mandibular fossa of the temporal bone, articular eminence, articular tubercle, and condyle of the mandible (Figure 9–1). Structures contributing to the integrity of the joint include the articular capsule, lateral ligament, sphenomandibular ligament, articular disc, and stylomandibular ligament. Of particular clinical significance is the articular disc, which is a thin, ovoid plate that lies between the mandibular condyle and fossa. Its upper surface is concavoconvex to accommodate to the shape of the mandibular fossa and articular tubercle. The lower surface of the disc is concave and in contact with the condyle. Around its circumference, the disc is connected to the articular capsule and tendon of the lateral pterygoid muscle. The disc also divides the joint into two cavities, each of which is furnished with a synovial membrane. Innervation of the joint is supplied from the auriculotemporal and masseteric branches of the mandibular division of the trigeminal nerve.

Movements about the joint are opening and closing of the jaws, as well as protrusion and lateral displacement of the mandible. With opening and closing of the jaws, movement occurs at both superior and inferior portions of the disc. The disc glides anteriorly on the articular tubercle while the condyle moves on the disc like a hinge. These actions cause the mandible to rotate about a center point near the middle of the ramus of the mandible. This movable center ac-

tion is caused, in part, by a sling formed from the masseter and medial pterygoid muscles. As the jaws open, the angle of the mandible moves posteriorly while the condyle glides forward as the short arm of a lever, and the chin moves like the long arm of the lever, collectively describing a wide arc. The motion between the condyle and articular disc accommodates the change in bony position.

MUSCLES ACTING ON THE TMJ

Muscles that open the jaw (depress the mandible) include the lateral pterygoid, with assistance from the mylohyoid, geniohyoid, and digastric. Closing of the jaw (elevation of the mandible) is accomplished through action of the temporalis, masseter, and medial pterygoid. Protrusion of the mandible is undertaken by concurrent contractions of both lateral pterygoid muscles and synergistic actions of the mandibular elevators. The jaw is drawn back by the posterior fibers of the temporalis, whereas lateral displacement (side-to-side motion) is accomplished by the lateral pterygoid of the opposite side.

RETHINKING TMJ DYSFUNCTION

For years clinicians have assumed that most, if not all, TMJ dysfunction was caused by problems in the integrity of the joint or its interspersed disc. A recent review of the literature,

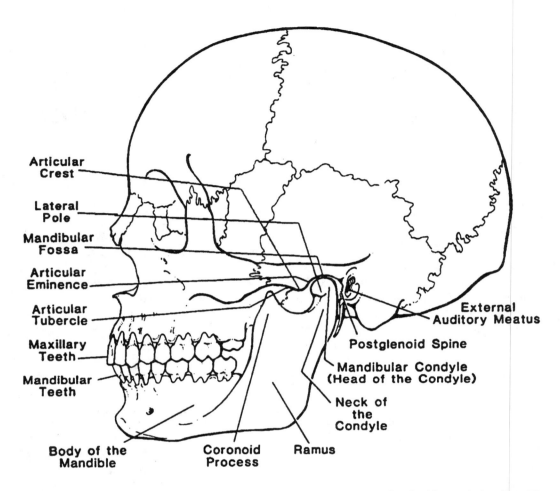

Figure 9–1 Bony anatomy of the TMJ and related structures. *Source:* Reprinted with permission from The Saunders Group, Inc., 1997.

however, brings this notion into some degree of suspect. Efforts to alter activity of masticatory muscles that act about the joint by using surface electromyography (SEMG) applications have not always been successful, nor have efforts to eliminate TMJ clicks necessarily been associated with SEMG changes. These realities have encouraged researchers and clinicians to look elsewhere besides the joint space and intervening disc to find the cause of TMJ problems. In reality, a more accurate description of TMJ dysfunction may well be embedded in other problems affecting the face or other structures about the cervical spine. Accordingly, it seems more reasonable to refer to this collective array of problems as myofacial pain.

The source of discomfort requiring clinical attention with occasional SEMG interventions may not necessarily emanate from the TMJ, but may be secondary to postural problems, abnormalities within the trigeminal nervous system, oral pathology, visual difficulties, or any combination of these sites or problems. This idea has been discussed by Glaros and Gevirtz[1] who speculate that what might be perceived as TMJ pain by some clinicians may be derived from neck, forehead, or other facial muscles. They observed that detailed assessments of patients whose primary complaints seem to highlight TMJ difficulties often reveal concomitant problems that may have been deemed insignificant by other clinicians. This important observation indicates that a detailed clinical assessment, including that with SEMG, should be attempted when clinicians examine patients whose alleged chief complaint may be TMJ pain. The clinician's attempt to achieve improvement in muscle patterns elsewhere in the face, neck, or axial skeleton may ameliorate the problem.

Within the past few years, several studies have addressed EMG, biomechanical, and behavioral variables related to myofacial dysfunction. Glaros and coworkers[2] demonstrated that there is no relationship between SEMG readings from masticatory muscles in individuals with and without measurable overbite, thus minimizing the possibility that myofacial dysfunction may be due primarily to overbite. These findings seem to corroborate those of Grechko and colleagues[3] and others,[4] who failed to identify a relationship between clinical patterns of myofacial dysfunction syndrome and SEMG changes in masticatory muscles. Therefore clinicians should exercise some caution in following guidelines for the use of SEMG as a primary tool to treat myofacial pain, as advocated by Hudzinski and Walters,[5] because the primary factor contributing to the pain may not necessarily reside in mandibular muscle dysfunction. Relaxing the masseter or temporal muscles bilaterally should not be the clinician's sole strategy. Clinicians should consider other muscle sites and training strategies.

Results of recent studies indicate that it may be important to develop clinical evaluation and retraining procedures for proprioceptive deficits in certain patients with myofacial pain. Flor and associates[6] found decrements in muscle perception by using discriminative tension tasks and SEMG measurements in patients with chronic temporomandibular pain. Glaros[7] found an in-

teraction between proprioceptive awareness and psychologic stress variables in a carefully selected subpopulation with myofacial pain. Thus thoughtful screening may help clinicians determine the most suitable candidates for SEMG feedback training. Feedback techniques that facilitate kinesthetic awareness should be considered during treatment planning.[8] Awareness of muscle tension may not necessarily be linked to relaxation ability (see Chapter 3), again suggesting a broad approach to symptom management that addresses idiosyncratic mechanical and psychodynamic issues.

In attempting to identify parameters that are most predictive of asymmetric (unilateral) chewing, SEMG is very reliable.[9] Ferrario and colleagues[10] examined 92 healthy subjects and found gender differences in SEMG activity generated during centric contractions, with women showing greater quantified SEMG amplitudes from the temporalis, and men having greater activity in the masseter. Furthermore, greater asymmetries were observed at low SEMG levels (less centric effort). A biomechanical model proposed by Ferrario and Sforza[11] indicated that reaction forces acting on the TMJ during unilateral biting do not always load the balancing side of the jaw more than the working side of the jaw. Modifications of an asymmetry index changed with the relative load between each TMJ, and greater temporalis SEMG activity was associated with increased loading force on both sides. These results suggest that bilateral activation of temporalis muscles might lead to symmetry in the bite.

From a psychologic perspective, Peterson and coworkers[12] explored the use of behavior therapy to reduce teeth clenching and grinding among three subjects with myofacial pain. This approach was successful in two of the three patients, as measured by pain scales, muscle palpation for pain, and mandibular–maxillary separation. The degree to which this approach affected nocturnal behavior was not identified.

Interestingly, many contemporary approaches to the treatment of myofacial pain disorders have not addressed the use of SEMG specifically.

Clark, Koyano, and Browne[13] have attempted to treat orofacial motor disorders affecting the jaw and neck musculature by using contingent afferent electrical stimulation of the lip. This procedure involves cutaneous electrical stimulation about the orbicularis oris when increased compressive forces between the maxilla and mandible are detected by force transducers. The technique has led to control over bruxism and enhanced endurance and recovery capabilities in jaw protrusive muscles, as well as fostered an interest in using this method in conjunction with botulism toxin injections to treat orofacial dystonia and dyskinesia. The role of integrating SEMG with these electrical stimulation approaches to enhance patient awareness and control is an inviting one to explore. By using a threshold level of SEMG from masseter or temporalis to trigger an auditory tone or other relevant reminder, the approach may be less intrusive and facilitate patient compliance. In fact, Turk and coworkers[14] have demonstrated that a combination of intraoral devices, SEMG feedback, and stress reduction may reduce pain symptoms for more than 6 months.

Patients with craniomandibular disorders treated either with mock occlusal adjustment or by manual adjustments to minimize mandibular sliding show no difference in improvements of signs and symptoms, suggesting that some occlusal procedures might not be beneficial.[15] The development of experimental occlusal devices designed to change the translatory motion patterns of the mandible, as well as information from Christensen and Rassouli,[16] demonstrate that SEMG activity is profoundly affected during the early phases of occlusal application. These changes are associated with short-term clinical signs of jaw muscle fatigue, pain, and TMJ clicking. Yoshida[17] showed that TMJ click is not associated by itself with changes in EMG recorded from the superior and inferior heads of the lateral pterygoid, anterior digastric, or temporalis muscles. Yet Vallon and coworkers[18] found a specific occlusal technique that reduced orofacial pain in patients for more than three months, compared with findings in a control

group. Clearly the specificity of the clinical problem and the skill or type of occlusal procedure used can affect the outcome measures. In both situations, SEMG can be used in an evaluative mode to see how signal behavior changes over time.

Moss and coworkers[19] have advanced a multifactorial theory for facial pain etiology. In a study spanning only 7 days among groups of patients with and without facial pain and with and without clinical symptoms of TMJ dysfunction, an interaction was found between TMJ dysfunction and facial pain for biting the lips and mouth. In addition, most control subjects without pain but with TMJ dysfunction stated they never bruxed their teeth. Further contention for the need to specify the etiology of orofacial pain comes from Hapak and associates.[20] They identified different pain scale values for patients with pain from neurologic causes (trigeminal neuralgia, tension-type headache, atypical facial pain), dentoalveolar pain, and musculoligamentous pain. One must deduce that the modality efficacy for the treatment of myofacial pain must await a clearer delineation of diagnoses and factors contributing to discomfort.

CONCLUSION

Although much is still to be learned about the etiologies of TMJ dysfunction, a prevailing notion is that difficulties may exist in more than just the joint, and myofacial pain may be a better descriptor of the problems. The development of comparative SEMG standards for this region is complicated by normal variation in facial morphology. A consistent expectation for the proportionate contribution of masseter and temporalis muscles to mandibular elevation has proven to be elusive. In addition, the function of each subject's left and right TMJs are mechanically linked. It remains unclear as to how pathology on one side affects muscle activity on the contralateral side. There is a role for SEMG in evaluation of appliances for particular individuals and in re-education of masticatory, facial, postural, and even respiratory muscles. SEMG feedback training can help correct proprioceptive deficits and psychophysiologic problems that subserve destructive parafunctional behaviors. Thus SEMG can be used to increase comprehension of each patient's issues and to improve function. SEMG training must ultimately facilitate patients in relating muscle activity, symptoms, and self-directed psychologic and kinesiologic treatment strategies.

REFERENCES

1. Glaros AG, Gevirtz R. AAPB white paper: temporomandibular disorders. In: Amar P, Schneider C, eds. *Clinical Applications of Biofeedback and Applied Psychophysiology*. Wheat Ridge, CO: Association for Applied Psychophysiology and Biofeedback; 1995;52–56.

2. Glaros AG, Brockman DL, Ackerman RJ. Impact of overbite on indicators of temporomandibular joint dysfunction. *Cranio*. 1992;10:277–281.

3. Grechko VE, Filiuk AI, Turbina LR, Semenov IL. Changes in the bioelectrical activity of the masticatory muscles and temporomandibular joint pathology in the myofascial dysfunction syndrome. *Zh Nevropatol Psikhiatr*. 1994;94:67–70.

4. Lund JP, Widmer CG. An evaluation of the use of surface electromyography in the diagnosis, documentation, and treatment of dental patients. *J Craniomandibular Disord Facial Oral Pain*. 1989;3:125–137.

5. Hudzinski LG, Walters PJ. Myofacial pain and TMJ. In: *Electromyography in Physical Therapy and Dentistry*. Paper 7. Montreal, Canada: Thought Technology, Ltd; 1993.

6. Flor H, Schugens M, Birbaumer N. Discrimination of muscle tension in chronic pain patients and healthy controls. *Biofeedback Self Regul*. 1992;17:165–177.

7. Glaros AG. Awareness of physiological responding under stress and nonstress conditions in temporomandibular disorders. *Biofeedback Self Regul*. 1996;21:261–272.

8. Hijzen TH, Siangen JL, Van Houweligan HC. Subjective, clinical, and EMG effects of biofeedback and splint treatment. *J Oral Rehabil*. 1986;13:529–539.

9. Balkhi KM, Tallents RH, Katzberg RW, Murphy W, Proskin H. Activity of anterior temporalis and masseter muscles during deliberate unilateral mastication. *J Orofacial Pain*. 1993;7:89–97.

10. Ferrario VF, Sforza C, Miani A Jr, D'Addona A, Barbini E. Electromyographic activity of human masticatory muscles in normal young people: statistical evaluation of reference values for clinical applications. *J Oral Rehabil*. 1993;20:271–280.

11. Ferrario VF, Sforza C. Biomechanical model of the human mandible in unilateral clench: distribution of temporomandibular joint reaction forces between working and balancing sides. *J Prosthet Dent*. 1994;72:169–176.

12. Peterson AL, Dixon DC, Talcott GW, Kelleher WJ. Habit reversal treatment of temporomandibular disorders: a pilot investigation. *J Behav Ther Exp Psychiatry*. 1993;24:49–55.

13. Clark GT, Koyano K, Browne PA. Oral motor disorders in humans. *J Calif Dent Assoc*. 1993;21:19–30.

14. Turk D, Hussein Z, Rudy T. Effects of intraoral appliance and biofeedback/stress management alone and in combination in treating temporomandibular disorders. *J Prosthet Dent*. 1993;70:158–164.

15. Tsolka P, Morris RW, Preiskel HW. Occlusal adjustment therapy for craniomandibular disorders: a clinical assessment by a double-blind method. *J Prosthet Dent*. 1992;68:957–964.

16. Christensen LV, Rassouli NM. Experimental occlusal interferences. *J Oral Rehabil*. 1995;22:515–520.

17. Yoshida K. The electromyographic activity of the masticatory muscles during temporomandibular joint clicking. *Schsweiz Monatsschr Zahnmed*. 1995;105:24–29.

18. Vallon D, Ekberg E, Nilner M, Kopp S. Occlusal adjustment in patients with craniomandibular disorders including headaches: a 3- and 6-month follow-up. *Acta Odontol Scand*. 1995;53:55–59.

19. Moss RA, Lombardo TW, Villarosa GA, Cooley JE, Simkin L, Hodgson JM. Oral habits and TMJ dysfunction in facial pain and non-pain subjects. *J Oral Rehabil*. 1995;22:79–81.

20. Hapak L, Gordon A, Locker D, Shandling M, Mock D, Tenenbaum HC. Differentiation between musculoligamentous, dentoalveolar, and neurologically based craniofacial pain with a diagnostic questionnaire. *J Orofac Pain*. 1994;8:357–368.

SEMG Program for Temporomandibular Joint Dysfunction and Myofacial Pain

Refer to the discussion in Chapter 9 for a review of intervention approaches. The suggestions that follow are derived from those resources. Descriptions and operational definitions are provided to clarify optional practice patterns.

CANDIDATES

Implement for patients
- with chronic myofacial pain. Candidates should display soft tissue tenderness, trigger points, apparent muscle hypertrophy, perception of tension or other evidence of chronic muscle dysfunction
- who may present with history of
  1. traumatic facial impact
  2. cervical injury
  3. motor vehicle accident
  4. orocranialfacial surgery
  5. immobilization
  6. malocclusion
  7. degenerative joint disease
  8. chronic bruxism
  9. insidious symptom onset

EVALUATION OBJECTIVES

- Identify elevated muscle tension at the mandibular elevators related to habitual clenching and grinding.
- Identify dysfunctional muscle activity patterns during mandibular and cervical movements.

- Assess effects of postural dysfunction on mandibular muscle activity.
- Assess the effects of orthotic appliances on muscle activity.
- Assess the relative contribution of psychophysiologic factors in the precipitation of excessive muscle tension.

FEEDBACK TRAINING OBJECTIVES

- Resolve habitual clenching, grinding, or other parafunctional behaviors.
- Restore optimal mechanical relationships between cervical and masticatory muscles and TMJ function.
- Improve postural function.
- Decouple psychologic stressors and muscle tension responses.
- Retain and generalize improved motor control to functional contexts.
- Resolve or reduce functional limitations and disability.

RECORDING SITES

- Judge the utility of each recording site on the basis of history and physical examination results.
- Include muscles that
  1. underlie the pain distribution
  2. potentially refer symptoms to the patient's area of complaint

3. reproduce the patient's symptoms when stretched, resisted, or palpated
- Consider use of a SEMG scan procedure (see Chapters 5 and 6 in the companion book *Introduction to Surface Electromyography*) to qualify sites for detailed postural and psychophysiologic assessments.
- Consult Chapter 14 in the companion book for specific electrode placement considerations.
- Confirm optimal sites from the following list by observation and palpation during isometric contraction:
  1. temporalis
  2. masseter
  3. sternomastoid, cervical paraspinal, lateral cervical, and trapezius groups if associated cervical dysfunction is suspected

EVALUATION PROCEDURES

- Select procedures that correspond to exacerbating and alleviating factors revealed by history and clinical examination.
- Refer to Chapter 2 for detailed discussion of evaluation methods.
- Perform at least five repetitions of each movement task to assess response consistency (consider discarding the results of the first one to two repetitions and averaging the results of the remaining repetitions). Many more repetitions may be needed to assess SEMG responses with reproduction of symptoms.
- Select relevant procedures from the following:
  1. psychophysiologic stress profile
  2. postural analysis
  3. active range of motion (AROM), observe for consistent excursion and velocity across test repetitions
     mandibular:
     –elevation
     –depression
     –left lateral deviation
     –right lateral deviation

–protrusion
–retrusion
4. isometric contractions:
   –bilateral clenching
   –unilateral biting with wadded gauze
5. repeated chewing, biting, speech
6. deep inspiration, upper chest versus abdominal breathing pattern
7. tension recognition thresholds
8. preapplication/postapplication of orthotic appliance
9. cervical AROM:
   –protraction
   –retraction
   –flexion
   –extension
   –side bending
   –rotation
10. analysis of masseter/temporalis and cervical synergy patterns during the above procedures

ASSESSMENT

- Refer to Chapter 2 for detailed discussion of SEMG assessment.
- Refer to Chapter 6 in the companion book for representative SEMG tracings of normal function, as well as for benchmark values for each site.
- Select SEMG assessment parameters from the following:
  1. Amplitude and variance of each channel during baseline. Activity during baseline should be stable and relatively quiescent. Mean amplitude values from nonpostural muscles should be close to internal noise levels of the recording device. Postural muscles may show low-level activity with the patient, in weight-bearing positions (typically, about 2–6 μV RMS).
  2. Peak or average amplitude of each channel during activation. Also observe for consistent amplitude elevations or depressions during a painful portion of the AROM arc.

3. Return to baseline amplitude after muscle activation. Qualitatively, recovery can be stated as prompt and complete versus elevated and delayed. Satisfactory baseline recovery is quantitatively defined (with a smoothing time constant of 0.1 second or less) as a return to an SEMG amplitude within two standard deviations of the original baseline mean, within 3 seconds of movement cessation, and maintenance within that amplitude range for at least 30 seconds or until the next movement is initiated. Recovery can be characterized by the latency to achieve this criterion. More simply, the amplitude (expressed as percentage of baseline) observed 3 seconds after movement termination can be reported.

4. Quiescence of cervical paraspinal activity in full flexion, the flexion–relaxation response.

5. Left/right peak amplitude symmetry for sagittal plane movements (eg, jaw opening/closing). Satisfactory symmetry is operationally defined as left/right scores within 35% as calculated [(higher value –lower value)/higher value] × 100. Symmetry assessment assumes an equivalent left/right AROM excursion and velocity.

6. Left/right timing symmetry for sagittal plane movements (ie, coincident recruitment, peak, and decruitment patterns; symmetric duration). When comparing the timing symmetry of synergist action, observe for changes in the recruitment order of muscles from one side to the other. For most clinical purposes, timing issues can be observed with rectified line tracings with a smoothing time constant of 0.1 second or less, SEMG sampling at 100 Hz or faster, frequency bandwidth filter low cutoff of 25 Hz or less, and a high resolution display with variable sweep speed. A graphic printout is useful for documentation of subtle timing differences. Documentation can be quantified with calculations of average slope, time to peak activity, or time to some percentage of maximal volitional isometric contraction activity that is clinically meaningful. Onset time can be reported simply as the latency to achieve a microvolt value equivalent to two standard deviations above the baseline mean. Duration may be noted as the amount of time between onset and baseline recovery as defined above.

7. Normal pattern of asymmetry for asymmetric plane movements (eg, jaw lateral deviation). Reciprocal symmetry of the SEMG patterns should be observed for reciprocal left/right tasks. Reciprocal asymmetry greater than 35% (assuming equal AROM excursion and velocity) is operationally an aberrant finding. Within a single side unilateral movement, similar levels of left/right co-activation are an aberrant finding.

8. Symmetrically proportionate left/right masseter and temporalis amplitude patterns during evaluation procedures.

9. Symmetrically proportionate left/right sternomastoid, cervical paraspinal, lateral cervical, and trapezius amplitude patterns during evaluation procedures.

COMMON PATIENT PRESENTATIONS

Chronic Bruxism

Bruxism is clenching, gritting, or grinding of the teeth. It is associated with mechanically destructive forces and can contribute to pathologic wear patterns on the teeth, gingival inflammation, and articular dysfunction. Chronic bruxism may also provoke tension-related myalgia from the temporalis and masseter muscles. Faulty posture or psychophysiologic stressors (or both) may be contributory in certain individuals (Figures 9–A–1 and 9–A–2). Aberrant hyperactivity from the masseter and temporalis can be identified with SEMG evaluation.

Bruxism may be suspected as a significant issue but be difficult to assess in the clinic setting. The clinician can note abnormal wear patterns on occlusal surfaces as a clue that bruxism is occurring. Observations from sleep partners or workmates may also help identify bruxing habits if the patient is unaware of them. Some portable SEMG units can record activity for many hours in the home or workplace. Data can be downloaded later to a printer or personal computer at the clinic. In this way, the clinician can look for habitually elevated patterns of muscle activity that occur during sleep or other functional activities. To eliminate the effects of artifact and inconsequential movements, the clinician defines a significant event as some minimal number of microvolts, maintained for some minimal length of time.

Asymmetric Masseter/Temporalis Activity

Asymmetric muscle recruitment during mandibular elevation can be a secondary consequence of asymmetric mobility in the TMJs. For example, if the left TMJ is hypomobile relative to the right, then the right condyle may translate a greater distance during opening and closing. Recruitment of the right masseter might then be considerably greater than that of the left. In this case, treatment would need to be directed to the left TMJ. It would be entirely inappropriate, and likely unsuccessful, to implement feedback training to reduce recruitment of the right masseter muscle unless and until joint function is improved. If the left joint dysfunction is subsequently resolved and the clinician believes that excessive right masseter activity persists, then SEMG feedback intervention would be appropriate.

TRAINING PROGRESSION

- Refer to Chapters 3 and 4 for detailed discussion of SEMG display setups and feedback structure.
- Refer to Chapter 5 for detailed discussion of SEMG feedback training techniques.
- As skill develops, generally
  1. Shape desired responses up or down.
  2. Add distractions.

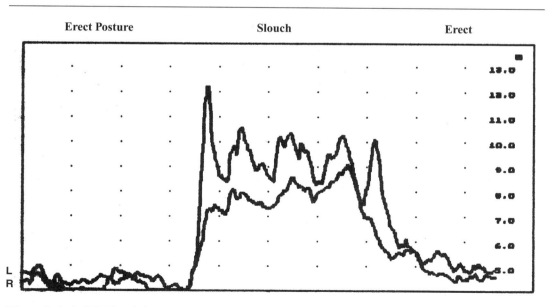

Figure 9–A–1 SEMG activity of the left (**L**) and right (**R**) masseter during assumption of erect retracted head posture versus slouched forward head posture, recorded from a patient with chronic myofacial pain.

A

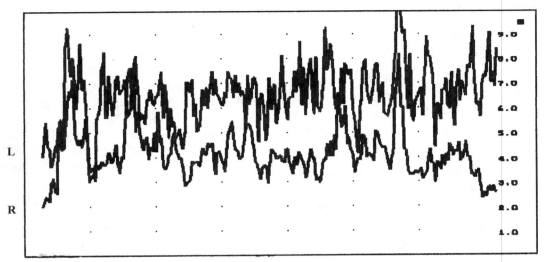

B

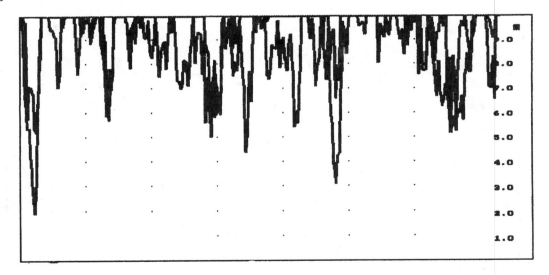

continues

Figure 9–A–2 SEMG activity of the left (**L**) and right (**R**) masseter, recorded from a patient with an acute flare of chronic myofacial pain. (**A**) Baseline activity in quiet sitting. (**B**) Activity with emotional stress-related imagery. (**C**) Activity after relaxation-based downtraining with SEMG feedback.

Figure 9–A–2 continued

C

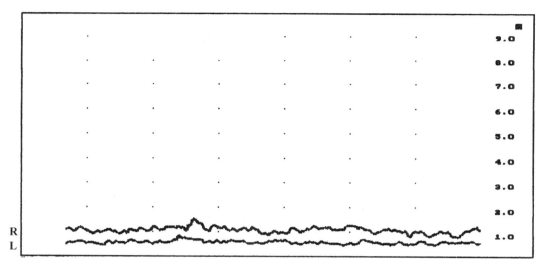

3. Randomize training activities.
4. Withdraw continuous audio/visual feedback.
• Select relevant SEMG feedback training tasks from the following:
   1. isolation of target muscle activity
   2. postural training with SEMG feedback
   3. relaxation-based downtraining
   4. threshold-based downtraining
   5. tension recognition threshold training
   6. tension discrimination training
   7. deactivation training
   8. left/right equilibration training
   9. motor copy training
   10. functional activity performance with SEMG feedback
• Integrate SEMG feedback training into a comprehensive approach to patient management:
   1. Ensure that the patient consults with a dentist for the current problem and as part of ongoing health maintenance.
   2. Refer the patient to a mental health practitioner if psychologic stressors seem to be contributory.

3. Consider consultation with a therapist or physician for adjunctive manual treatment techniques:
   –exercise prescription
   –physical agents
   –functional activity modification
4. Advise the patient to avoid
   –forward head postures
   –habitual lip biting or sucking
   –clenching
   –habitual gum chewing
   –repeated chewing on stringy, hard, or crunchy foods
5. Encourage soft foods, small bites of foods, and conscious awareness of jaw position.
6. Instruct the patient that in the absence of chewing and speech, a few millimeters of space should separate opposing teeth.
7. Ask the patient to self-monitor jaw status six to eight times per day.
8. Instruct the patient to check/correct head posture and rest the mandible with the teeth slightly apart, with the tongue gently touching the roof of the mouth.

Accompany this with a conscious shift to rhythmic abdominal breathing.
- Promote transfer of relaxation skills to functional environments:
  1. Instruct the patient in other related therapies, such as
     –systematic desensitization
     –stress inoculation
     –positive self-talk
     –relaxation trigger words
     –hand positions
     (Refer to Chapter 5.)
  2. Have the patient practice an abbreviated relaxation technique in work, home, and recreational settings.
  3. Use frequent trials with the tension discrimination training procedure for muscle awareness training.
  4. Once basic competence is demonstrated in the clinic, have the patient practice at home without SEMG, simply by estimating SEMG scores from the masseter and temporal muscles as if he or she were connected to the feedback machine.

- Consult other Application Guides in this book on tension-type headache and cervical dysfunction for associated problems.
- If nocturnal bruxism persists, consider use of a home SEMG feedback trainer:
  1. Ensure the device can provide continuous monitoring through the night.
  2. Set the unit to audio alarm if muscle activity exceeds a threshold of at least two to three times greater than the waking resting baseline for 20 seconds or longer. These settings will avoid spurious alarms if the patient rolls over.
  3. Instruct the patient in unit operation and what he or she should expect to experience. The method requires a high degree of patient (and sleep partner) commitment.
  4. Prescribe a home unit after the patient is practiced in the recognition and reduction of jaw muscle tension in the clinic and other underlying mechanical and psychologic issues have been addressed.
  5. Have the patient continue on a nightly course for at least 1 month.

SUGGESTED READINGS

Barker GR, Wastell DG, Duxbury AJ. Spectral analysis of masseter and anterior temporalis: an assessment of reliability for use in the clinical situation. *J Oral Rehabil.* 1989;16:309–313.

Cannistraci AJ, Fritz G. Dental applications of biofeedback. In: Basmajian JV, ed. *Biofeedback: Principles and Practice for Clinicians.* 3rd ed. Baltimore, MD: Williams & Wilkins; 1989;289–305.

Dahlstrom L. Electromyographic studies of craniomandibular disorders: a review of the literature. *J Oral Rehabil.* 1989;16:1–20.

Ferrario VF, Sforza C, Miani A Jr, D'Addona A, Barbini E. Electromyographic activity of human masticatory muscles in normal young people: statistical evaluation of reference values for clinical applications. *J Oral Rehabil.* 1993;20:271–280.

Gervitz RN, Glaros AG, Hopper D, Schwartz MS. Temporomandibular disorders. In: Schwartz MS, ed. *Biofeedback:*

A Practitioner's Guide. 2nd ed. New York: Guilford Press; 1995;411–428.

Glaros AG, Gervitz R. AAPB white paper: temporomandibular disorders. In: Amar P, Schneider C, eds. *Clinical Applications of Biofeedback and Applied Psychophysiology.* Wheat Ridge, CO: Association for Applied Psychophysiology and Biofeedback; 1995;52–56.

Hijzen TH, Slanger JL, Van Houweligan HC. Subjective, clinical and EMG effects of biofeedback and splint treatment. *J Oral Rehabil.* 1986;13:529–539.

Hudzinski LG, Lawrence GS: Myofacial pain and the temporo-mandibular joint. In: Cram JR, ed. *Clinical EMG for Surface Recordings.* Vol 2. Nevada City, CA: Clinical Resources, 1990;329–351.

Turk D, Hussein Z, Rudy T. Effects of intraoral appliance and biofeedback/stress management alone and in combination in treating temporomandibular disorders. *J Prosthet Dent.* 1993;70:158–164.

CHAPTER 10

Cervical Dysfunction

PATHOPHYSIOLOGY AND ASSESSMENT OF CERVICAL DYSFUNCTION

Cervical dysfunction and pain have many causes, including trauma, infection, tumors, congenital malformations, and inflammatory and degenerative disorders.[1] After an individual sustains traumatic injury to muscle and connective tissue, protective postures and altered patterns of muscle contraction develop so he or she can avoid pain. These short-term avoidance strategies may lead to long-term habitual compensatory postures and muscle patterns, causing reduced muscle length, strength, and endurance as well as chronic pain.[2] Abnormal postures unrelated to trauma can develop through degenerative or inflammatory processes, congenital malformations, or repetitive activities. Faulty posturing increases mechanical loading on joints and changes muscle length–tension relationships, resulting in compensatory movement patterns. Prolonged use of alternative movement patterns produces overuse and fatigue in some muscle groups and weakness related to disuse in others. The relationship among muscle overuse, localized muscle fatigue, and pain is well documented.[3,4] Localized muscle fatigue from prolonged contraction results in reduced adenosine triphosphate formation and blood flow, leading to an accumulation of metabolic byproducts[5] symptomatically expressed as muscle pain.

Maintenance of cervical pain may be attributed to dysfunctional patterns of muscle use and posture and to disturbances in locomotor control.[6] Chronic dysfunction may develop into myofascial pain syndrome, characterized by trigger points. A trigger point is defined as a hyperirritable spot, which on compression gives rise to referred pain in a characteristic pattern, tenderness, and an autonomic response.[7] In this case, function is impaired by pain and abnormal autonomic nervous system responses.

Many resources are available for assessment of the painful cervical spine. Those most commonly recommended include past medical history, description of neck pain and associated symptoms, observation of functional tasks relevant to the patient, postural assessment, passive and active cervical–thoracic and shoulder range of motion, manual muscle testing, testing for neurologic signs, bony and soft tissue palpation of the upper quadrant, and joint accessory play testing.[2,7–11] Surface electromyography (SEMG) has also been used as an adjunct for assessment of muscle dysfunction in the cervical region.

SEMG ASSESSMENT

SEMG analysis of the cervical spine is best performed by monitoring muscle groups that function simultaneously during cervical motion (flexion–extension, rotation, side-bending) by using four or more channels of SEMG, although bilateral comparisons with two channels of SEMG are also acceptable. Muscle groups recommended for assessment are cervical paraspinal muscles paired with upper trapezius, and cervical paraspinal muscles paired with sternomastoid.[12] Muscle monitoring of cervical superficial muscle groups during movement will also detect activity from deep cervical muscle groups.[13]

During symmetric movements (flexion–extension), muscle activity tends to be symmetric in pain-free individuals and asymmetric in certain patients with pain.[12] Asymmetric movement patterns (rotation and side-bending) produce asymmetric muscle activity in pain-free individuals and may be associated with symmetric activity, or an exaggerated asymmetry, in patients with pain. SEMG amplitude and timing differences can also be found in pain-free subjects with postural asymmetries and cervical hypomobility.[14,15] There are no follow-up studies correlating asymmetric movement patterns from asymptomatic individuals with potential (or later confirmed) cervical spine pain. Degrees of asymmetric muscle imbalance seem to exist in all persons during movement. The key is to determine whether motor impairments and pain are related to the patient's functional limitations and disability.

Sometimes movement patterns are normal with respect to left/right symmetry, but inappropriate activity is present in the form of a compensatory movement strategy. With compensatory movement patterns, muscles that are usually active at low levels shift to robust recruitment patterns, and typical prime movers are less active.[12] Assessing movement in various functional positions becomes important in establishing a baseline for each patient. Recording locations that show unbalanced muscle activity may be associated with underlying myofascial pathology.[16]

Clinically, isometric muscle testing against resistance is used to evaluate muscle function and localization of pain.[2] Using SEMG, Schuldt and Harms-Ringdahl[17] suggested certain isometric test contractions can be used to isolate target muscle groups in the cervical spine. Optimal isolation of the cervical erector spinae was accomplished by neck extension with resistance at the occiput, and lateral neck flexion best isolated levator scapulae and splenius capitis. This information supports the use of SEMG by clinicians during manual muscle testing, as well as for students learning manual muscle testing as an augmentative tool.

SEMG is also used to measure localized muscle fatigue by extracting the slope of the median frequency during sustained maximal volitional isometric contraction (MVIC). Evidence of greater fatigue in anterior neck muscles (sternomastoid) at 50%, 80%, and 100% MVIC and posterior neck muscles (upper trapezius) at 80% and 100% MVIC was demonstrated in patients with osteoarthritis of the cervical spine as compared to normal subjects.[18] Clinically, this finding supports the need for endurance training of anterior and posterior neck muscles. Overuse of muscles can also contribute to fatigue, as implied by Middaugh and coworkers[19] while studying headache patients for whom the upper trapezius continued to contract excessively during the rest portion of work/rest activity cycles, compared with findings in control subjects. Another investigation in normal subjects demonstrated fatigue of the upper trapezius and supraspinatus muscles within 1 to 5 minutes of continuous contraction at 11% MVIC, as measured by mean SEMG voltage and power frequency.[20] During study of prolonged low-load continuous contractions (5% MVIC), evidence of fatigue occurred in 1 hour.[21] Moreover, work tasks alternated with pauses increased work capacity and endurance,[22] suggesting rest breaks between repetitive low-load tasks may be beneficial.

SEMG also seems to have a place in ergonomic assessments in screening workers at risk for cervical pain and determining worksite modifications. Bilateral SEMG monitoring of upper trapezius activity in female workers during standardized tasks at a packing machine showed higher levels of static muscle activity and fewer low amplitude "gaps" in SEMG recordings from workers with prior musculoskeletal complaints.[23] These gaps are also known as "micromomentary" rests or "microrests," and can be as short as 0.2 second. The transient rests are not consciously perceived by the worker. Preventive microrest training of musculature during packing tasks at a conscious level may prevent musculoskeletal pain and injury.

Results of further studies with female production workers and manual laborers verified a consistent association between increased static muscle activation and fewer pauses in SEMG patterns with cervical pain.[14,24,25] Interestingly, the correlation was not found in office workers.[14,24] Veiersted and coworkers[25] reviewed new female production line employees in a chocolate manufacturing plant on hiring and every tenth week by using SEMG to measure the amount of static muscle activity and pauses in SEMG during repetitive work tasks. Increased static muscle activity and fewer gaps in SEMG tracings, measured prospectively, correlated with future complaints of trapezius myalgia, again suggesting preventive relaxation training during repetitive tasks may be beneficial.

Worksite modifications can also be helpful in injury prevention. Factory workstations were examined in a longitudinal study by Aaras.[26] SEMG activity of the upper trapezius was correlated with posture, limb positions, upper quarter loading, lifestyle, and sick leave for musculoskeletal problems. Higher or prolonged loading of the upper trapezius was associated with increased frequencies of sick leave related to musculoskeletal complaints. Redesigning a work station reduced static loading of upper trapezius from 4.5% MVIC to 1.5% MVIC and correlated with a reduction in sick leave for musculoskeletal problems. Aaras concluded that static loading of the upper trapezius at 1% MVIC was safest, in conjunction with rest breaks—a finding that contradicted previous recommendations of 2% to 5% MVIC by Jonsson.[27]

In a test of the utility of ergonomic modification with SEMG monitoring of neck and shoulder muscle activity in assembly line workers, two upper extremity aids each reduced muscle activity.[28] This finding suggests that ergonomic

aids may assist in prevention of cervical or shoulder muscle pain. Yates and Karwowski[29] analyzed static and dynamic lifting tasks with individuals in seated and standing positions by using SEMG monitoring of the muscles in the upper back, shoulder, abdomen, and low back. They found that seated lifts required greater amounts of muscle activity. On the basis of this study, it seems that job tasks requiring static and dynamic lifting would be best performed in standing position. Analysis of SEMG activity in cervical and thoracic erector spinae, levator scapulae, trapezius, and infraspinatus of female cashiers using conventional keyboards, scanners, and pen readers also showed less activity in standing versus seated positions.[30]

Middaugh and associates[6] considered both ergonomic and motor programming issues in several studies of patients with and without chronic pain. They found that patients with pain had increased SEMG activity in the upper trapezius in quiet sitting. In addition, this increased activity could not be deactivated after brief voluntary contractions. When pain-free subjects were positioned in ergonomically incorrect postures while they typed on a computer keyboard, a gradual increase in mean SEMG activity for the upper trapezius occurred over a 15-minute period. This effect was not seen when pain-free subjects used a more ergonomically correct alignment. Thus muscle overuse seems to be fostered in individuals assuming ergonomically incorrect keyboard postures. These investigators also noted that forward head posture increases mechanical loading on joints and alters patterns of muscle firing. They concluded that prolonged muscle overuse and fatigue can be clinically expressed as headache and cervical pain, and they also considered the effects of altered breathing patterns that seem to accompany muscle overuse.

Despite the body of work described above, controversy continues to exist as to whether heightened activity of the upper trapezius correlates with cervical pain. Vasseljen and associates[31] evaluated change in activity of the upper trapezius and perceived general tension before, at the conclusion of, and at 6 months after physiotherapy intervention in women workers with shoulder and neck pain. They found that in all groups pain decreased, whereas activity of this muscle site increased. Carlson and colleagues[32] monitored the upper trapezius with SEMG in patients with and without cervical pain during ambulation for 3 consecutive days. The investigators were not able to identify group differences between SEMG recording levels and self-reports of perceived muscle tension. It seems probable that aberrant muscle activity is but one factor contributing to neck pain. The extent to which muscle tension patterns become problematic probably depends on musculoskeletal comorbidities and psychologic issues. Experimental results will tend to vary with the types of SEMG measurements used, patient populations included, and environmental contexts studied.

Integration into Treatment Paradigms

SEMG can be incorporated into treatment programs for the cervical spine on the basis of observations of recruitment patterns that frequently correlate with pain. When insufficient recruitment exists, uptraining of muscle activity is appropriate. With excessive activity, downtraining needs to occur. Training for changes in recruitment patterns may incorporate psychotherapy, thermal and electrical agents, manual therapy, and exercise prescription.[12]

Training in movement patterns functionally relevant to the patient is imperative for motor learning to occur.[33] Ettare and Ettare[16] have labeled this "Muscle Learning Therapy," with the understanding that pain originates from pathologic tissue in need of re-education. Training to contract and quickly relax muscles during movement with SEMG is critical in decreasing muscle overuse, in giving proprioceptive cues to the patient, and in regaining muscle control. The movement patterns for training are simulated from daily activities and work conditions. Patients can wear portable SEMG units during the day to provide relaxation cues during the treatment phase. Middaugh and coworkers[6] also rec-

ommend that treatment of cervical hypertonicity be initiated with relaxation of the upper trapezius while the patient is in quiet sitting, with a progression to quick relaxation after repeated contract/relax cycles and, finally, to functional tasks.

Feedback to the clinician regarding effects of various treatment strategies may be useful in determining the optimal intervention for individual patients,[34] as well as in reporting to third-party payers. Monitoring of muscles during cervical traction and stretching activities used for muscle relaxation has been investigated. In healthy subjects, DeLacerda[35] found intermittent cervical traction with the subject in supine position resulted in greater myoelectric activity in the upper trapezius when the traction was pulling than when it was released. The larger the angle of pull, the greater the myoelectric activity displayed. In another study, Jette and coworkers[36] found no statistically significant difference in myoelectric activity of the upper trapezius before, during, or after intermittent cervical traction for patients with neck pain in supine position at a force of 8% body weight. Hence, use of intermittent cervical traction for muscle relaxation was not supported.

Murphy[37] monitored scalene activity in the posterior triangle of the neck in patients with and without pain. Results showed that for both groups SEMG levels for this site were elevated during and immediately after supine intermittent cervical traction, also suggesting that muscle relaxation did not occur. Patients with pain did, however, report relief of neck pain up to 12 hours after traction.

Osteopathic manipulation for more than 3 months in four patients with chronic cervical spine injury showed beneficial results, as evidenced by SEMG findings as well as patient complaints and physician examination results.[38] Prolonged treatment interventions, however, have become increasingly difficult to justify to third-party payers. A similar study would be useful to determine whether shortened treatment regimens involving manipulation would affect SEMG patterns in cervical patients.

Kendall and colleagues[2] have suggested that postural deviations are a cause of pain and should be addressed in treatment plans. Specifically, pain in the upper quadrant has been associated with faulty cervical posture.[2,39] Forward head posture has been associated with spasm in the upper trapezius and with neck pain. Correction of forward head posture includes axial extension and neutral neck position. Comparison of these two head positions in healthy subjects showed reduced SEMG activity of the upper trapezius in both corrective positions, although subjects reported greater difficulty in maintaining axial extension versus a neutral neck position.[40] Results of another comparative study of flexed and neutral neck positions while subjects performed assembly work in sitting position showed reduced activity in the cervical–thoracic erector spinae and trapezius with a neutral versus forward head position.[41] Clinically, SEMG can be used to monitor cervical muscle activity during postural correction in particular individuals, with rapid identification of postural changes that are likely to have an impact on each patient's cervical function. Use of SEMG feedback cues by the patient is further presumed to be highly reinforcing of change compliance.

SEMG feedback has also been used successfully in treatment of spasmodic torticollis through initial downtraining of both sternomastoid muscles in tandem.[42] In a controlled study with the use of television-monitored relaxation with and without SEMG feedback from the sternomastoid muscles, Duddy and McLellan[43] found no significant difference between cervical range of motion and ability to inhibit involuntary movements in the two groups. Therefore relaxation training by itself does not seem to be effective in treatment of spasmodic torticollis.

CONCLUSION

Applications of SEMG in the cervical spine are valuable as adjunctive assessment and treatment tools. The upper trapezius and cervical paraspinal muscles have been studied extensively, and reports with lateral and anterior cervical recording sites have been generated to a lesser extent. Levels of static and dynamic activity, %MVICs, and microrest pauses in SEMG tracings have been analyzed during movement, isometric testing, and work tasks. Efficacy of therapeutic and ergonomic treatment interventions has also been investigated with SEMG. The available literature provides a foundation for clinicians seeking to use SEMG to assess common and idiosyncratic patterns of muscle activity, as well as to use SEMG feedback to retrain posture and movement strategies.

REFERENCES

1. Sherk H, Watters W, Zeiger L. Evaluation and treatment of neck pain. *Orthop Clin North Am.* 1982;13:439–452.

2. Kendall F, McCreary E, Provance P. *Muscles Testing and Function with Posture and Pain.* 4th ed. Baltimore: Williams & Wilkins; 1993.

3. Enoka R, Stuart D. Neurobiology of muscle fatigue. *J Appl Physiol.* 1992;72:1631–1648.

4. Hagberg M. Occupational musculoskeletal stress disorders of the neck and shoulder: a review of possible pathophysiology. *Int Arch Occup Environ Health.* 1984;53:269–278.

5. Guyton A. Contraction of skeletal muscle. In: Guyton A, ed. *Textbook of Medical Physiology.* 5th ed. Philadelphia: WB Saunders Co; 1981;122–137.

6. Middaugh SJ, Kee WG, Nicholson JA. Muscle overuse and posture as factors in the development and maintenance of chronic musculoskeletal pain. In: Grzesiak RC, Ciccone DS, eds. *Psychological Vulnerability to Chronic Pain.* New York: Springer Publishing Co; 1994;55–89.

7. Travell J, Simons D. *Myofascial Pain and Dysfunction.* Baltimore: Williams & Wilkins; 1983.

8. Cyriax J, Cyriax P. The cervical spine. In: Cyriax J, Cyriax P, eds. *Illustrated Manual of Orthopaedic Medicine.* London: Butterworth; 1983;145–166.

9. Greenman P. Cervical spine technique. In: Greenman P, ed. *Principles of Manual Medicine.* Baltimore: Williams & Wilkins; 1989;125–149.

10. Hoppenfeld S. Physical examination of the cervical spine and temporomandibular joint. In: Hoppenfeld S, ed. *Physical Examination of the Spine and Extremities.* New York: Appleton-Century-Crofts; 1976;105–132.

11. Lewis C, McNerney T. Cervical spine complications: a rehabilitation perspective. In: Lewis C, Knortz K, eds. *Orthopedic Assessment and Treatment of the Geriatric Patient.* St Louis, MO: CV Mosby; 1993;89–100.

12. Donaldson S, Donaldson M. Multi-channel EMG assessment and treatment techniques. In: Cram JR, ed. *Clinical EMG for Surface Recordings.* Vol 2. Nevada City, CA: Clinical Resources; 1990;143–173.

13. Perry J, Easterday S, Antonelli D. Surface versus intramuscular electrodes for electromyography of superficial and deep muscles. *Phys Ther.* 1981;61:7–15.

14. Jensen C, Nilsen K, Hansen K, et al. Trapezius muscle load as a risk indicator for occupational shoulder–neck complaints. *Int Arch Occup Environ Health.* 1993; 64:415–423.

15. Vorro J, Johnston W. Clinical biomechanic correlates for cervical function, part II: a myoelectric study. *J Am Osteopath Assoc.* 1987;87:353–367.

16. Ettare DL, Ettare R. Muscle learning therapy: a treatment protocol. In: Cram, JR, ed. *Clinical EMG for Surface Recordings.* Vol 2. Nevada City, CA: Clinical Resources; 1990;197–233.

17. Schuldt K, Harms-Ringdahl K. Activity levels during isometric test contractions of neck and shoulder muscles. *Scand J Rehabil Med.* 1988;20:117–127.

18. Gogia P, Sabbahi M. Electromyographic analysis of neck muscle fatigue in patients with osteoarthritis of the cervical spine. *Spine.* 1994;19:502–506.

19. Middaugh SJ, Kee WG, Nicholson JA, Allenback G. Upper trapezius overuse in chronic headache and correction with EMG biofeedback training. *Proceedings of the Association for Applied Psychophysiology and Biofeedback (AAPB) 26th Annual Meeting, Cincinnati, Ohio, March 1995.* Wheat Ridge, CO: AAPB; 1995;89–92.

20. Hagberg M. Electromyographic signs of shoulder muscular fatigue in two elevated arm positions. *Am J Phys Med Rehabil.* 1981;60:522–525.

21. Jorgenson K, Falletin N, Krogh-Lund C, et al. Electromyography and fatigue during prolonged low-level static contractions. *Eur J Appl Physiol.* 1988;57:316–321.

22. Hagberg M. Muscular endurance and surface electromyogram in isometric and dynamic exercise. *J Appl Physiol.* 1981;51:1–7.

23. Veiersted KB, Westgaard RH, Andersen P. Pattern of muscle activity during stereotyped work and its relation to muscle pain. *Int Arch Occup Environ Health.* 1990;62:31–41.

24. Vasseljen O, Westgaard R. A case-control study of trapezius muscle activity in office and manual workers with shoulder and neck pain and symptom-free controls. *Int Arch Occup Environ Health.* 1995;67:11–18.

25. Veiersted KB, Westgaard RH, Andersen P. Electromyographic evaluation of muscular work pattern as a predictor of trapezius myalgia. *Scand J Work Environ Health.* 1993;19:284–290.

26. Aaras A. *Postural Load and the Development of Musculo-Skeletal Illness.* Oslo, Norway: Ministry of Local Government and Labour; 1987.

27. Jonsson B. Measurement and evaluation of local muscular strain in the shoulder during constrained work. *J Hum Ergol (Tokyo).* 1982;11:73–88.

28. Schuldt K, Ekholm J, Harms-Ringdahl K, et al. Effects of arm support or suspension on neck and shoulder muscle activity during sedentary work. *Scand J Rehabil Med.* 1987;19:77–84.

29. Yates J, Karwowski W. An electromyographic analysis of seated and standing lifting tasks. *Ergonomics.* 1992;35:889–898.

30. Lannersten L, Harms-Ringdahl K. Neck and shoulder muscle activity during work with different cash register systems. *Ergonomics.* 1990;33:49–65.

31. Vasseljen O, Johansen B, Westgaard R. The effect of pain reduction on perceived tension and EMG recorded trapezius muscle activity in workers with shoulder and neck pain. *Scand J Rehabil Med.* 1995;27:243–252.

32. Carlson C, Wynn K, Edwards J, et al. Ambulatory electromyogram activity in the upper trapezius region: patients with muscle pain vs. pain-free control subjects. *Spine.* 1996;21:595–599.

33. Schmidt R. *Motor Control and Learning: A Behavioral Emphasis.* 2nd ed. Champaign, IL: Human Kinetics; 1988.

34. Wolf S, Edwards D, Shutter L. Concurrent assessment of muscle activity (CAMA): a procedural approach to assess treatment goals. *Phys Ther.* 1986;66:218–244.

35. DeLacerda F. Effect of angle of traction pull on upper trapezius muscle activity. *J Orthop Sports Phys Ther.* 1980;1:205–209.

36. Jette D, Falkel J, Trombly C. Effect of intermittent, supine cervical traction on the myoelectric activity of the upper trapezius muscle in subjects with neck pain. *Phys Ther.* 1985;65:1173–1176.

37. Murphy M. Effects of cervical traction on muscle activity. *J Orthop Sports Phys Ther.* 1985;13:220–225.

38. Beal M, Vorro J, Johnston W. Chronic cervical dysfunction: correlation of myoelectric findings with clinical progress. *J Am Osteopath Assoc.* 1989;89:891–900.

39. Greigel-Mooris P, Larson K, Mueller-Klaus K, et al. Incidence of common postural abnormalities in the cervical, shoulder, and thoracic regions and their association with pain in two age groups of healthy subjects. *Phys Ther*. 1992;72:26–32.

40. Enwemeka C, Bonet I, Jayanti A, et al. Postural correction in persons with neck pain, II: integrated electromyography of the upper trapezius in three simulated neck positions. *J Orthop Sports Phys Ther*. 1986;8:240–242.

41. Schuldt K. On neck muscle activity and load reduction in sitting postures: an electromyographic and biomechanical study with applications in ergonomics and rehabilitation. *Scand J Rehabil Med Suppl*. 1988;19:1–49.

42. Jankel W. Electromyographic feedback in spasmodic torticollis. *Am J Clin Biofeedback*. 1978;1:28–29.

43. Duddy J, McLellan D. Lack of influence of EMG biofeedback in relaxation training for spasmodic torticollis. *Clin Rehabil*. 1995;9:297–303.

SEMG Program for Cervical Dysfunction

Refer to the discussion in Chapter 10 for a review of intervention approaches. The suggestions that follow are derived from those resources. Descriptions and operational definitions are provided to clarify optional practice patterns.

CANDIDATES

Implement for patients
- with chronic neck pain in whom muscle dysfunction is suspected
- who may present with history of
  1. motor vehicle accident
  2. work injury
  3. athletic trauma
  4. insidious symptom onset

Neck pain can occur in conjunction with headache, temporomandibular joint problems, or shoulder girdle dysfunction.

Candidates should relate subjective remarks regarding inappropriate tension sensations about the neck and proximal shoulder girdle. Psychologic stressors—such as posttraumatic stress syndrome after motor vehicle accident—may seem to trigger aberrant muscle tension. Alternatively, physical examination should reveal faulty posture, palpable hypertonicity, trigger points, or imbalances in muscle flexibility and strength.

EVALUATION OBJECTIVES

- Assess the effects of posture and dynamic movement on cervical muscle activity.
- Identify aberrant patterns of muscle activity about the neck, potentially contributing to musculoskeletal pain:
  1. myalgia due to excessive levels or duration of muscle tension
  2. imbalanced muscle activity that potentially results in soft tissue or joint dysfunction
- Assess psychophysiologic factors in the precipitation of excessive muscle tension.

FEEDBACK TRAINING OBJECTIVES

- Reduce excessive or imbalanced muscle tension.
- Resolve underlying cervical mechanical dysfunction; improve postural function and ergonomic alignment.
- Decouple psychologic stressors and muscle tension responses.
- Retain and generalize improved motor control to functional contexts.
- Resolve or reduce functional limitations and disability.

RECORDING SITES

- Judge the utility of each recording site on the basis of history and physical examination results.
- Include muscles that
  1. underlie the pain distribution
  2. potentially refer symptoms or are mechanically related to the patient's area of complaint
  3. reproduce the patient's symptoms when stretched, resisted, or palpated
- Consider use of an SEMG scan procedure (see Chapters 5 and 6 in the companion book, *Introduction to Surface Electromyography*) to qualify sites for detailed postural and psychophysiologic assessments.
- Consult Chapter 14 in the companion book for specific electrode placement considerations.
- Confirm optimal sites from the following list by observation and palpation during isometric contraction:
  1. cervical paraspinal groups (trapezius, splenius, semispinalis, erector spinae, suboccipitals, levator scapulae, rhomboids)
     –upper cervical
     –middle cervical
     –lower cervical/upper thoracic
  2. sternomastoid
  3. lateral cervical region (scalenes, levator scapulae)
  4. upper trapezius
  5. middle interscapular region (middle trapezius, rhomboids, erector spinae)
  6. lower interscapular region (lower trapezius is the intended target, some degree of cross-talk from rhomboids and erector spinae is likely)
  7. lower fibers of serratus anterior

EVALUATION PROCEDURES

- Select procedures that correspond to exacerbating and alleviating factors revealed by history and clinical examination.

- Refer to Chapter 2 for detailed discussion of evaluation methods.
- Perform at least five repetitions of each movement task to assess response consistency (consider discarding the results of the first one to two repetitions and averaging the results of the remaining repetitions). Many more repetitions may be needed to assess SEMG responses with reproduction of symptoms.
- Select relevant procedures from the following:
  1. psychophysiologic stress profile
  2. postural analysis
  3. cervical active range of motion (AROM), observe for consistent excursion and velocity across test repetitions
     –flexion
     –extension
     –side-bending
     –rotation
     –protraction
     –retraction
  4. shoulder girdle AROM, observe for consistent excursion and velocity across test repetitions: Test left side, right side, simultaneous bilateral movements; concentric versus eccentric phases through
     –scapular elevation, retraction
     –shoulder flexion, abduction, scaption (elevation in the scapular plane, between flexion and abduction)
  5. deep inhalation
  6. isometric contractions of target recording muscles:
     –maximal
     –submaximal, progressively graded
  7. tension recognition thresholds
  8. analysis of muscle synergy patterns and reciprocal activity (eg, cervical paraspinals and sternomastoid during cervical rotation and side-bending; upper trapezius with lower trapezius and serratus anterior during arm elevation)
  9. functional activity analysis
     –job
     –home
     –recreation

For example, reproduce exacerbating and alleviating lifting tasks, overhead maneuvers, prolonged typing, and sports-specific movements.

ASSESSMENT

- Refer to Chapter 2 for detailed discussion of SEMG assessment.
- Refer to Chapter 14 in the companion book for representative SEMG tracings of normal function, as well as for baseline benchmark values for each site.
- Select SEMG assessment parameters from the following:
  1. Amplitude and variance of each channel during baseline. Activity during baseline should be stable and relatively quiescent. Mean amplitude values from nonpostural muscles should be close to internal noise levels of the recording device. Postural muscles may show low-level activity in weight-bearing positions (typically, about 2–6 µV RMS).
  2. Peak or average amplitude of each channel during activation. Activity can appear to be unremarkable, grossly excessive and erratic, or markedly depressed. Association of aberrant magnitude or erratic activity with a painful portion of the AROM arc should be noted.
  3. Return to baseline amplitude after muscle activation. Qualitatively, recovery can be stated as prompt and complete versus elevated and delayed. Satisfactory baseline recovery is quantitatively defined (with a smoothing time constant of 0.1 second or less) as a return to an SEMG amplitude within two standard deviations of the original baseline mean, within 3 seconds of movement cessation, and maintenance within that amplitude range for at least 30 seconds or until the next movement is initiated. Recovery can be characterized by the latency to achieve this criterion. More simply, the amplitude (expressed as percentage of baseline) observed 1 to 3 seconds after movement termination can be reported.
  4. Quiescence of cervical paraspinal activity in full flexion, the flexion-relaxation response (Figure 10–A–1).
  5. Left/right peak amplitude symmetry for sagittal plane movements of the spine or bilateral symmetric movements of the extremities (eg, cervical flexion–extension and bilateral shoulder flexion, respectively). Satisfactory symmetry is operationally defined as left/right scores within 35% as calculated [(higher value – lower value)/higher value] × 100. Symmetry assessment assumes an equivalent left/right AROM excursion and velocity. Asymmetries recorded from electrodes placed over multiple muscle layers can be difficult to define. It may be possible to approximate the activity of a particular muscle within a group by observing the SEMG display while the patient performs the isolated isometric action of that muscle. For example, an asymmetric pattern recorded from the middle interscapular region could be secondary to middle trapezius dysfunction, rhomboid dysfunction, or both. Cross-talk and co-activation are likely for most patients during arm elevation tasks. However, occasionally the asymmetry is reproduced only during manual muscle test of the middle trapezius[1,2] and not during that for the rhomboid, or vice versa. Thus asymmetries observed from nonspecific recording sites during movement may be compared with findings on selective manual muscle tests. The process sometimes yields insight as to the offending muscle, but true confirmation requires intramuscular electrode placement.
  6. Left/right timing symmetry for sagittal plane or bilateral symmetric movements (ie, coincident recruitment, peak, and

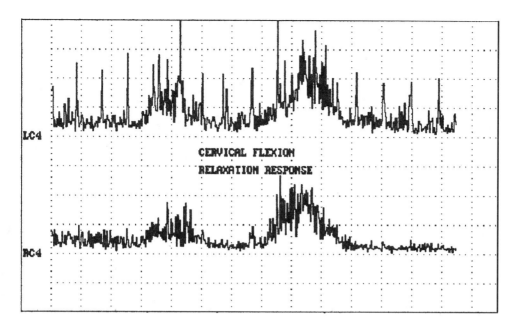

Figure 10–A–1 SEMG activity of the (**L**) left and (**R**) right (**C4**) cervical paraspinals at the level of the fourth vertebra. The cervical flexion–relaxation response is illustrated. Rising activity corresponds to initiation of eccentric cervical flexion (first rise); maintenance of full cervical flexion, the flexion–relaxation response (trough between rises); and concentric return to neutral (second rise). Cardiac artifact is seen as a series of spikes throughout the tracing, especially in left side signal.

decruitment patterns; symmetric duration). When comparing the timing symmetry of synergist action, observe for changes in the recruitment order of muscles from one side to the other. For most clinical purposes, timing issues can be observed with rectified line tracings with a smoothing time constant of 0.1 second or less, SEMG sampling at 100 Hz or faster, frequency bandwidth filter low cutoff of 25 Hz or less, and a high resolution display with variable sweep speed. A graphic printout is useful for documentation of subtle timing differences. Documentation can be quantified with calculations of average slope, time to peak activity, or time to some percentage of MVIC activity that is clinically meaningful. Onset time can be reported simply as the latency to achieve a microvolt value equivalent to two standard deviations above the baseline mean. Duration may be noted as the amount of time between onset and baseline recovery as defined above.

7. Normal pattern of SEMG asymmetry for asymmetric or unilateral movements (eg, cervical rotation and unilateral shoulder flexion). Reciprocal symmetry of the SEMG patterns should be observed for reciprocal left/right tasks. Reciprocal asymmetry greater than 35% (assuming equal AROM excursion and velocity) is operationally an aberrant finding. Within a single side unilateral movement, similar levels of left/right co-activation are an aberrant finding.

8. Proportionate cervical and scapular muscle amplitude patterns that are symmetric from left to right:

–contralateral cervical paraspinal and sternomastoid activity during rotation, ipsilateral activity during side-bending

–ipsilateral upper and lower portions of trapezius, serratus anterior activity during arm elevation tasks

For comparisons across nonhomologous muscles, amplitudes may be expressed as a:

–percentage of MVIC amplitude by using standard manual muscle tests (test activity amplitude/MVIC amplitude × 100)

–percentage of some submaximal contraction obtained with a standardized force intensity, joint angle, and body posture

9. Low-amplitude gaps or microrests in each channel display during functional tasks (obtained with use of a rectified moving line tracing display with a smoothing time constant of 0.1 second or less, SEMG sampling at 100 Hz or faster, and a frequency bandwidth filter low cutoff of 25 Hz or less) can be identified by setting a visible threshold marker at a microvolt value of about 5% MVIC for that muscle. This value should be above the range of the patient's postural baseline tracing. If the patient's postural baseline range exceeds 5% MVIC, the assessment should be deferred. Instruct the patient to perform continually a functional task that tends to exacerbate symptoms. With suitable precautions for patient safety, maintain task performance until the patient reports reproduction or exacerbation of symptoms. At the outset and every 2 to 3 minutes of task performance thereafter, save or freeze and print a copy of a 30- to 60-second display sweep. Count the number of threshold crossings. Microrests are typically produced in a range of approximately 0.2 second to several seconds, without conscious patient effort. Observe for a minimal presence of microrests throughout the course, as well as for changes in microrest frequency and duration as symptoms are produced. Compare left with right microrest frequencies/durations if the functional task involves symmetric movements and patient has unilateral involvement (Figure 10–A–2).

10. Tonic amplitude during repeated task trials or a continuous functional activity. With use of the same type of display as in No. 9 above, observe the lowest level of activation consistently produced during performance of a continuous functional task. This tonic amplitude level appears as the continually running baseline from which the muscle is phasically activated (Figure 10–A–3). Assuming a satisfactory, low noise recording setup, the tonic amplitude should be less than 5% to 10% MVIC for tasks that are functionally performed for about 1 hour or longer. Note the tonic amplitude at the outset and every 2 to 3 minutes of task performance thereafter. Compare left with right sides if the functional task involves symmetric movements and patient has unilateral symptoms.

11. Change in average activity level for a particular muscle and task across treatment sessions. To document this parameter a normalization procedure is preferred to enhance reliability. A reliable maximal manual muscle test effort or a standardized submaximal contraction is required. For example, the average upper trapezius SEMG amplitude produced during typing can be expressed as a percentage of upper trapezius activity while maintaining 90 degrees of shoulder abduction. The average amplitude during the test task is divided by that day's reference contraction amplitude, and the quotient is multiplied by 100.

12. Frequency spectral analysis for fatigue assessment. This analysis requires spe-

A

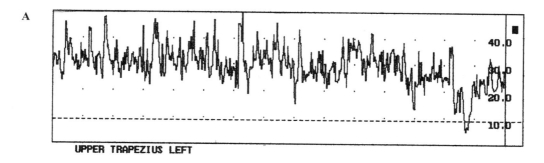

B

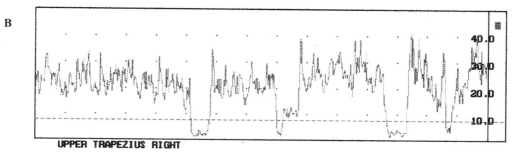

Figure 10–A–2 SEMG activity of the (**A**) left and (**B**) right upper trapezius during performance of a bilateral typing task recorded from a patient with chronic left posterolateral neck pain. Fewer microrest gaps are produced on the left compared with the right, despite that the patient's hands were bilaterally paused during each gap period apparent on the right. Dashed markers correspond to about 5% MVIC amplitude for each recording site.

cialized equipment and technique. Observe the median frequency during a standardized isometric contraction of at least 50% MVIC. Observe the rate of decline in median frequency values (indicative of increased fatigue) during a prolonged effort contraction, comparing left and right side muscle performance. To track fatigue during a dynamic functional task, obtain SEMG frequency data during a high-level isometric contraction before initiation of the functional activity. Then have the patient perform the functional task for a duration expected to induce fatigue or increase symptoms. Repeat the standardized isometric test, extract median frequency values, and compare these values with initial levels for indications

of fatigue. Have the patient rest for 1 to 3 minutes, and then repeat the isometric test and frequency analysis. Continue a rest period:frequency test sequence to assess for recovery to initial median frequency values.

COMMON PATIENT PRESENTATIONS

Postural Dysfunction

Postural-related pain is frequently encountered in the neck region. Forward head postures tend to be accompanied by increased activity at cervical paraspinal and upper trapezius sites (Figure 10–A-4). This posture may be further associated with low-level sternocleidomastoid recruitment during cervical side-bending or rotation (Figure 10–A–5).

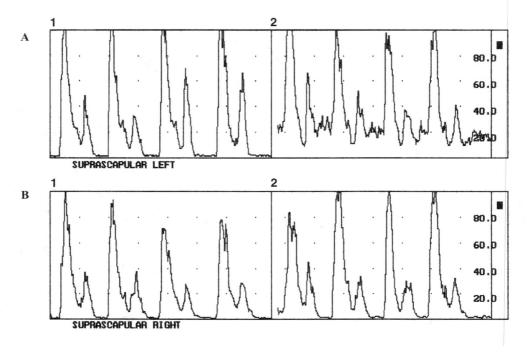

Figure 10–A–3 SEMG activity from the (**A**) left and (**B**) right suprascapular sites during repeated trials of a bilateral upper extremity martial arts maneuver recorded from a patient with cumulative left suprascapular pain. Each doublet of activity corresponds to one trial. (**A1, B1**) Initiation of task repetitions. (**A2, B2**) A series of repetitions after 30 intervening trials. The tonic amplitude increases on the left but not on the right.

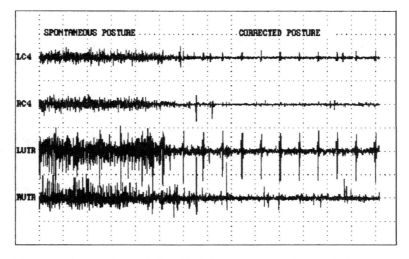

Figure 10–A–4 SEMG activity of the (**L**) left and (**R**) right (**C4**) cervical paraspinals at the level of the fourth vertebra and (**UTR**) upper trapezius recorded from a patient with bilateral cervical and suprascapular pain during sitting work tasks. Effects of the patient's spontaneous forward head posture (leading half of tracings) and a corrected postural alignment (second half of tracings) are illustrated. Cardiac artifact is seen as a series of spikes, especially in **LC4** and **LUTR** signals.

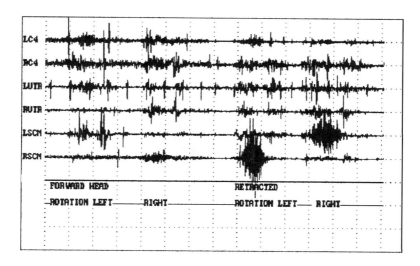

Figure 10–A–5 SEMG activity of the (**L**) left and (**R**) right (**C4**) cervical paraspinals at the level of the fourth vertebra, (**UTR**) upper trapezius, and (**SCM**) sternomastoids recorded from a patient with bilateral cervical and suprascapular pain during sitting work tasks. Effects of head rotational movements to the left and right during forward versus retracted head posture are illustrated. Note the change in SCM recruitment pattern and relative C4:SCM activity between postures.

Training Progression for Postural Dysfunction

- Refer to Chapters 3 and 4 for detailed discussion of SEMG display setups and feedback structure.
- Refer to Chapter 5 for detailed discussion of SEMG training techniques.
- As skill develops, generally
  1. Shape desired responses up or down.
  2. Incorporate multijoint control.
  3. Add distractions.
  4. Randomize training activities.
  5. Withdraw continuous audio/visual feedback.
- Select relevant SEMG feedback training tasks from the following:
  1. isolation of target muscle activity
  2. postural training with SEMG feedback
  3. integration with functional activities:
     –home
     –work
     –driving
     –recreation

- Integrate SEMG training into a comprehensive approach to patient management.
  1. Include home exercises and adjunctive manual therapies as indicated. Suboccipital, sternomastoid, scalene, upper trapezius, pectoralis major, pectoralis minor, and latissimus muscles, among others, may be shortened.
  2. Provide simple strategies for the patient to use to check and correct posture throughout the day, as well as to practice in a variety of functional settings.

Neck Pain with Upper Trapezius Hyperactivity

Upper trapezius hyperactivity is perhaps the most usual finding in cervical patients. The syndrome can be associated with muscle responsiveness to psychologic stressors, as well as with kinesiologic dysfunction (Figure 10–A–6). Tight passive extensibility of the upper trapezius and elevated scapular position at rest or during shoulder movements may be observed. Postural

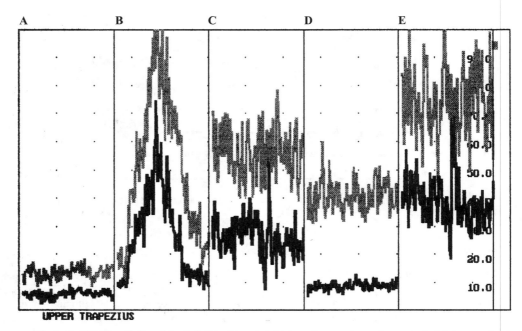

Figure 10–A–6 SEMG activity of the left (black) and right (gray) upper trapezius recorded from a patient with chronic neck pain and muscle hyperactivity on the right. (**A**) Baseline activity in quiet sitting. (**B**) Bilateral symmetric arm abduction. (**C**) Bilateral typing task. (**D**) Emotionally stressful imagery. (**E**) Typing and stressful imagery. Muscle hyperactivity is affected by both mechanical and psychologic factors.

dysfunction is commonly seen in conjunction with hyperactivity of the upper trapezius. Hyperactivity may be present unilaterally or bilaterally.

Training Progression for Neck Pain with Upper Trapezius Hyperactivity

- Refer to Chapters 3 and 4 for detailed discussion of SEMG display setups and feedback structure.
- Refer to Chapter 5 for detailed discussion of SEMG training techniques.
- As skill develops, generally
  1. Shape desired responses up or down.
  2. Incorporate multijoint control.
  3. Add distractions.
  4. Randomize training activities.
  5. Withdraw continuous audio/visual feedback.

- Select relevant feedback training tasks from the following:
  1. isolation of target muscle activity
  2. relaxation-based downtraining
  3. threshold-based downtraining
  4. deactivation training
  5. tension recognition thresholds
  6. tension discrimination training
  7. generalization to progressively dynamic movement
  8. left/right equilibration training
  9. postural training with SEMG feedback
  10. therapeutic exercises with SEMG feedback. Emphasize
      −exercise selection and relaxation/stretching for shortened muscles
      −isolation and conditioning for weak or easily fatigued muscles
  11. functional activity performance with SEMG feedback

- Integrate SEMG training into a comprehensive approach to patient management:
  1. Refer the patient to a mental health practitioner if psychologic stressors seem to be contributory.
  2. Counsel patient for wellness. Include concepts relating to
     –general relaxation
     –modification of stressful cognitive appraisals
     –maintenance of appropriate postures and ergonomic setups
     –sensible pacing of activities
     –nutritional balance
     –aerobic fitness
     –general conditioning
     –body weight management
- Promote transfer of relaxation skills to functional environments:
  1. Instruct the patient in other related therapies, such as
     –systematic desensitization
     –stress inoculation
     –positive self-talk
     –relaxation trigger words
     –hand positions
     (Refer to Chapter 5.)
  2. Have the patient practice an abbreviated relaxation technique in work, home, and recreational settings.
  3. Instruct the patient in postural self-checks to use throughout the day.
  4. Combine tactics in the three recommendations above with
     –abdominal breathing
     –cervical stretching
     –adaptation of muscle deactivation and tension discrimination training procedures
  5. Once basic competence is demonstrated with tension discrimination training in the clinic, have the patient practice at home without SEMG feedback, simply by estimating SEMG scores from the target muscles as if he or she were connected to the feedback machine.

- Prescribe frequent, brief practice sessions and adjunctive therapies for the patient with muscle asymmetries.
  1. Emphasize repetition of muscle equilibration procedures and stretching throughout the day.
  2. Develop a careful plan to implement indicated changes in ergonomic setups and functional motor habits.
  3. Consider consultation with a therapist or physician for
     –adjunctive manual treatments
     –exercise prescription
     –physical agents
     –taping techniques
     –functional activity modification
- Consider uptraining recruitment of the lower trapezius or serratus anterior to balance the upper trapezius (see below, as well as Application Guide 11–A, SEMG Program for Shoulder Girdle Dysfunction).

Neck Pain with Asymmetric Sternomastoid/ Cervical Paraspinal Balance

Left/right asymmetries in sternomastoid and cervical paraspinal function are seen after whiplash injuries. Imbalances between the two muscles are also observed. Head rotation is produced in part by a force couple generated by the ipsilateral superficial cervical paraspinal muscles and contralateral sternomastoid. In side-bending, the ipsilateral cervical paraspinal and sternomastoid muscles act together. For flexion–extension movements, the left and right of each homologous muscle pair function as synergists. Asymmetries recorded from these two muscle sites are often contralaterally paired. For example, the left side cervical paraspinal and right sternomastoid muscles might each be consistently elevated in activity throughout AROM. Reciprocal symmetry would be expected for reciprocal side-bending and rotation movements. Instead the left cervical paraspinal muscles could generate greater activity during movement to the left than that of the right cervical paraspinal muscles during motion to the right. The left cervical paraspinal muscles could also continue to fire in an inappropriate co-contraction pattern during reciprocal motion to the right. Further, the left cervical paraspinal muscles might obviously predominate over the right side during flexion–extension. The right sternomastoid muscle would show an analogous pattern of dysfunction, predominating during flexion–extension, showing reciprocally greater activity during right side–bending and left rotation movements, and inappropriately co-contracting. The syndrome tends to be associated with range of motion and muscle length imbalances on physical examination, faulty postures, multiple trigger points, and movement-related anxiety. Examples of imbalanced, nonreciprocating function are illustrated in Figures 10–A–7 through 10–A–10.

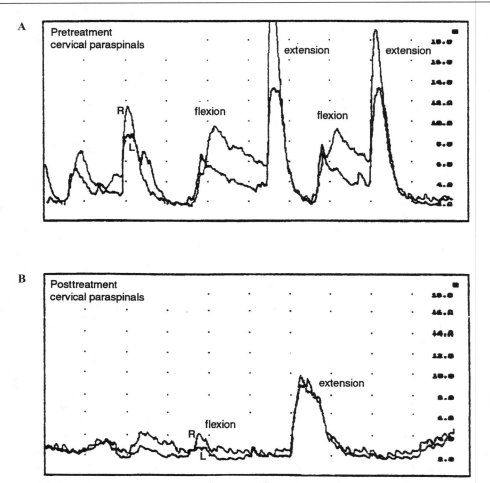

Figure 10–A–7 SEMG activity of the (**L**) left and (**R**) right cervical paraspinal muscles during repeated cervical flexion and extension recorded from a patient with right greater than left chronic neck pain. (**A**) Activity at initial presentation, before therapy. Range of motion (not shown) was well within normal limits. (**B**) Activity approximately 4 weeks later, after a course of manual therapy, postural and work station modification, exercise prescription, and SEMG feedback training. Pain symptoms were largely resolved by this point. The degree of left/right asymmetry, as well as absolute levels of recruitment, are considerably reduced, and a normal flexion–relaxation response has emerged.

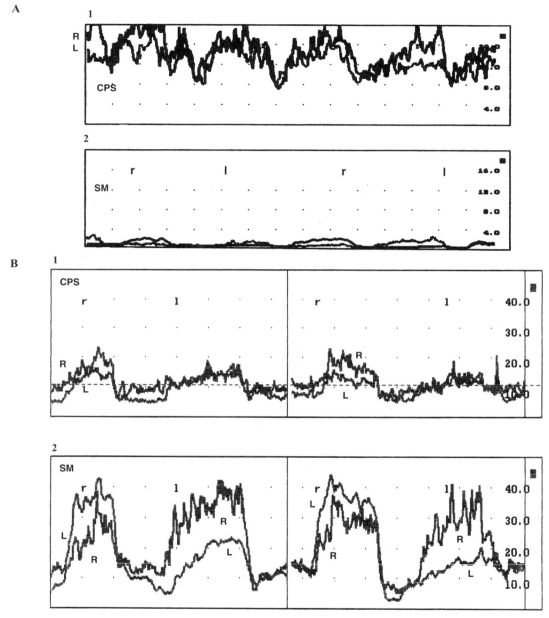

Figure 10–A–8 SEMG activity of (**L**) left and (**R**) right (**CPS**) cervical paraspinal and (**SM**) sternomastoid muscles during repeated head rotation (**r**) right and (**I**) left, recorded from a patient with persistent pain 6 weeks after C-4–C-5 surgical fusion. (**A1, A2**) Activity at initial presentation, before feedback training. Note co-activation of (**L**) left and (**R**) right cervical paraspinals (**A1**) and minimal sternomastoid (**A2**) activity levels. (**B1, B2**) Activity at the conclusion of the second SEMG feedback training session, 2 days later, with diminished pain and improved range of motion. Emphasis was placed on postural correction and sternomastoid uptraining. Note increased sternomastoid activity (**B2**), diminished cervical paraspinal activity (**B1**), and beginning emergence of left/right muscle reciprocation.

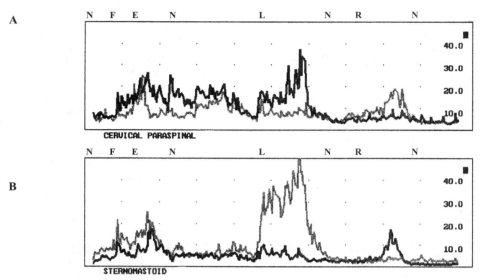

Figure 10–A–9 SEMG activity of left (thicker line) and right (thinner line) (**A**) cervical paraspinal and (**B**) sternomastoid muscles recorded from a patient with chronic bialteral neck pain after a motor vehicle accident. Activity is illustrated during seated (**N**) neutral head position and active cervical (**F**) flexion, (**E**) extension, (**L**) left rotation, and (**R**) right rotation. Muscle responses appear asymmetric and erratic during flexion-extension and reciprocally asymmetric during left-right rotation through a roughly equivalent excursion.

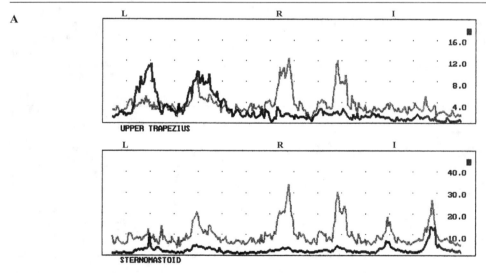

continues

Figure 10–A–10 SEMG activity of left (thicker line) and right (thinner line) upper trapezius and sternomastoid muscles recorded from a patient with chronic right neck pain after a motor vehicle accident. Activity is illustrated during two repetitions each of seated (**L**) left shoulder shrug, (**R**) right shoulder shrug, and (**I**) deep inspiration. At the (**A**) start of treatment, baseline muscle responses are asymmetric and left shoulder shrug is accompanied by inappropriate co-activation of the right upper trapezius. Right sternomastoid activity is present during shoulder shrugs whereas left side activity is quiescent. Asymmetric activity patterns are further manifested during deep inspiration. The patient was treated with manual therapies, SEMG feedback training, and home exercise prescription. At the (**B**) conclusion of therapy, pain has largely resolved and SEMG activity appears stable and symmetric.

Figure 10–A–10 continued

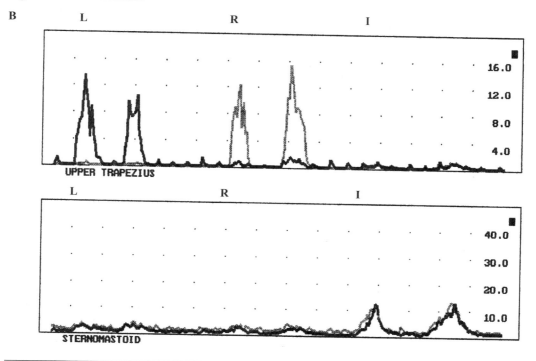

Training Progression for Neck Pain with Asymmetric Sternomastoid/Cervical Paraspinal Balance

- Refer to Chapters 3 and 4 for detailed discussion of SEMG display setups and feedback structure.
- Refer to Chapter 5 for detailed discussion of SEMG training techniques.
- As skill develops, generally
    1. Shape desired responses up or down.
    2. Incorporate multijoint control.
    3. Add distractions.
    4. Randomize training activities.
    5. Withdraw continuous audio/visual feedback.
- Select relevant SEMG feedback training tasks from the following:
    1. isolation of target muscle activity
    2. postural training with SEMG feedback
    3. tension discrimination training
    4. therapeutic exercises with SEMG feedback

5. left/right equilibration training. Downtraining the high amplitude side is an option, but often it is easier to uptrain the low amplitude side.
6. generalization to progressively dynamic movements. Work for symmetric recruitment for sagittal plane movements and asymmetric recruitment during rotation or side-bending motions, with reciprocal symmetry from the left to right movement planes.
7. motor copy training
8. promotion of correct muscle synergies and related coordination patterns between sternomastoid and cervical paraspinal muscles. Postural correction and sternomastoid uptraining will generally decrease cervical paraspinal muscle activity. As the amplitude of a low side sternomastoid is uptrained, a hyperactive contralateral cervical paraspinal group will tend to decrease spontaneously in activity.

9. functional activity performance with SEMG feedback

- Integrate SEMG feedback training into a comprehensive approach to patient management:
  1. Emphasize repetition of muscle equilibration procedures, stretching, and postural correction throughout the day.
  2. Develop a careful plan to implement indicated changes in ergonomic setups and functional motor habits.
  3. Consider consultation with a therapist or physician for
     —manual treatments
     —exercise prescription
     —physical agents
     —functional activity modification

Cervical–Scapular Muscle Imbalance

Cervical–scapular muscle imbalances can be observed after work injury, or athletic trauma, as well as with insidious onset of neck pain. The upper trapezius, middle trapezius, lower trapezius, and lower fibers of the serratus anterior act synergistically to produce upward rotation of the scapula during arm elevation. In some patients the upper trapezius appears hyperactive, whereas the lower trapezius and serratus anterior appear hypoactive (each relative to the contralateral side). SEMG feedback training includes uptraining the lower trapezius or serratus anterior as well as downtraining the upper trapezius. Uptraining generally begins with isometrics and prime scapular movements and progresses to training during shoulder flexion and abduction. This syndrome and related syndromes are discussed in greater detail in Application Guide 11–A, SEMG Program for Shoulder Girdle Dysfunction.

Thoracic Outlet Syndrome with Cervical Muscle Hyperactivity

Thoracic outlet syndrome refers to mechanical compression of portions of the brachial plexus and associated vascular bundle. It is a far less frequent problem than other cervical dysfunction presentations described earlier. When thoracic outlet syndrome is suspected, however, assessment and treatment can be troublesome. Compression is thought to occur at the outlet between the anterior and middle scalenes, at the passage of the neurovascular bundle between the clavicle and possibly anomalous first rib, or between the pectoralis minor and upper ribs.

Clinical presentation includes radiating cervical, pectoral, and upper extremity pain, parasthesias, and numbness. Differential diagnosis is difficult and includes cervical root impingement due to a herniated disc, degenerative facet disease and lateral canal stenosis, soft tissue trigger points, dural tension and upper extremity neural entrapment syndromes, obstruction due to tumor, and other medical problems. Diagnosis is made by clinical examination, radiologic studies, and laboratory procedures. Some patients diagnosed with thoracic outlet syndrome show patterns of scalene tightness and SEMG hyperactivity. Others demonstrate diffuse hyperactivity from ipsilateral upper trapezius, lateral cervical, and sternomastoid recording sites. Diffuse hyperactivity may be caused by pain-mediated reflexes or reactive guarding to preserve subclavicular and subpectoral space. Psychologic stress, coupled with muscle tension responses, may exacerbate symptoms in those anatomically predisposed to the problem (Figure 10–A–11).

Training Progression for Thoracic Outlet Syndrome and Cervical Muscle Hyperactivity

- Refer to Application Guide 11–A regarding training progression for cervical–scapular muscle imbalance.
- Refer to Chapters 3 and 4 for detailed discussion of SEMG display setups and feedback structure.
- Refer to Chapter 5 for detailed discussion of SEMG feedback training techniques.
- As skill develops, generally
  1. Shape desired responses up or down.

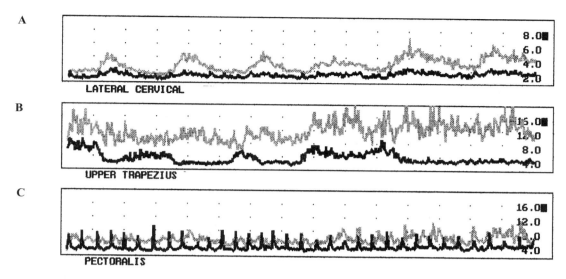

Figure 10–A–11 SEMG activity from the left (black) and right (gray) (**A**) lateral cervical, (**B**) upper trapezius, and (**C**) clavicular pectoralis sites recorded from a patient with right lateral cervical, pectoral, and upper extremity pain and parasthesias, and suspected thoracic outlet syndrome. Tracings were recorded while the patient was guided through visualization of emotionally stressful events. Note the progressive tendency toward right greater than left asymmetry. Waxing and waning of the right lateral cervical signal is coupled to respiratory inspiration and expiration, respectively. Cardiac artifact is seen in the (**C**) left pectoral signal as a series of recurrent spikes throughout the sweep.

2. Incorporate multijoint control.
3. Add distractions.
4. Randomize training activities.
5. Withdraw continuous audio/visual feedback.

• Select relevant SEMG feedback training tasks from the following:
   1. isolation of target muscle activity:
      –cervical paraspinals
      –upper trapezius
      –scalenes
      –sternomastoid
      –pectoralis group
   2. relaxation-based downtraining
   3. threshold-based downtraining
   4. postural training with SEMG feedback
   5. therapeutic exercises with SEMG feedback:
      –patient specific, based on physical examination findings
      –usually for assistance with stretching of scalene and pectoral groups
   6. *after* structural issues have been addressed, provide SEMG training with:
      –left/right equilibration training
      –motor copy training
      –promotion of correct (ie, symmetric) muscle synergies and related coordination patterns for cervical–scapular–pectoral area

Patients with structural dysfunction require careful exercise prescription, skilled adjunctive manual therapies, and counseling on posture and functional activity modification.

REFERENCES

1. Hislop HJ, Montgomery J. *Daniels and Worthingham's Muscle Testing: Techniques of Manual Examination.* 6th ed. Philadelphia: WB Saunders Co; 1995.

2. Kendall F, McCreary E, Provance P. *Muscles Testing and Function with Posture and Pain.* 4th ed. Baltimore: Williams & Wilkins; 1993.

SUGGESTED READINGS

Donaldson S, Donaldson M. Multi-channel EMG assessment and treatment techniques. In: Cram JR, ed. *Clinical EMG for Surface Recordings.* Vol 2. Nevada City, CA: Clinical Resources; 1990;143–173.

Ettare DL, Ettare R. Muscle learning therapy: a treatment protocol. In: Cram JR, ed. *Clinical EMG for Surface Recordings.* Vol 2. Nevada City, CA: Clinical Resources, 1990;197–233.

Jonsson B. The static load component in muscle work. *Eur J Appl Physiol.* 1988;57:305–310.

Middaugh SJ, Kee WG, Nicholson JA. Muscle overuse and posture as factors in the development and maintenance of chronic musculoskeletal pain. In: Grzesiak RC, Ciccone DS, eds. *Psychological Vulnerability to Chronic Pain.* New York: Springer Publishing Co; 1994;55–89.

Nitz AJ, Carlson CR. Differentiation of neck pain vs. no-pain conditions using paraspinal iEMG and flexion–extension cervical ROM. *J Orthop Sports Phys Ther.* 1995;21:59.

Schuldt K, Ekholm J, Harms-Ringdahl K, Nemeth G, Arborelius UP. Effects of changes in sitting work posture on static neck and shoulder muscle activity. *Ergonomics.* 1988;29:1525–1537.

Skubick DL, Clasby R, Donaldson CCS, Marshall WM. Carpal tunnel syndrome as an expression of muscular dysfunction in the neck. *J Occup Rehabil.* 1993;3:31–44.

Veiersted KB, Westgaard RH, Andersen P. Electromyographic evaluation of muscular work pattern as a predictor of trapezius myalgia. *Scand J Work Environ Health.* 1993;19:284–290.

Veiersted KB, Westgaard RH, Andersen P. Pattern of muscle activity during stereotyped work and its relation to muscle pain. *Int Arch Occup Environ Health.* 1990;62:31–41.

Winkel J, Westgaard R. Occupational and individual risk factors for shoulder–neck complaints: part II: the scientific basis (literature review) for the guide. *Int J Industrial Ergonomics.* 1992;10:85–104.

CHAPTER 11

Shoulder Girdle and Upper Extremity Dysfunction

PATHOPHYSIOLOGY AND ASSESSMENT OF SHOULDER GIRDLE DYSFUNCTION

The shoulder girdle complex is composed of four joints: sternoclavicular, acromioclavicular, scapulothoracic, and glenohumeral articulations.[1] Electromyography has been used to analyze muscles of the shoulder girdle during movement.[2] Normal, pain-free shoulder motion requires adequate mobility and muscle activity around each of the component joints. Changes in joint or soft tissue structures may lead to pain, muscle spasm and substitution patterns, and dysfunction of the upper extremity.[3–5]

A common problem in shoulder girdle and upper extremity dysfunction is related to pathologic changes in the rotator cuff. Changes and resulting sequelae can be associated with impingement or tearing of the cuff that can result from the normal aging process,[6] as well as from cumulative trauma as in athletes who perform repetitive overhead throwing activities.[7,8] Shoulder impingement syndrome is characterized by repetitive microtrauma to structures such as the subacromial bursa.[7] Structural (abnormal shape of the acromion, thickening of tendons) and functional (rotator cuff weakness, poor scapular–humeral rhythm, and capsular tightness) factors contribute to subacromial impingement.[9]

Neer[10] identified three stages of rotator cuff impingement. Stage I is a reversible process characterized by edema and hemorrhage and commonly found in athletes younger than 25 years of age. Clinically, findings reveal palpable tenderness over structures around the anterior aspect of the acromion; a painful arc of abduction between 60 and 120 degrees; and pain occurring at night as well as during resistive movements and functional activities. Fibrosis and tendinitis due to repeated mechanical inflammation are features of stage II; at this point the impingement process is no longer reversible. Patients are typically 25 to 40 years of age, complain of recurrent pain with activity and at night, and have mild active and passive range of motion limitations. Stage III lesions are typically found in adults older than 40 years of age with complete or partial tears of the rotator cuff and possibly the biceps tendon. Clinical presentation includes a painful arc of motion during eccentric contraction of the shoulder from 120 to 70 degrees of abduction, increased subacromial crepitus, muscle weakness (particularly in the external rotators), and positive findings on impingement tests.

Signs of impingement can also be present in an unstable shoulder, coupled with capsular laxity and weakness of the rotator cuff muscles.[11] Frank anterior instabilities are associated with weakness of the subscapularis, pectoralis major, coracobrachialis, and long head of the biceps.[12] Infraspinatus, teres minor, and posterior deltoid weakness is associated with posterior instabilities. Multidirectional instability and inferior instability or subluxation can also occur. Inferior subluxation is accompanied by weakness of deltoid and supraspinatus muscles.

Shoulder impingement and instabilities related to the glenohumeral articulation are also associated with scapular weakness. The serratus anterior, rhomboid, trapezius, levator scapulae, and pectoralis minor muscles are primary stabilizers of the scapula during glenohumeral motion.[9,13] Normal patterns of surface electromyography (SEMG) activity from the upper, middle, and lower aspects of the trapezius as well as the serratus anterior during arm elevation in the scapular plane have been reported by Bagg and Forrest.[14] Abnormal force coupling between scapular muscles leads to glenohumeral pain and dysfunction. Periscapular pain is often accompanied by hyperactivity of the upper scapular stabilizers (upper and middle portions of the trapezius as well as pectoralis minor and, potentially, rhomboid muscles) and hypoactivity of the lower stabilizers (lower aspect of the trapezius as well as serratus anterior muscles.)[15] Stabilization of the shoulder girdle by upper stabilizers also increases stress on the cervical spine. In addition, faulty scapular muscle action can lead to postural dysfunction and compression of anterior chest wall structures, clinically manifested as impaired respiration or thoracic outlet syndrome.[16] Joint angles and loading tasks—coupled with postural abnormalities, shortened or elongated soft tissue structures, reduced muscle strength, and uncoordinated joint motion—interact to cause and exacerbate shoulder problems.

Successful treatment of shoulder girdle syndromes depends on an accurate diagnosis. It is critical for the clinician to obtain a careful history and physical examination. Important aspects of the physical examination include inspection of posture, bony positioning, and muscle symmetry. Palpation of bony and soft tissue structures; evaluation of cervical, thoracic, and scapulohumeral range of motion; tests of shoulder and scapular strength; as well as other tests and vascular examination may be part of a comprehensive evaluation.[17–20] Analysis of shoulder and scapular muscle function can be augmented by using SEMG.

SEMG MONITORING DURING FUNCTIONAL TASKS

SEMG monitoring of shoulder muscles in ergonomics has been used to prevent injury and modify activities. Simulated work studies of healthy women performing repeated maximal shoulder flexion for 150 repetitions at two angular velocities showed that SEMG mean power frequency decreased during the initial 40 to 60 contractions and then stabilized, suggesting fatigue of fast twitch motor units.[21] Sundelin and Hagberg[22] monitored cervical portions of the upper trapezius and infraspinatus during performance of simulated repetitive work tasks for 1 hour in healthy women. Muscle fatigue, measured by reduction in SEMG mean power frequency and increase in root-mean-square amplitude, occurred in both muscle groups. Patterns of fatigue varied between muscles and subjects. Thus highly repetitive, short-cycle work tasks may cause cervical dysfunction in vulnerable individuals. In a follow-up study, Sundelin[23] assessed continuous and paused repetitive work tasks for 1 hour. Although perceived exertion and discomfort were similar and muscle fatigue occurred during both forms of work, there was less myoelectric change when work was integrated with pauses. Prevention or reduction of muscle fatigue may be possible through varied work pace and muscle use patterns.

Carryover of fatigue patterns in simulated work occurs during actual work tasks. Measurement of bilateral trapezius SEMG activity in female industrial sewing machine operators during a typical 8-hour day reveals changes in mean power frequency and zero crossing frequency rate, indicative of fatigue.[24] Heavy loading of shoulder muscles in elevated positions leads to overuse of supraspinatus and infraspinatus muscles, and overhead static work tasks seem to be correlated with abnormalities of the rotator cuff of the shoulder at an earlier age.[24]

In reviewing numerous studies with the use of SEMG and other measurements, Winkel and Westgaard[25] extensively discuss position, load, and duration of exposure to work to prevent injury. They review percentage of maximal volitional isometric contraction (MVIC) work levels, primarily for the trapezius, relative to pacing demands. The investigators recommend exposure of less than 4 hours per day for seated work with a static load of less than 5% MVIC. With shoulder elevation and static loading of the trapezius muscle at 10% MVIC, exposure of 1 hour or less may be necessary to decrease injury. They also recommend an exposure period of less than 1 hour for work requiring large excursions and forces (60% MVIC).

Shoulder EMG with the use of intramuscular electrodes has been implemented during sporting activities for injury prevention and design of therapeutic exercise programs to enhance performance. In swimmers, normal and painful shoulder muscle activity has been reviewed by using fine wire electrodes and cinematography during freestyle and butterfly strokes. Healthy subjects during freestyle[26] and butterfly[27] strokes robustly activate subscapularis and serratus anterior muscles, making them susceptible to fatigue. Swimmers with painful shoulders show significantly different patterns of EMG activity across multiple muscles, compared with findings in healthy subjects, during both strokes.[28,29] Different muscle patterns are present for each stroke. Strengthening and endurance training of subscapularis and serratus anterior muscles should be part of a routine exercise program to prevent injury. In other EMG studies, pitching,[30] golf,[31] rowing,[32] and tennis[33] have been assessed in healthy subjects. Common to all sports discussed is the need for scapular stability, so that optimal glenohumeral motion will occur.

In addition, shoulder muscles of patients with paraplegia have been monitored with SEMG to reduce rotator cuff injury during functional wheelchair tasks. Wheelchair transfers,[34,35] pressure relief,[36] and propulsion have been assessed,[16] and muscles for preventive strengthening have been identified.

INTEGRATION OF SEMG INTO TREATMENT PARADIGMS

Traditional shoulder rehabilitation programs for impingement syndrome focus on strengthening of rotator cuff muscles with minimal emphasis on scapulothoracic musculature. More recently the importance of the scapulothoracic muscles during glenohumeral motions has been recognized.[9] Muscle strengthening, endurance training, and timing of muscle patterns in rotator cuff and scapulothoracic muscles should be part of a comprehensive shoulder rehabilitation program for impingement syndrome. SEMG feedback can be used to assist patients to develop more efficient movement patterns and perform corrective exercise programs. Feedback training can also be integrated with exercise to address glenohumeral instabilities, focusing on obtaining a balance between anterior and posterior muscles.[37,38]

The effectiveness of therapeutic exercise interventions in isolating shoulder muscles for any problem can be verified with SEMG. For example, proprioceptive neuromuscular facilitation patterns of the upper extremity have been used for facilitating and strengthening particular muscle groups. Sullivan and Portney[39] tested this premise and verified the existence of optimal patterns of recruitment with SEMG. Other investigators[4,40,41] have used fine wire electrodes to evaluate the effects of standard and modified shoulder rehabilitation exercises on specific muscles. Their recommendations can be adapted for use with surface electrode monitoring for the larger, superficial muscles and incorporated in noninvasive feedback training regimens.

CONCLUSION

Movement through the shoulder results from coordination of complex kinematic and kinetic relationships. There is evidence that impingement syndromes, instabilities, and periscapular pain syndromes are accompanied by muscle imbalances in the shoulder. Monitoring of shoulder girdle muscles with SEMG is most challenging for the clinician because of the difficulty in isolating many of the key muscles. Nevertheless, surface recordings have proved to be a highly effective and noninvasive vehicle for studying functional muscle control. Recommendations for occupational injury prevention have been defined with SEMG. As one component of a comprehensive intervention strategy, these guidelines can be adapted for clinical assessment and feedback training. SEMG can also be incorporated into orthopaedic assessment and athletic training programs for the upper quadrant.

There is a paucity of literature relating SEMG to more distal upper extremity problems. Many of the same principles identified for shoulder impairments, however, will likely prove relevant for distal repetitive strain injuries. In view of associated financial and social costs, this is a ripe area for research.

REFERENCES

1. Calliet R. *Shoulder Pain*. 3rd ed. Philadelphia: FA Davis; 1991.
2. Basmajian J, DeLuca C. *Muscles Alive: Their Functions Revealed by Electromyography*. 5th ed. Baltimore: Williams & Wilkins; 1985.
3. Babyar S. Excessive scapular motion in individuals recovering from painful and stiff shoulders: causes and treatment strategies. *Phys Ther*. 1996;76:226–238.
4. Moseley B, Jobe F, Pink M, Perry J, Tibone J. EMG analysis of the scapular muscles during a shoulder rehabilitation program. *Am J Sports Med*. 1992;20:128–134.
5. Peat M, Grahame R. Electromyographic analysis of soft tissue lesions affecting shoulder function. *Am J Phys Med*. 1977;56:223–240.
6. Yost J, Schmoll D. Shoulder disorders: an orthopedic perspective. In Lewis C, Knortz K, eds. *Orthopedic Assessment and Treatment of the Geriatric Patient*. St Louis, MO: CV Mosby; 1993;101–111.
7. Corso G. Impingement relief test: an adjunctive procedure to traditional assessment of shoulder impingement syndrome. *J Orthop Sports Phys Ther*. 1994;22:183–192.
8. McLeod W, Andrews J. Mechanisms of shoulder injuries. *Phys Ther*. 1986;66:1901–1911.
9. Kamkar A, Irrgang J, Whitney S. Nonoperative management of secondary shoulder impingement syndrome. *J Orthop Sports Phys Ther*. 1993;17:212–224.
10. Neer C. Impingement lesions. *Clin Orthop*. 1983; 173:70–77.
11. Warner J, Lyle M, Arslanizn L. Patterns of flexibility, laxity, and strength in normal shoulders and shoulders with instability and impingement. *Am J Sports Med*. 1990;18:366–375.
12. Jobe F, Moynes D, Brewster C. Rehabilitation of shoulder joint instabilities. *Orthop Clin North Am*. 1987; 18:473–482.
13. Paine R, Voight M. The role of the scapula. *J Orthop Sports Phys Ther*. 1993;18:386–391.
14. Bagg SD, Forrest WJ. Electromyographic study of the scapular rotators during arm abduction in the scapular plane. *Am J Phys Med*. 1986;65:111–124.
15. Taylor W. Dynamic EMG biofeedback in assessment and treatment using a neuromuscular re-education model. In: Cram JR, ed. *Clinical EMG for Surface Recordings*. Vol 2. Nevada City, CA: Clinical Resources; 1990;175–196.
16. Masse L, Lamontagne M, O'Riain M. Biomechanical analysis of wheelchair propulsion for various seating positions. *J Rehabil Res Dev*. 1992;29:12–28.
17. Boublik M, Hawkins R. Clinical examination of the shoulder complex. *J Orthop Sports Phys Ther*. 1993; 18:379–385.
18. Cyriax J, Cyriax P. The shoulder. In: Cyriax J, Cyriax P, eds. *Illustrated Manual of Orthopaedic Medicine*. London: Butterworth; 1983;29–46.
19. Hoppenfeld S. Physical examination of the shoulder. In: Hoppenfeld S, ed. *Physical Examination of the Spine and Extremities*. New York: Appleton-Century-Crofts: 1976;1–34.
20. Sobel J. Shoulder injuries: a rehab perspective. In: Lewis C, Knortz K, eds. *Orthopedic Assessment and Treatment of the Geriatric Patient*. St Louis: CV Mosby; 1993;89–100.
21. Elert J, Gerdle B. The relationship between contraction and relaxation during fatiguing isokinetic shoulder flexions: an electromyographic study. *Eur J Appl Physiol*. 1989;59:303–309.
22. Sundelin G, Hagberg M. Electromyographic signs of shoulder muscle fatigue in repetitive arm work paced by the methods-time measurement system. *Scand J Work Environ Health*. 1992;18:262–268.

23. Sundelin G. Patterns of electromyographic shoulder muscle fatigue during MTM-paced repetitive arm work with and without pauses. *Int Arch Occup Environ Health*. 1993;64:485–493.

24. Jensen B, Schibye B, Sogaard K, Simonsen E, Sjogaard G. Shoulder muscle load and muscle fatigue among industrial sewing-machine operators. *Eur J Appl Physiol*. 1993;57:467–475.

25. Winkel J, Westgaard R. Occupational and individual risk factors for shoulder neck complaints; part II: the scientific basis (literature review) for the guide. *Int J Indust Ergo*. 1992;10:85–104.

26. Pink M, Perry J, Browne A, Scovazzo ML, Kerrigan J. The normal shoulder during freestyle swimming: an electromyographic and cinematographic analysis of twelve muscles. *Am J Sports Med*. 1991;19:569–576.

27. Pink M, Jobe F, Perry J, Kerrigan J, Browne A, Scovazzo ML. The normal shoulder during the butterfly swim stroke: an electromyographic and cinematographic analysis of twelve muscles. *Clin Orthop*. 1992;288:48–59.

28. Pink M, Jobe F, Perry J, Browne A, Scovazzo ML, Kerrigan J. The painful shoulder during the butterfly stroke: an electromyographic and cinematographic analysis of twelve muscles. *Clin Orthop*. 1992;288:60–72.

29. Scovazzo ML, Browne A, Pink M, Jobe FW, Kerrigan J. The painful shoulder during freestyle swimming: an electromyographic cinematographic analysis of twelve muscles. *Am J Sports Med*. 1991;19:577–582.

30. Jobe F, Moynes D, Tibone J, Perry J. An EMG analysis of the shoulder in throwing and pitching: a second report. *Am J Sports Med*. 1984;12:218–220.

31. Pink M, Jobe F, Perry J. Electromyographic analysis of the shoulder during the golf swing. *Am J Sports Med*. 1990;18:137–140.

32. Rodriguez R, Rodriguez R, Cook S, Sandborn P. Electromyographic analysis of rowing stroke biomechanics. *J Sports Med Phys Fitness*. 1990;30:103–108.

33. Ryu R, McCormick J, Jobe FW, et al. An electromyographic analysis of shoulder function in tennis players. *Am J Sports Med*. 1988;16:481–485.

34. Perry J, Gronley J, Newsam C, Reyes M, Mulroy S. Electromyographic analysis of the shoulder muscles during depressions transfers in subjects with low-level paraplegia. *Arch Phys Med Rehabil*. 1996;77:350–355.

35. Wang Y, Kim C, Ford H, et al. Reaction force and EMG analyses of wheelchair transfers. *Percept Mot Skills*. 1994;79:763–766.

36. Reyes M, Gronley J, Newsam C, Mulroy S. Electromyographic analysis of shoulder muscles of men with low-level paraplegia during a weight relief raise. *Arch Phys Med Rehabil*. 1995;76:433–439.

37. Beall S, Diefenbach G, Allen A. Electromyographic biofeedback in the treatment of voluntary posterior instability of the shoulder. *Am J Sports Med*. 1987;15:175–178.

38. Young M. Electromyographic biofeedback use in the treatment of voluntary posterior dislocation of the shoulder: a case study. *J Orthop Sports Phys Ther*. 1994;20:171–175.

39. Sullivan P, Portney L. Electromyographic activity of shoulder muscles during unilateral upper extremity proprioceptive neuromuscular facilitation patterns. *Phys Ther*. 1980;60:283–288.

40. Ballantyne BT, O'Hare SJ, Paschall JL, et al. Electromyographic activity of selected shoulder muscles in commonly used therapeutic exercises. *Phys Ther*. 1993;73:668–682.

41. McCann PD, Wootten ME, Kadaba MP, Bigliani LU. A kinematic and electromyographic study of shoulder rehabilitation exercises. *Clin Orthop*. 1993;288:179–188.

SEMG Program for Shoulder Girdle Dysfunction

Refer to the discussion in Chapter 11 for a review of intervention approaches. The suggestions that follow are derived from those resources. Descriptions and operational definitions are provided to clarify optional practice patterns.

CANDIDATES

Implement for patients with chronic
- glenohumeral instability
- shoulder impingement syndrome
- shoulder or periscapular pain and in whom muscle dysfunction is suspected.
  Patients may present with a variety of diagnoses, including
  1. posttraumatic and postsurgical deficits
  2. fibromyalgia
  3. fibrositis
  4. tendinitis
  5. bursitis
  6. overuse syndromes
  7. psychophysiologic stress syndromes
  Problems can occur in close conjunction with cervical dysfunction syndromes.

Candidates should relate subjective remarks regarding inappropriate tension sensations and potentially contributory psychologic stressors. Alternatively, physical examination should reveal

- faulty posture and scapular alignment
- aberrant scapulohumeral rhythm
- palpable hypertonicity
- trigger points
- imbalances in muscle flexibility and strength

EVALUATION OBJECTIVES

- Assess the effects of posture and dynamic movement on muscle activity.
- Identify aberrant patterns of muscle activity about the shoulder girdle, potentially contributing to musculoskeletal pain:
  1. myalgia due to excessive levels or duration of muscle tension
  2. imbalanced muscle activity that potentially results in soft tissue or joint dysfunction
- Assess psychophysiologic factors in the precipitation of excessive muscle tension.

FEEDBACK TRAINING OBJECTIVES

- Reduce excessive muscle tension.
- Improve postural function and ergonomic alignment.
- Increase recruitment and strength of dynamic shoulder stabilizers.
- Re-educate normal patterns of scapulohumeral muscle synergy.
- Resolve underlying mechanical dysfunction.
- Decouple psychologic stressors and muscle tension responses.

- Retain and generalize improved motor control to functional contexts.
- Resolve or reduce functional limitations and disability.

RECORDING SITES

- Judge the utility of each recording site on the basis of history and physical examination results.
- Include muscles that
  1. Underlie the pain distribution.
  2. Potentially refer symptoms or are mechanically related to the patient's area of complaint.
  3. Reproduce patient's symptoms when stretched, resisted, or palpated.
- Consult Chapter 14 in the companion book, *Introduction to Surface Electromyography*, for specific electrode placement considerations.
- Confirm optimal sites from the following list by observation and palpation during isometric contraction.
  1. upper trapezius
  2. upper trapezius/supraspinatus
  3. middle interscapular region (middle trapezius, rhomboids, erector spinae)
  4. lower interscapular region (lower trapezius is the intended target, some degree of cross-talk from rhomboids and erector spinae is likely)
  5. lower fibers of serratus anterior
  6. infraspinatus
  7. anterior deltoid
  8. lateral deltoid
  9. posterior deltoid
  10. pectoralis major
  11. thoracic paraspinal group

EVALUATION PROCEDURES

- Select procedures that correspond to exacerbating and alleviating factors revealed by history and clinical examination.
- Refer to Chapter 2 for detailed discussion of evaluation methods.
- Perform at least five repetitions of each

movement task to assess response consistency (consider discarding the results of the first one to two repetitions and averaging the results of the remaining repetitions). Many more repetitions may be needed to assess SEMG responses with reproduction of symptoms.
- Select relevant procedures from the following:
  1. psychophysiologic stress profile
  2. postural analysis
  3. shoulder active range of motion (AROM); observe for consistent excursion and velocity across test repetitions. Test left side, right side, simultaneous bilateral movements, concentric versus eccentric phases through:
     –flexion
     –abduction
     –scaption (elevation in the scapular plane, between flexion and abduction)
     –medial rotation
     –lateral rotation
     –horizontal adduction/abduction
  4. isometric contractions. Test maximal and progressively graded submaximal effort levels for:
     –flexors
     –abductors with arm at side, arm abducted
     –medial rotators
     –lateral rotators with arm at side, arm abducted
  5. dynamic contractions at progressive intensities. Select exacerbating movement planes from no. 3 above.
  6. dynamic contractions at progressive velocities. Select exacerbating movement planes from no. 3 above.
  7. analysis of scapular muscle function for postural recruitment versus prime scapular movements versus scapular stabilization for overhead activity
  8. analysis of muscle synergy patterns:
     –upper trapezius–lower trapezius–lower fibers of serratus anterior for upward scapular rotation

-infraspinatus–lateral deltoid for humeral abduction

9. functional activity analysis:
   –push/pull
   –overhead reach/lift
   –other job, home, sports-specific activities

10. repeat of any of the above procedures,
    as appropriate, with corrections for the
    following:
    –posture
    –sports technique
    –equipment, work station modification
    –orthotic taping

ASSESSMENT

- Refer to Chapter 2 for detailed discussion
  of SEMG assessment.
- Refer to Chapter 14 in the companion book
  for representative SEMG tracings of normal function, as well as for benchmark
  baseline values for each site.
- Select SEMG assessment parameters from
  the following:

  1. Amplitude and variance of each channel
     during baseline. Activity during base-
     line should be stable and relatively qui-
     escent. Mean amplitude values from
     nonpostural muscles should be close to
     internal noise levels of the recording de-
     vice. Postural muscles may show low-
     level activity with the patient in weight-
     bearing positions (typically, about 2–6
     μV RMS).

  2. Peak or average amplitude of each chan-
     nel during activation. Activity can ap-
     pear to be unremarkable, grossly exces-
     sive and erratic, or markedly depressed.

  3. Relationship of salient SEMG events to
     particular range of motion arcs. Observe
     for consistent amplitude elevations or
     depressions during a painful portion of
     the AROM arc.

  4. Quiescence of thoracic paraspinal activ-
     ity in full flexion, the flexion–relaxation
     response.

5. Return to baseline amplitude after
   muscle activation. Qualitatively, recovery can be stated as prompt and
   complete versus elevated and delayed.
   Satisfactory baseline recovery is quantitatively defined (with a smoothing time
   constant of 0.1 second or less) as a return to an SEMG amplitude within two
   standard deviations of the original
   baseline mean, within 3 seconds of
   movement cessation, and maintenance
   within that amplitude range for at least
   30 seconds or until the next movement is
   initiated. Recovery can be characterized
   by the latency to achieve this criterion.
   More simply, the amplitude (expressed
   as percentage of baseline) observed 1 to
   3 seconds after movement termination
   can be reported.

6. Left/right peak amplitude symmetry for
   bilateral symmetric movements (eg, bilateral shoulder flexion) and reciprocal
   movements (eg, left shoulder flexion followed by reciprocal right shoulder flexion). Satisfactory symmetry is operationally defined as left/right scores within
   35% as calculated [(higher value – lower
   value)/higher value] × 100. Symmetry
   assessment assumes an equivalent left/
   right AROM excursion and velocity.
   Asymmetries recorded from electrodes
   placed over multiple muscle layers can
   be difficult to define. It may be possible
   to approximate the activity of a particular
   muscle within a group by observing the
   SEMG display while the patient performs the isolated isometric action of that
   muscle. For example, an asymmetric pattern recorded from the middle interscapular region could be caused by dysfunction of the middle trapezius,
   rhomboid, or both. Cross-talk and co-activation are likely for most patients during arm elevation tasks. However, occasionally the asymmetry is reproduced
   only during manual muscle test of the
   middle trapezius[1,2] and not during that for

the rhomboid, or vice versa. Thus asymmetries observed from nonspecific recording sites during movement may be compared with findings on selective manual muscle tests. The process sometimes yields insight as to the offending muscle, but true confirmation requires intramuscular electrode placement.

7. Left/right amplitude asymmetry for unilateral movements (eg, left shoulder flexion with right arm at rest). Within a single side unilateral movement, similar levels of left/right co-activation are an aberrant finding.

8. Left/right timing symmetry for bilateral symmetrical movements (ie, coincident recruitment, peak, decruitment patterns; symmetrical duration). When comparing the timing symmetry of synergist action, observe for changes in the recruitment order of muscles from one side to the other. For most clinical purposes, timing issues can be observed with rectified line tracings with a smoothing time constant of 0.1 second or less, SEMG sampling at 100 Hz or faster, frequency bandwidth filter low cutoff of 25 Hz or less, and a high resolution display with variable sweep speed. A graphic printout is useful for documentation of subtle timing differences. Documentation can be quantified with calculations of average slope, time to peak activity, or time to some percentage of MVIC activity that is clinically meaningful. Onset time can be reported simply as the latency to achieve a microvolt value equivalent to two standard deviations above the baseline mean. Duration may be noted as the amount of time between onset and baseline recovery as defined above.

9. Proportionate amplitude patterns among muscular synergists that are symmetric from left to right:
   –infraspinatus and deltoid
   –upper trapezius, lower trapezius, and serratus anterior

–other muscular synergists as indicated
For comparisons across nonhomologous muscles, amplitudes may be expressed as a:
–percentage of MVIC amplitude by using standard manual muscle tests (test activity amplitude/MVIC amplitude × 100)
–percentage of some submaximal contraction with a standardized force intensity, joint angle, and body posture.

10. Low-amplitude gaps or microrests in each channel display during functional tasks (obtained with use of a rectified moving line tracing display with a smoothing time constant of 0.1 second or less, SEMG sampling at 100 Hz or faster, and a frequency bandwidth filter low cutoff of 25 Hz or less) can be identified by setting a visible threshold marker at a microvolt value of about 5% MVIC for that muscle. This value should be above the range of the patient's postural baseline tracing. If the patient's postural baseline range exceeds 5% MVIC, the assessment should be deferred. Instruct the patient to perform continually a functional task that tends to exacerbate symptoms. With suitable precautions for patient safety, maintain task performance until the patient reports reproduction or exacerbation of symptoms. At the outset and every 2 to 3 minutes of task performance thereafter, save or freeze and print a copy of a 30- to 60-second display sweep. Count the number of threshold crossings. Low-amplitude microrests are typically produced in a range between approximately 0.2 second and several seconds, without conscious patient effort. Observe for a minimal presence of microrests throughout the course, as well as for changes in microrest frequency and duration as symptoms are produced. Compare left with right microrest frequencies/dura-

tions if the functional task involves symmetric movements and patient has unilateral involvement (see Figure 10–A–2 in Application Guide 10–A).

11. Tonic amplitude during repeated task trials or a continuous functional activity. With use of same type of display as in no. 10 above, observe the lowest level of activation consistently produced during performance of a continuous functional task. This tonic amplitude appears as the continually running baseline from which the muscle is phasically activated (see Figure 10–A–3 in Application Guide 10–A). Assuming a satisfactory, low-noise recording setup, the tonic amplitude should be less than 5% to 10% MVIC for tasks that are functionally performed for about 1 hour or longer. Note the tonic amplitude at the outset and every 2 to 3 minutes of task performance thereafter. Compare left with right sides if the functional task involves symmetric movements and patient has unilateral involvement.

12. Change in average activity level for a particular muscle and task across treatment sessions. To document this parameter a normalization procedure is preferred to enhance reliability. A reliable maximal manual muscle test effort or a standardized submaximal contraction is required. For example, the average upper trapezius SEMG amplitude produced during typing can be expressed as a percentage of upper trapezius activity while maintaining 90 degrees of shoulder abduction. The average amplitude during the test task is divided by that day's reference contraction amplitude, and the quotient is multiplied by 100.

13. Frequency spectral analysis for fatigue assessment. This analysis requires specialized equipment and technique. Observe the median frequency during a standardized isometric contraction of at least 50% MVIC. Observe the rate of decline in median frequency values (indicative of increased fatigue) during a prolonged effort contraction, comparing left and right side muscle performance. To track fatigue during a dynamic functional task, obtain SEMG frequency data during a high-level isometric contraction before initiation of the functional activity. Then have the patient perform the functional task for a duration expected to induce fatigue or increase symptoms. Repeat the standardized isometric test, extract median frequency values, and compare these values to initial levels for indications of fatigue. Have the patient rest for 1 to 3 minutes, and then repeat isometric test and frequency analysis. Continue a rest period:frequency test sequence to assess for recovery to initial median frequency values.

COMMON PATIENT PRESENTATIONS

Glenohumeral Instability

Glenohumeral instability is excessive motion in the form of subluxation or frank dislocation of the humeral head relative to the glenoid fossa. Contributory factors include structural and positional faults, capsular and ligamentous laxities, and faulty dynamic muscle control. Instability can occur in an anterior and, less commonly, a posterior direction. SEMG feedback is used to help retrain dynamic muscle stabilization during movements that might threaten joint integrity. Because access to the rotator cuff with surface electrodes is limited, SEMG training focuses on the infraspinatus, regardless of the direction of instability. The intent is that contraction of the infraspinatus will limit aberrant anterior gliding of the humeral head, act as a dynamic wall for posteriorly directed stress, and facilitate the coordinated action of other portions of the rotator cuff. In addition, the anterior deltoid and pectoralis major can be uptrained for anterior instability, and the posterior deltoid can be uptrained for posterior instability. Patterns of asymmetry from the involved to the uninvolved side can be used to guide electrode site selection. The training sequences described below—the first for anterior and the second for posterior glenohumeral instability—are appropriate for nonsurgical and postsurgical patients.

Training Progression for Anterior Instability

- Refer to Chapters 3 and 4 for detailed discussion of SEMG display setups and feedback structure.
- Refer to Chapters 5 and 6 for detailed discussion of SEMG feedback training techniques.
- As skill develops, generally
  1. Shape desired responses up or down.
  2. Incorporate multijoint control.
  3. Add distractions.
  4. Randomize training activities.
  5. Withdraw continuous audio/visual feedback.
- Select relevant SEMG feedback training tasks from the following:
  1. isolation of target muscle activity:
     - Begin with isometric contractions with the patient's arm at his or her side.
     - Use gently resisted lateral rotation for the infraspinatus.
     - Use flexion/medial rotation for the anterior deltoid or pectoralis major as indicated.
  2. threshold based uptraining:
     - Begin with isometric contractions with the patient's arm at his or her side.
     - Progress to lateral rotation AROM, uptraining the infraspinatus.
  3. generalization to progressively dynamic movement:
     - Position the patient's arm in about 30 degrees of flexion, and uptrain infraspinatus by actively performing medial to lateral rotation repetitions.
     - Repeat the sequence with the patient's arm at 60 degrees and then 90 degrees of flexion.

- Transition to shoulder flexion AROM, uptraining infraspinatus and anterior deltoid as indicated. Consider positioning the patient close to a wall or door frame, sliding his or her arm against the surface with modest lateral pressure through a flexion arc.
- Progress to larger movement arcs.
- Progress to faster movement speeds.
- Transition to infraspinatus uptraining or infraspinatus/anterior deltoid cocontraction during horizontal abduction.
- Carefully approach the combined movement planes that threaten stability (eg, flexion/abduction/lateral rotation).
- Continue infraspinatus uptraining or infraspinatus/anterior deltoid co-contraction training.
- Repeat the sequence with pectoralis major uptraining if indicated.
- Add posterior deltoid downtraining through above sequence if indicated.
  4. motor copy training. Acquire a template from the uninvolved side for any target muscle.
  5. functional performance activity with SEMG feedback. Select work, sports-specific activities that threaten stability, and practice muscle stabilization.
  6. therapeutic exercises with SEMG feedback for home. Instruct the patient in conditioning of the infraspinatus and any other shoulder muscles desired.
  7. SEMG-triggered neuromuscular electrical stimulation. Consider use of this training technique for the infraspinatus during the above listed activities.
- At all times, avoid positions that generate a patient perception of pending subluxation, and progress accordingly:
  1. Modify movement planes and sequencing to match patient needs. The idea is to begin uptraining procedures with movements that are opposite to those that provoke instability, or are otherwise nonprovocative.

2. As skill is gained, carefully approach the combined movement planes that have previously been associated with instability.

- Integrate SEMG feedback training with a comprehensive treatment plan for shoulder girdle rehabilitation.
- Consider consultation with a therapist or physician for adjunctive interventions, such as
  1. physical agents
  2. manual treatments
  3. taping techniques
  4. exercise prescription
  5. functional activity modification
- Consider needs for scapular muscle training as described later.

Training Progression for Posterior Instability

- Refer to Chapters 3 and 4 for detailed discussion of SEMG display setups and feedback structure.
- Refer to Chapters 5 and 6 for detailed discussion of SEMG feedback training techniques.
- As skill develops, generally
  1. Shape desired responses up or down.
  2. Incorporate multijoint control.
  3. Add distractions.
  4. Randomize training activities.
  5. Withdraw continuous audio/visual feedback.
- Select relevant SEMG feedback training tasks from the following:
  1. isolation of target muscle activity:
     –Begin with isometric contractions with the patient's arm at his or her side.
     –Use gently resisted lateral rotation for the infraspinatus.
     –Use extension/lateral rotation for the posterior deltoid.
  2. threshold based uptraining:
     –Begin with isometric contractions with the patient's arm at his or her side.

–Progress to lateral rotation AROM, uptraining infraspinatus and posterior deltoid.

3. generalization to progressively dynamic movement:
   –Uptrain infraspinatus and posterior deltoid with abduction AROM in lateral rotation.
   –Progress to larger movement arcs.
   –Progress to faster movement speeds.
   –Transition to elevation in the scapular plane (between abduction and flexion) and then to flexion, possibly positioning the patient close to a wall or door frame, sliding his or her arm against the surface with modest lateral pressure through the movement arc.
   –Carefully approach combined movement planes that potentially threaten stability (eg, flexion/medial rotation).
   –Continue infraspinatus or infraspinatus/deltoid uptraining.
4. motor copy training. Acquire a template from the uninvolved side for any target muscle.
5. functional activity performance with SEMG feedback. Select work, sports-specific activities that threaten stability, and practice infraspinatus/posterior deltoid stabilization.
6. therapeutic exercises with SEMG feedback for home. Instruct the patient in conditioning of infraspinatus and any other shoulder muscles desired.
7. SEMG-triggered neuromuscular electrical stimulation. Consider use of this training technique for the infraspinatus during the above-listed activities.

- At all times, avoid positions that generate a patient perception of pending subluxation and progress accordingly.
  1. Modify movement planes and sequencing to match patient needs. The idea is to begin uptraining procedures with movements that are opposite to those that provoke instability or are otherwise non-provocative.

2. As skill is gained, carefully approach the combined movement planes that have previously been associated with instability.
- Integrate SEMG feedback training with a comprehensive treatment plan for shoulder girdle rehabilitation.
- Consider consultation with a therapist or physician for adjunctive interventions, such as
  1. physical agents
  2. manual treatments
  3. taping techniques
  4. exercise prescription
  5. functional activity modification
- Consider the need for scapular muscle training as described later.

Postural-Related Thoracic Pain: Paraspinal Muscle Hypoactivity

Postural pain in the thoracic region tends to be associated with accentuated thoracic kyphosis; rounded shoulders; forward head; and tightness at the sternomastoid, suboccipital, pectoral, and latissimus muscles. Pain is presumably related to chronic spinal ligamentous stretch and faulty intervertebral alignment. The patient's discomfort increases throughout the day with maintenance of static upright postures. Baseline activity on SEMG about the thoracic paraspinal and interscapular regions may be of exceptionally low amplitude. Activity during movement can appear relatively unremarkable or aberrant with scapular muscle imbalances (see below). Upper cervical paraspinal SEMG activity tends to be elevated throughout test procedures. The treatment emphasis is on improved postural alignment with patient education and corrective exercises.

Training Progression for Postural-Related Thoracic Pain: Paraspinal Muscle Hypoactivity

- Refer to Chapters 3 and 4 for detailed discussion of SEMG display setups and feedback structure.

- Refer to Chapters 5 and 6 for detailed discussion of SEMG feedback training techniques.
- As skill develops, generally
  1. Shape desired responses up or down.
  2. Incorporate multijoint control.
  3. Add distractions.
  4. Randomize training activities.
  5. Withdraw continuous audio/visual feedback.
- Select relevant SEMG feedback training tasks from the following:
  1. postural training with SEMG feedback:
     –Be aware that paraspinal SEMG magnitudes will become greater as the patient uses muscle activity to hold corrected thoracic positioning.
     –Cue the minimal increase necessary to hold the corrected posture. With proper training and exercise, SEMG values tend to decrease over time.
     –Train the patient in sitting, standing, and functional activity positions as appropriate.
  2. therapeutic exercises with SEMG feedback:
     –Emphasize feedback during stretch of pectoralis and latissimus muscles, or passive thoracic extension mobilization as indicated.
     –Consider feedback during prone exercises of paraspinal and middle/lower trapezius for power and endurance.
- Provide cues to promote postural recognition and correction throughout the day.
- Monitor the patient's compliance with corrective exercise performance.

Interscapular Pain: Diffuse Hyperactivity

SEMG activity from upper trapezius and all interscapular recording sites tends to be hyperactive in this syndrome, during both postural baseline assessment and movement. Asymmetric symptoms and ipsilateral, diffuse SEMG hyperactivity are commonly recorded after traumatic injury, although symptoms can be bilaterally present and of insidious origin. The scapulae are often posturally held in an elevated and adducted position. Rhomboid and levator scapulae contours can appear prominent during observation of the patient's alignment. Soft tissue dysfunction may be related to overuse of the trapezius, rhomboid, and levator scapulae muscles for scapular stabilization during upper extremity function. Other contributory factors are postural dysfunction and passive myofascial tightness. In some patients, manual muscle tests show weakness at middle and lower trapezius. Thus there may be imbalances between the middle trapezius and rhomboids/levator scapulae in some persons and more generalized hyperactivity in others. Manual muscle tests can be used in speculative attempts to isolate asymmetric SEMG responses to a particular muscle. However, the actions of these muscles cannot be reliably isolated with surface electrodes, and imbalance cannot be confirmed on the basis of SEMG results. Psychophysiologic stress-related responses can also be contributory in this region. An illustration of asymmetric interscapular activity is provided in Figure 11–A–1.

Training Progression for Interscapular Pain: Diffuse Hyperactivity

- Refer to Chapters 3 and 4 for detailed discussion of SEMG display setups and feedback structure.
- Refer to Chapter 5 for detailed discussion of SEMG feedback training techniques.
- As skill develops, generally
  1. Shape desired responses up or down.
  2. Incorporate multijoint control.
  3. Add distractions.
  4. Randomize training activities.
  5. Withdraw continuous audio/visual feedback.
- Select relevant SEMG feedback training tasks from the following:
  1. isolation of target muscle activity. Use shoulder shrugs and scapular retraction to help patient gain familiarity with voluntary muscle activation of scapular muscles.

2. postural training with SEMG feedback
3. relaxation-based downtraining
4. threshold-based downtraining
5. deactivation training after scapular elevation and retraction movements
6. tension recognition threshold training
7. tension discrimination training
8. left/right equilibration training. Downtraining the high amplitude side is an option, but it is often easier to uptrain the low amplitude side.
9. generalization to progressively dynamic movement. Decrease recruitment of the upper trapezius and interscapular muscles during arm elevation. Find minimum recruitment levels necessary to accomplish each assigned task, and train for prompt and complete deactivation. Progress from:
   –small AROM arcs to larger arcs
   –shoulder AROM with elbow bent to elbow straight to progressive extrinsic resistance
   –flexion to diagonal and combined movement planes
   –slow to faster speeds
   –unilateral movement to bilateral simultaneous symmetric movement to bilateral reciprocal movement to bilateral asymmetric movement
10. functional activity performance with SEMG feedback
- Integrate SEMG feedback training into a comprehensive approach to patient management:
  1. Refer the patient to a mental health practitioner if psychologic stressors seem to be contributory.
  2. Counsel patient for wellness. Include concepts related to
     –relaxation
     –modification of stressful cognitive appraisals
     –maintenance of appropriate postures and ergonomic setups
     –sensible pacing of activities
  3. Provide instruction in
     –nutritional balance

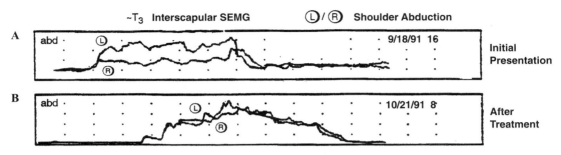

Figure 11–A–1 SEMG activity from the (**L**) left and (**R**) right interscapular sites at the (**T**$_3$) level of the third thoracic vertebra during performance of a symmetric work task. Signals were recorded from a patient with left interscapular pain 4 weeks after on-the-job work injury involving pushing and pulling a heavy cart and overhead lifting. (**A**) Activity at initial presentation. (**B**) Activity approximately 5 weeks later after a treatment program involving physical agents, manual soft tissue mobilization, and SEMG feedback training. Symptoms were largely resolved by this point. Note the reduction in left/right asymmetry as well as absolute recruitment levels for the same functional task. The display range is 0–16 μV in (**A**) compared with 0–8 μV in (**B**).

–aerobic fitness and general conditioning

–body weight management

• Promote transfer of relaxation skills to functional environments:

1. Instruct the patient in other related therapies, such as

    –systematic desensitization

    –stress inoculation

    –positive self-talk

    –relaxation trigger words

    –hand positions

    (Refer to Chapter 5.)

2. Have the patient practice an abbreviated relaxation technique in work, home, and recreational settings.

3. Instruct the patient in postural self-checks to use throughout the day.

4. Combine tactics in the three recommendations above with

    –abdominal breathing

    –cervical stretching

    –adaptation of muscle deactivation and tension discrimination training procedures

5. Once basic competence is demonstrated with tension discrimination training in the clinic, have the patient practice at home without SEMG feedback, simply by estimating SEMG scores from the target muscles as if he or she were connected to the feedback machine.

• Prescribe frequent, brief practice sessions and adjunctive therapies for the patient with muscle asymmetries.

1. Emphasize repetition of muscle equilibration procedures and stretching throughout the day.

2. Develop a careful plan to implement indicated changes in ergonomic setups and functional motor habits.

3. Consider consultation with a therapist or physician for adjunctive

    –manual treatments

    –exercise prescription

    –physical agents

    –functional activity modification

Shoulder Impingement Syndrome: Infraspinatus Hypoactivity

Shoulder impingement syndrome involves compression and cumulative trauma of the subacromial soft tissues between the humeral head and acromial arch occurring during arm elevation. The syndrome may develop as a result of structural and alignment faults, inefficient coordination patterns between shoulder girdle muscles, and passive tightness or laxity. Several approaches to adjunctive SEMG feedback treatment are offered below. Careful physical examination and SEMG assessment guide the clinician in selection of the best treatment plan.

Infraspinatus hypoactivity is seen in some cases of shoulder impingement syndrome, especially after old rotator cuff trauma, surgical repair, and immobilization. The infraspinatus muscle contributes to the rotator cuff action of limiting superior gliding of the humeral head as the arm is raised. This counteracts the component force of the deltoid, which would tend to compress the humeral head against the acromial arch. SEMG hypoactivity is judged relative to the uninvolved side. Deltoid activity can be correspondingly increased on the involved relative to the uninvolved side during shoulder abduction. Infraspinatus hypoactivity may manifest throughout shoulder elevation AROM, only during the eccentric phase, or during concentric and eccentric portions of a painful arc. SEMG feedback is used for uptraining the infraspinatus while impingement maneuvers are avoided.

Training Progression for Shoulder Impingement Syndrome: Infraspinatus Hypoactivity

- Refer to Chapters 3 and 4 for detailed discussion of SEMG display setups and feedback structure.
- Refer to Chapters 5 and 6 for detailed discussion of SEMG feedback training techniques.
- As skill develops, generally:
  1. Shape desired responses up or down.
  2. Incorporate multijoint control.
  3. Add distractions.
  4. Randomize training activities.
  5. Withdraw continuous audio/visual feedback.
- Select relevant SEMG feedback training tasks from the following:
  1. isolation of target muscle (ie, infraspinatus) activity. Use shoulder lateral rotation with the patient's arm at his or her side.

2. Threshold-based uptraining:
   -Begin with isometric contractions with the patient's arm at his or her side.
   -If anterior, lateral, or posterior deltoid activity is asymmetrically hyperactive, use a second channel and threshold marker for that site.
   -Cue selective isolation and uptraining of infraspinatus relative to the hyperactive deltoid.
3. generalization to progressively dynamic movement:
   -Continue with lateral rotation AROM with the patient's arm at his or her side.
   -Perform lateral rotation movements in progressively greater amounts of isometric shoulder flexion.
   -Consider beginning each new flexion position with the patient's arm supported on pillows; then withdraw support as skill is demonstrated.
   -Continue infraspinatus deltoid uptraining during shoulder flexion AROM.
   -Consider positioning the patient close to a wall or door frame, sliding his or her arm against the surface with modest lateral pressure through the movement arc.
   -Emphasize eccentric as well as concentric control.
   -Progress to larger movement arcs.
   -Progress to faster movement speeds.
   -Progress to increased loads (eg, lifting dumbbells).
4. motor copy training. Acquire a template from the uninvolved infraspinatus.
5. therapeutic exercises with SEMG feedback for home. Instruct the patient (as indicated) in
   -infraspinatus uptraining
   -SEMG feedback as adjunct to pectoralis or latissimus stretching
6. postural training with SEMG feedback
7. SEMG-triggered neuromuscular electrical stimulation. Consider use of this training technique for the infraspinatus during the above-listed activities.

8. functional activity performance with SEMG feedback. Continue training with performance of home, work, sports-specific activities that were previously exacerbating.

• Integrate SEMG feedback training with a comprehensive treatment plan for shoulder girdle rehabilitation:
   1. Consider consultation with a therapist or physician for adjunctive interventions, such as
      –physical agents
      –manual treatments
      –taping techniques
      –exercise prescription
      –functional activity modification
   2. Consider also SEMG monitoring of the pectoralis major, working toward decreasing hyperactive responses from the involved side if present.

• Note that in some cases of shoulder impingement syndrome the infraspinatus on the involved side appears hyperactive relative to the activity displayed on the uninvolved side. If the infraspinatus on the involved side generates asymmetrically higher SEMG activity at submaximal contraction intensities, but lower activity at maximal contraction intensities, muscle deconditioning may be a primary component (see Chapter 7). In this case, the patient may still respond well to a rotator cuff conditioning exercise program.

• Note that infraspinatus hyperactivity can be seen at all contraction intensities (and be associated with subtle compensatory shoulder motions). Patterns of scapular muscle activity should then be investigated for associated imbalance (see below).

Scapular Muscle Imbalance: Periscapular Pain and Shoulder Impingement Syndrome

The upper trapezius, middle trapezius, and lower trapezius contract with the lower fibers of the serratus anterior to produce upward rotation of the scapula during arm elevation movements.

Inefficient coupling of forces from these muscles leads to faulty scapulothoracic control. The result is mechanical overload of cervical and interscapular myofascial tissue. Because the scapulothoracic and glenohumeral articulations function as part of a coordinated kinetic chain, normal scapulohumeral rhythm is also disturbed. Suboptimal length–tension relationships of the rotator cuff may be produced. When combined, these factors bring about deviations of joint surface accessory motions, surface velocities, and instantaneous joint centers of rotation. As the humeral head is inadequately depressed away from the acromial arch, impingement syndromes are created. Assessment of scapular muscle imbalances with SEMG has garnered much attention in educational and conference settings. Problems with scapular muscle balance are believed to be associated with many cervical and shoulder girdle problems. Issues related to practical guidance are therefore discussed in greater detail than with the previous syndromes. Descriptions of the syndromes are speculative, however, and require confirmation with kinematic techniques, as well as with systematic intramuscular and SEMG study.

A popular clinical belief is that the peak SEMG amplitude of the lower trapezius should be about double that of the upper trapezius during full range shoulder abduction. Figure 11–A–2 shows an example of imbalanced, asymmetric SEMG activity from the upper and lower trapezius. The ratiometric point at which aberrant imbalance occurs is contentious because nonnormalized data from these sites tend to be inherently variable across patients. Even if a mean upper trapezius to lower trapezius ratio score was defined at about 2:1, the distribution of individual scores around this mean in healthy subjects would probably be wide, making it difficult to discriminate abnormal from normal variation. Also, electrode placement for the lower trapezius tends not to be uniform across clinicians. Cross-talk from neighboring muscles is perhaps inevitable at lower trapezius recording sites with standard commercial electrode configurations and processing equipment. Nor-

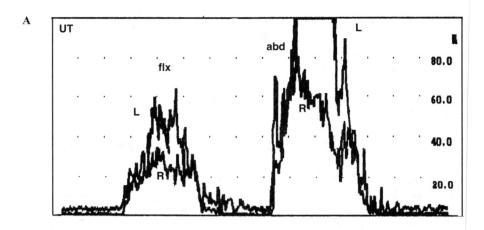

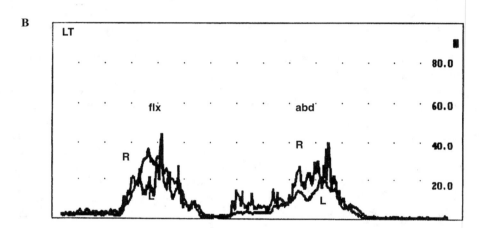

Figure 11–A–2 Bilateral SEMG activity of the (**A**) upper trapezius (**UT**) and (**B**) lower trapezius (**LT**) during bilateral symmetric shoulder (**flx**) and abduction (**abd**). Signals were recorded from a patient with 3-year history of (**L**) left greater than (**R**) right neck and interscapular pain. Note tendencies toward left greater than right upper trapezius activity, left less than right lower trapezius activity, and bilaterally diminished lower trapezius activity compared with upper trapezius activity.

malization to 100% MVIC is fraught with difficulties for this reason, and although alternatives are feasible, they are complex for the typical clinician to execute. Without a rigorous quantitative standard, it may be prudent for the clinician to use a more conservative criterion. A widely accepted consensus point is that the peak amplitude of the lower trapezius during abduction should be as great as, or greater than, that of the upper trapezius.

The authors have observed rare cases in which the peak lower trapezius amplitude is four to five times that of the upper trapezius, with relatively low absolute levels of upper trapezius activity. This tends to be accompanied by observations of scapular upward rotation, but also by scapular depression and adduction, the latter of which are opposite to findings normally expected during arm elevation. Often the shoulder girdles seem more downward sloped in standing posture, the upper trapezius of good passive length, and the contours of the lower trapezius quite obvious. In other words, an imbalance is suspected with the lower trapezius acting in a hyperactive manner and the upper trapezius acting in a hypoactive fashion.

In another variation, the upper trapezius appears asymmetrically or bilaterally hypoactive; the middle interscapular region, hyperactive; and the lower interscapular site variably hyperactive or hypoactive. The scapula visually appears to show decreases in elevation, abduction, and upward rotation during arm elevation. Rhomboid and levator scapulae contours may appear prominent during observation of the patient's alignment. Soft tissue dysfunction may be related to underuse of the trapezius in general, along with overuse of the rhomboids and levator scapulae for scapular stabilization during upper extremity function. It is suspected that increased electrical activity from the deeper muscle layer is detected by surface electrodes through relatively thin middle and lower portions of the trapezius, thus generating apparent SEMG hyperactivity at middle and lower interscapular sites. This type of patient needs general trapezius uptraining. Thus, although downtraining of the upper trapezius and uptraining of the lower trapezius have become popular clinical vehicles, training protocols that rigidly call for such approaches may not always be appropriate. The upper trapezius may sometimes function in a hypoactive fashion, and the lower trapezius can function in a hyperactive manner. SEMG assessment and careful physical examination should always precede feedback training.

There are wide variations in impedance and muscle geometry at the serratus anterior recording site. A good quality signal is obtainable in relatively slender, reasonably well-conditioned persons. However, a satisfactory recording can be virtually impossible to achieve in obese, deconditioned individuals. There is no standardized amplitude comparison of serratus anterior with upper trapezius recording sites, nor any prevailing clinical belief as to satisfactory signal amplitudes. Peak activity for the serratus ante-

rior site is almost always of a much lower microvolt value than that for upper and lower trapezius sites. The best that can be done is to compare left with right sides, or to normalize to 100% MVIC and use clinical judgment in combination with physical examination findings to gauge insufficiency.

Scapular signals can also be normalized as a percentage of the maximum value recorded during elevation in the scapular plane, from 0 to 180 degrees. For example, the SEMG amplitude for the upper trapezius at each point in the range of motion arc is divided by the peak amplitude during that same movement, and the quotient is multiplied by 100. When so expressed and visualized with high-temporal resolution, the expected activation sequence can be approximated as upper trapezius–serratus anterior–lower trapezius. This means that as the arm is raised, the upper trapezius tends to be significantly recruited first, followed by the serratus anterior, and then by the lower trapezius. The reverse pattern tends to be observed during eccentric return. Variable timing relationships can be observed with commercially available equipment (Figures 11–A–3 through 11–A–5). There are cases in which the serratus anterior appears delayed in recruitment as shoulder flexion or scaption proceeds. The lower trapezius may generate substantial activity but only toward the end of the concentric arc and with rapid termination as the eccentric phase begins. This pattern seems to be associated with general lower trapezius hypoactivity, noticeable weakness on manual muscle test, and winging of the scapula during the terminal eccentric return from elevation.

Training Progression for Upper Trapezius Hyperactivity and Lower Trapezius or Serratus Anterior Hypoactivity

- Consider the following issues in planning implementation of this training program:
  1. Scapular motion during active arm elevation may give the appearance of excessive elevation and insufficient superior rotation.

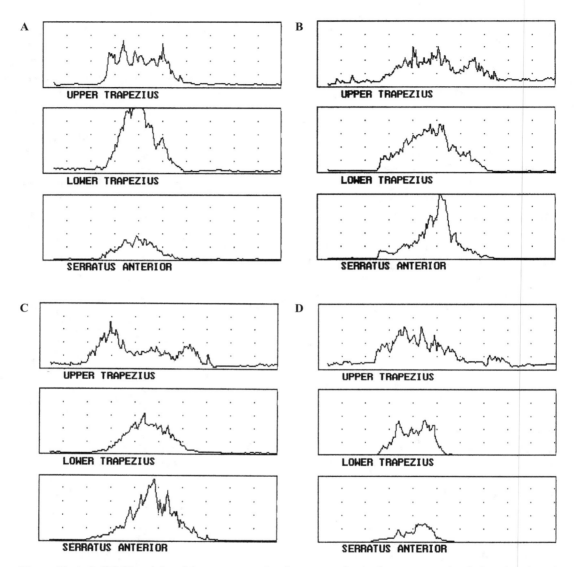

Figure 11–A–3 SEMG activity of the upper trapezius, lower trapezius, and serratus anterior during elevation of the patient's arm in the scapular plane. (**A**) Typical pattern in a symptom-free individual. (**B–D**) Variations from patients with shoulder impingement and/or periscapular pain syndromes.

2. The syndrome can be associated with tight passive extensibility of the upper trapezius, as well as weakness of the lower trapezius and serratus anterior on manual muscle tests.

3. There can also be hypertrophy of the rhomboids and levator scapulae. Hyper-

activity from these muscles can potentially contribute to increased SEMG amplitudes detected from superior and middle interscapular electrodes, although the effects cannot be reliably isolated from middle trapezius activity. Persons with rhomboid/levator scapulae

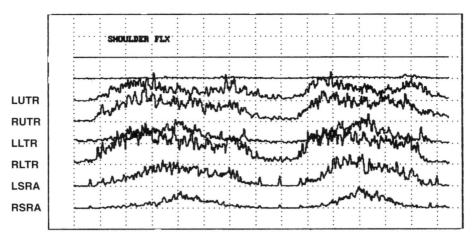

Figure 11–A–4 SEMG activity from the **(L)** left and **(R)** right **(UTR)** upper trapezius, **(LTR)** lower trapezius, and **(SRA)** serratus anterior during two repetitions of bilateral simultaneous symmetric full-range shoulder flexion **(FLX)**. Signals were recorded from a patient with right cervical, suprascapular, interscapular pain and shoulder impingement syndrome. Note increased right compared with left upper trapezius activity, increased right compared with left lower trapezius activity, and altered timing of right compared with left serratus anterior activity.

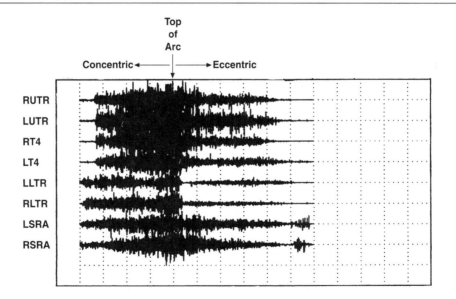

Figure 11–A–5 SEMG activity from the **(L)** left and **(R)** right **(UTR)** upper trapezius, interscapular recording sites at the **(T4)** level of the fourth thoracic vertebra, and **(LTR)** lower trapezius, and **(SRA)** serratus anterior during bilateral simultaneous symmetric full-range shoulder abduction. Signals were recorded from a patient with bilateral shoulder impingement syndrome. Winging of the medial border of the scapula was observed only during the eccentric movement phase. Although all signals are diminished in amplitude during the eccentric compared with the concentric phase, reduced lower trapezius activity is dramatic and atypical. Feedback uptraining (not shown) of lower trapezius activity during the eccentric phase was followed by symptom resolution and normalization of activity patterns.

overuse may appear posturally to hold the scapulae in a relatively adducted position. Other patients posturally maintain the scapulae in a relatively abducted position in association with forward head and rounded shoulders.

- Refer to Chapters 3 and 4 for detailed discussion of SEMG display setups and feedback structure.
- Refer to Chapters 5 and 6 for detailed discussion of SEMG feedback training techniques.
- As skill develops, generally
  1. Shape desired responses up or down.
  2. Incorporate multijoint control.
  3. Add distractions.
  4. Randomize training activities.
  5. Withdraw continuous audio/visual feedback.
- Select relevant SEMG feedback training tasks from the following:
  1. isolation of target muscle activity. Train isolation of the upper trapezius, lower trapezius, and serratus anterior, each independent of the other, as indicated:
     –isolate the upper trapezius with a pure shoulder shrug, instructing the patient to "gently shrug your shoulder straight up."
     –isolate the lower trapezius with conjoint scapular retraction and depression, instructing the patient to "pull your shoulder blade gently back and down."
     –isolate the serratus anterior with scapular protraction and depression, instructing the patient to "pull your shoulder blade gently forward and down from the back of the arm pit." If appropriate, use light manual pressure or a sweeping motion against the patient's skin overlying the target muscle. Initiating serratus anterior isolation tends to be more difficult than for the others.
     –observe for pectoral muscle substitution; consider pectoral SEMG feedback downtraining if suspected.

  2. relaxation-based downtraining and threshold-based downtraining. Use for the upper trapezius if hyperactivity is present at postural baseline.
  3. left/right equilibration training:
     –Use for the upper trapezius if hyperactivity is asymmetrically present at postural baseline.
     –Emphasize activation of the low amplitude side, then bilateral relaxation.
  4. postural training with SEMG feedback.
  5. tension discrimination training. Use isolating actions of the upper trapezius, lower trapezius, and serratus anterior as indicated.
  6. promotion of correct muscle synergies and related coordination patterns. Uptraining of the lower trapezius and serratus anterior relative to the upper trapezius.
     –Execute upper trapezius stretch with relaxation.
     –With the patient's arm resting on table, in about 30 degrees of shoulder flexion, isometrically activate lower trapezius or serratus anterior; relax the upper trapezius.
     –Repeat the sequence at higher degrees of flexion, with the patient's arm passively supported.
     –Increase the recruitment of lower trapezius relative to upper trapezius, or serratus anterior relative to upper trapezius through AROM.
     –Include flexion, scaption, and abduction planes as appropriate while avoiding symptom provocation.

A caution is warranted not to overtrain the lower trapezius. This can result by calling for scapular retraction/depression before arm elevation. The maneuver readily produces increased activity in the lower trapezius and decreased activity in the upper trapezius, but results in an unnatural movement pattern. Aberrant lower trapezius hyperactivity then produces excessive scapular depression. The scapular retraction/depression motion should be used to teach isolation. During arm elevation, the patient should be trained to consciously increase lower trapezius SEMG activity after motion has started (about 20 to 30 degrees of elevation) and continue increasing activity to the peak of the arc. Overtraining of the serratus anterior does not seem to pose an analogous risk.

7. generalization to progressively dynamic movement. Progressively increase
   –AROM excursion with emphasis of eccentric as well as concentric control
   –movement velocity
   –movement load
   –unilateral movement to bilateral simultaneous symmetric movement to bilateral reciprocal symmetric movement to bilateral asymmetric movement

8. therapeutic exercises with SEMG feedback. Consider specifically
   –cervical side-bending stretch with relaxation of the upper trapezius
   –conditioning of the lower trapezius
   Patient in prone position: hands clasped (a) over neck—gentle elbow lift, upper trapezius relaxed; (b) shoulder lateral rotation—abduction 90 degrees, forearm over edge of bench; (c) arm raise—shoulder at edge of bench, arm over edge of bench. Raise the arm forward toward ceiling, thumb pointed up, upper trapezius relaxed as much as possible. Begin with passive positioning, followed by slow withdrawal of support while asking for isometric hold of the lower trapezius. Progress by instructing the patient to raise his or her arm with a flexed elbow, to arm raises with a straight elbow, to arm raises with a straight elbow and 1 to 3 lb of free weight. Too much weight can cause substitution patterns.
   Patient sitting on a stool or standing: wall slide—spine lightly pressed flush

against a wall, from bottom to top, hands slide up above head while wall contact is maintained.
   –conditioning of serratus anterior muscle
   Patient in side-lying position: involved side up, arm supported on pillows. Glide the scapula into protraction with shoulder transitioning from passive to active-assisted movement. Progress to resistive movement, using flexion, and a piece of elastic tubing to increase concentric and eccentric loading.
   Patient in supine position: press—upper extremity active "punch" up toward the ceiling with a dumbbell; press plus—same as above but with conscious scapular protraction at the peak of the movement
   Patient in standing position: wall push-ups; wall push-ups plus—same as wall push-ups but with conscious scapular protraction at the peak of the movement
   Patient in prone position on floor: push-ups; push-ups plus

9. SEMG-triggered neuromuscular electrical stimulation. Use for the lower trapezius if there are no contraindications and difficulty persists with the above-described training sequence. SEMG-triggered neuromuscular electrical stimulation tends to be difficult to impossible for the serratus anterior. However, SEMG-triggered (nonmotor) electrical stimulation can be used as a cutaneous cue over the serratus anterior to aid in its facilitation.

10. motor copy training. Use with an uninvolved side serving as a template for the involved side.

11. functional activity performance with SEMG feedback. Continue training with home, work, sports-specific activities that were previously exacerbating.

• Integrate SEMG feedback training with a comprehensive treatment plan for shoulder girdle rehabilitation. Consider consultation with a therapist or physician for adjunctive interventions, such as

1. physical agents
2. manual treatment
3. taping techniques
4. exercise prescription
5. functional activity modification

• Some clinicians suspect that a shortened, hyperactive pectoralis minor may sometimes accompany these scapular syndromes. Note that it is not possible to isolate activity from the pectoralis minor with surface electrodes. However, activity for the pectoralis major muscle can be easily detected with SEMG. The operator can investigate potential left/right asymmetries, following with equilibration feedback training or modification of recruitment levels as the lower trapezius, serratus anterior, or infraspinatus is appropriately uptrained.

REFERENCES

1. Hislop HJ, Montgomery J. *Daniels and Worthingham's Muscle Testing: Techniques of Manual Examination.* 6th ed. Philadelphia: WB Saunders Co; 1995.

2. Kendall F, McCreary E, Provance P. *Muscles Testing and Function with Posture and Pain.* 4th ed. Baltimore: Williams & Wilkins; 1993.

SUGGESTED READINGS

Bagg SD, Forrest WJ. Electromyographic study of the scapular rotators during arm abduction in the scapular plane. *Am J Phys Med.* 1986;65:111–124.

Ballantyne BT, O'Hare SJ, Paschall JL, et al. Electromyographic activity of selected shoulder muscles in commonly used therapeutic exercises. *Phys Ther.* 1993;73:668–682.

Jobe FW, Tibone JE, Jobe CM, Kvitne RS. The shoulder in sports. In: Rockwood CA, Matsen FA, eds. *The Shoulder.* Philadelphia: WB Saunders Co; 1990;961–990.

Ludewig PM, Cook TM, Nawoczenski DA. Three-dimensional scapular orientation and muscle activity at selected positions of humeral elevation. *J Orthop Sports Phys Ther.* 1996;24:57–65.

McCann PD, Wooten ME, Kadaba MP, Bigliani LU. A kinematic and electromyographic study of shoulder rehabilitation exercises. *Clin Orthop.* 1992;288:179–188.

Moseley A, Jobe FW, Pink M, Perry J, Tibone JE. EMG analysis of the scapular muscles during a shoulder rehabilitation program. *Am J Sports Med.* 1992;20:128–134.

Pink M, Jobe F, Perry J, Browne A, Scovazzo ML, Kerrigan J. The painful shoulder during the butterfly stroke: an electromyographic and cinematographic analysis of twelve muscles. *Clin Orthop.* 1992;288:60–72.

Reid DC, Saboe LA, Chepeha JC. Anterior shoulder instability in athletes: comparison of isokinetic resistance exercises and an electromyographic biofeedback re-education program—a pilot program. *Physiother Can.* Fall 1996:251–256.

Saboe L, Chepena J, Reid D, Okamura G, Grace M. *Electromyography Applications in Physical Therapy: The Unstable Shoulder.* Monograph. Montreal, Canada: Thought Technology Ltd; 1990.

Scovazzo ML, Browne A, Pink M, Jobe FW, Kerrigan J. The painful shoulder during freestyle swimming: an electromyographic cinematographic analysis of twelve muscles. *Am J Sports Med.* 1991;19:577–582.

Taylor W. Dynamic EMG biofeedback in assessment and treatment using a neuromuscular re-education model. In: Cram JR, ed. *Clinical EMG for Surface Recordings.* Vol 2. Nevada City, CA: Clinical Resources; 1990;175–196.

Young MS. Electromyographic biofeedback use in the treatment of voluntary posterior dislocation of the shoulder: a case study. *J Orthop Sports Phys Ther.* 1994;20:171–175.

SEMG Program for Forearm and Wrist Dysfunction

CANDIDATES

Implement for patients with
- chronic elbow medial or lateral epicondylitis during work activities
- carpal tunnel syndrome and in whom proximal or distal muscle overuse patterns are suspected
- distal upper extremity chronic pain and in whom muscle dysfunction is suspected
Patients may present with a variety of diagnoses, including
1. posttraumatic and postsurgical deficits
2. fibromyalgia
3. tenosynovitis
Patient intake should indicate
1. high-demand emotional work stress
2. repetitive upper extremity loading with poor pacing
3. inadequate ergonomic setup
Physical examination should reveal
1. faulty posture
2. palpable hypertonicity
3. trigger points
4. imbalances in muscle flexibility and strength

EVALUATION OBJECTIVES

- Assess the effects of posture and dynamic movement on muscle activity.
- Identify aberrant patterns of muscle activity about the distal upper extremity, potentially contributing to musculoskeletal pain:
  1. myalgia due to excessive levels or duration of muscle tension
  2. imbalanced muscle activity that potentially results in soft tissue or joint dysfunction
- Assess psychophysiologic factors in the precipitation of excessive muscle tension.

FEEDBACK TRAINING OBJECTIVES

- Reduce excessive muscle intensity and duration.
- Improve postural function and ergonomic alignment.
- Balance recruitment of proximal cervical and shoulder stabilizers with distal motor function.
- Resolve underlying mechanical dysfunction.

313

- Decouple psychologic stressors and muscle tension responses.
- Retain and generalize improved motor control to functional contexts.
- Resolve or reduce functional limitations and disability.

RECORDING SITES

- Judge the utility of each recording site on the basis of history and physical examination results.
- Include muscles that
  1. underlie the pain distribution
  2. potentially refer symptoms or are mechanically related to the patient's area of complaint
  3. reproduce the patient's symptoms when stretched, resisted, or palpated
- Consult the companion book, *Introduction to Surface Electromyography*, for specific electrode placement considerations.
- Confirm optimal sites from the following list by observation and palpation during isometric contraction:
  1. forearm flexor compartment sites
  2. forearm extensor compartment sites
  3. hand sites
  4. upper trapezius
  5. sternomastoid
  6. lateral cervical
  7. cervical paraspinals
  8. middle interscapular
  9. lower interscapular
  10. anterior deltoid
  11. lateral deltoid
  12. posterior deltoid
  13. pectoralis major

EVALUATION PROCEDURES

- Select procedures that correspond to exacerbating and alleviating factors revealed by history and clinical examination.
- Refer to Chapter 2 for detailed discussion of evaluation methods.

- Perform at least five repetitions of each movement task to assess response consistency (consider discarding the results of the first one to two repetitions and averaging the results of the remaining repetitions). Many more repetitions may be needed to assess SEMG responses with reproduction of symptoms.
- Select relevant procedures from the following:
  1. psychophysiologic stress profile
  2. elbow, wrist, hand AROM as appropriate. Observe for consistent excursion and velocity across test repetitions.
  3. cervical AROM with patient seated, arms supported comfortably at rest. Observe for consistent excursion and velocity across test repetitions.
  4. functional activity analysis:
     - Test work activities associated with changes in symptoms.
     - Consider specifically tasks involving high loads, high velocities, repetitive loads, poor rest pacing, and awkward body alignment.
  5. analysis of muscular coordination patterns among cervical and upper extremity groups
  6. repeat of any of above procedures, as appropriate, with corrections for the following:
     - posture
     - task technique
     - equipment, work station modification
     - orthotic application

ASSESSMENT

- Refer to Chapter 2 for detailed discussion of SEMG assessment.
- Refer to Chapter 14 in the companion book for representative SEMG tracings of normal function.
- Select SEMG assessment parameters from the following:

1. Amplitude and variance of each channel during baseline. Activity during baseline should be stable and relatively quiescent. Mean amplitude values from nonpostural muscles should be close to internal noise levels of the recording device. Postural muscles may show low-level activity with the patient in weight-bearing positions (typically, about 2–6 μV RMS).

2. Peak or average amplitude of each channel during activation. Activity can appear to be unremarkable, grossly excessive and erratic, or markedly depressed.

3. Relationship of salient SEMG events to particular range of motion arcs. Observe for consistent amplitude elevations or depressions during a painful portion of the AROM arc.

4. Return to baseline amplitude after muscle activation. Qualitatively, recovery can be stated as prompt and complete versus elevated and delayed. Satisfactory baseline recovery is quantitatively defined (with a smoothing time constant of 0.1 second or less) as a return to an SEMG amplitude within two standard deviations of the original baseline mean, within 3 seconds of movement cessation, and maintenance within that amplitude range for at least 30 seconds or until the next movement is initiated. Recovery can be characterized by the latency to achieve this criterion. More simply, the amplitude (expressed as percentage of baseline) observed 1 to 3 seconds after movement termination can be reported.

5. Left/right peak amplitude symmetry for bilateral symmetric movements (eg, bilateral wrist extension) and reciprocal movements (eg, left wrist extension followed by reciprocal right wrist extension). Satisfactory symmetry is operationally defined as left/right scores within 35% as calculated [(higher value

– lower value)/higher value] × 100. Symmetry assessment assumes an equivalent left/right AROM excursion and velocity.

6. Left/right asymmetry for unilateral movements (eg, left wrist extension with right upper extremity at rest). Within a single side unilateral movement, similar levels of left/right co-activation may be an aberrant finding.

7. Symmetric left/right timing and amplitude relationships among muscular antagonists and synergists.

8. Quiescence of forearm and hand recording sites during seated cervical AROM. With patient's arms supported at rest, activation of forearm and hand muscles during gentle cervical AROM is an aberrant finding. Observe for low-amplitude discharges consistently time locked to cervical movement.

9. Low amplitude gaps or microrests during functional tasks (obtained with use of a rectified moving line tracing display with a smoothing time constant of 0.1 second or less, SEMG sampling at 100 Hz or faster, and a frequency bandwidth filter low cutoff of 25 Hz or less). Microrests can be identified by setting a visible threshold marker at a microvolt value of about 5% of MVIC for the distal upper extremity muscle. This value should be above the range of the patient's postural baseline tracing. If the patient's postural baseline range exceeds 5% MVIC, the assessment should be deferred. Instruct the patient to perform continually a functional task that tends to exacerbate symptoms. With suitable precautions for patient safety, maintain task performance until the patient reports reproduction or exacerbation of symptoms. At the outset and every 2 to 3 minutes of task performance thereafter, save or freeze and print a copy of a 30- to 60-second display

sweep. Count the number of threshold crossings. Microrests are typically produced in a range between approximately 0.2 second and several seconds without conscious patient effort. Observe for a minimal presence of microrests throughout the course, as well as for changes in microrest frequency and duration as symptoms are produced. Compare left with right microrest frequencies/durations if the functional task involves symmetric movements and patient has unilateral involvement (see Figure 10–A–2 in Application Guide 10–A).

10. Tonic amplitude during repeated task trials or a continuous functional activity. With use of the same type of display as in no. 9 above, observe the lowest level of activation consistently produced during performance of a continuous functional task. This tonic amplitude appears as the continually running baseline from which the muscle is phasically activated (see Figure 10–A–3 in Application Guide 10–A). Assuming a satisfactory, low-noise recording setup, the tonic amplitude should be less than 5% to 10% MVIC for tasks that are functionally performed for about 1 hour or longer. Note the tonic amplitude at the outset and every 2 to 3 minutes of task performance thereafter. Compare left with right sides if the functional task involves symmetric movements and the patient has unilateral involvement.

11. Change in activity level for a particular muscle and task across treatment sessions. To document this parameter, a normalization procedure is preferred to enhance reliability. A reliable maximal manual muscle test effort or a standardized submaximal contraction is required. The average amplitude during the test task is divided by that day's reference contraction and the quotient is multiplied by 100. For example, SEMG activity during a problematic work task

may be found initially to average 25% MVIC. With treatment, that value could drop to 5% MVIC and be associated with symptomatic improvement.

12. Frequency spectral analysis for fatigue assessment. This analysis requires specialized equipment and technique. Observe the median frequency during a standardized isometric contraction of at least 50% MVIC. Observe the rate of decline in median frequency values (indicative of increased fatigue) during a prolonged effort contraction, comparing left and right side muscle performance. To track fatigue during a dynamic functional task, obtain SEMG frequency data during a high-level isometric contraction before initiation of the functional activity. Then have the patient perform the functional task for a duration expected to induce fatigue or increase symptoms. Repeat the standardized isometric test, extract median frequency values, and compare these values with initial levels for indications of fatigue. Have the patient rest for 1 to 3 minutes, and then repeat the isometric test and frequency analysis. Continue a rest period:frequency test sequence to assess for recovery to initial median frequency values.

COMMON PATIENT PRESENTATIONS

Lateral and Medial Elbow Epicondylitis

Lateral and medial elbow epicondylitis are typically viewed as forms of tendinitis occurring at the proximal attachments of wrist extensors and flexors, respectively. Lateral epicondylitis (tennis elbow) is far more common and most often attributed to microtrauma involving extensor carpi radialis brevis, although other extensors may be compromised. Medial epicondylitis arises from recurrent microtrauma at the tenoperiosteal junction of the common flexor tendon. Although laypersons tend to associate epicondylitis with sports injuries, it can be produced from overuse in the workplace or around the home. Involvement is usually unilateral, and SEMG activity can appear asymmetrically elevated on the involved side, both at postural baseline and during dynamic movements, as well as with a delayed and incomplete deactivation after a repetitive movement series (Figure 11–B–1). Psychologic stressors may contribute to general upper extremity tone and inappropriate extensor/flexor co-activation in particular. The pathophysiology of these problems is uncertain because the evidence for acute inflammatory processes or tissue degeneration is inconsistent.

Training Progression for Lateral and Medial Elbow Epicondylitis

- Refer to Chapters 3 and 4 for detailed discussion of SEMG display setups and feedback structure.

- Refer to Chapter 5 for detailed discussion of training techniques.
- As skill develops, generally
  1. Shape desired responses up or down.
  2. Incorporate multijoint control.
  3. Add distractions.
  4. Randomize training activities.
  5. Withdraw continuous audio/visual feedback.
- Select relevant SEMG training tasks from the following:
  1. isolation of target muscle activity:
     –Beginning with the patient's forearm supported and wrist in a gravity-neutral position, instruct the patient to perform discrete wrist flexion and extension movements.
     –Work for isolation of extensors from flexors.
     –Repeat isolation training for flexors and extensors against gravity.

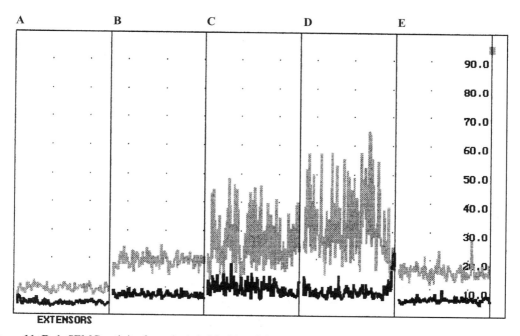

Figure 11–B–1 SEMG activity from the left (black) and right (gray) forearm extensor surfaces recorded from a patient with chronic right lateral epicondylitis. (**A**) Baseline activity, with the patient's arms relaxed in lap; supported sitting. (**B**) The patient positioned as in **A** but with emotionally stressful imagery. (**C**) Initiation of a bilateral typing task. (**D**) Continued typing after 20 minutes of typing. (**E**) One minute after cessation of the typing task.

2. postural training with SEMG feedback. Changes in head and trunk alignment may induce changes in baseline forearm muscle activity levels.
3. relaxation-based downtraining and threshold-based downtraining. Use if forearm hyperactivity is present at postural baseline.
4. deactivation training
5. tension recognition thresholds. Use isolating actions of extensors or flexors as indicated.
6. tension discrimination training
7. motor copy training. Use with an uninvolved side serving as a template for the involved side activity during extension or flexion movements.
8. therapeutic exercises with SEMG feedback. Train for
   –relaxation during performance of isolated extensor or flexor stretches
   –proper pacing of strength/endurance exercises
   –monitoring for complete baseline recovery between exercise repetitions and sets
9. functional activity performance with SEMG feedback. Modify workplace equipment, setups, technique, and pacing with adjunctive feedback. Train for appropriate levels of extensor/flexor co-activation and production of microrests.

• Integrate SEMG feedback training into a comprehensive approach to patient management.
• Refer the patient to a mental health practitioner if psychologic stressors seem to be contributory.
• Promote transfer of relaxation skills to functional environments:
  1. Instruct patient in other related therapies, such as
     –systematic desensitization
     –stress inoculation
     –positive self-talk
     –relaxation trigger words

–hand positions
(Refer to Chapter 5.)
  2. Have the patient practice an abbreviated relaxation technique in work, home, and recreational settings.
  3. Instruct the patient in postural self-checks to use throughout the day.
  4. Combine tactics in three recommendations above with
     –abdominal breathing
     –cervical stretching
     –adaptation of muscle deactivation and tension discrimination training procedures
• Develop a careful plan to implement indicated changes in ergonomic setups, functional motor habits, pacing, rotation of job tasks, and workplace exercise routines.
• Consider the potential utility of adjunctive physical agents, orthoses, and manual treatments.

Carpal Tunnel Syndrome

Carpal tunnel syndrome has emerged as a frequent, disabling, and expensive problem in office and industrial work settings. The syndrome involves compression of the median nerve within the carpal tunnel and is associated with tenosynovitis within the flexor group, dysplasia, and inefficient dissipation of biomechanical stress.

A degree of flexor/extensor muscle co-activation is to be expected for most functional activities. Some clinicians believe that co-activation imbalance contributes to carpal tunnel syndrome. The notion is that unopposed overuse of the flexor muscles results in hypertrophic thickening of the associated tendons and flexor retinaculum. These events are believed to be accompanied by inflammation and further reduction of available space within the carpal tunnel. Insufficient antagonistic action by the extensor muscles is viewed by some as contributing to a wrist alignment that raises pressure within the carpal tunnel, as well as leading to an efficient length-tension relationship for the flexor muscles. Conversely, excessive extensor muscle activity can be predicted to produce similar outcomes and disturb normal force relationships within the carpal tunnel. Another line of thinking holds that tonic, higher intensity muscle contractions result in altered blood flow relationships that disrupt normal tissue metabolism or retard repair. Although these pathophysiologic mechanisms are speculative, patterns of muscle activity can be clinically investigated with SEMG.

Faulty SEMG findings tend to be of two types. One is dysfunction of the forearm musculature in patterns similar to that described above for epicondylitis. The second type relates to production of low-amplitude discharges from the forearm musculature during neck movements, with the upper extremities ostensibly at rest (Figure 11–B–2). Aberrant forearm activity is accompanied by clearly identifiable SEMG asymmetries or co-activations in cervical and shoulder girdle muscles during those test movements. Cervical and shoulder girdle asymmetries also appear during exacerbating functional tasks, and some clinicians hypothesize they are causally related to the carpal tunnel syndrome. That is, the proximal muscles fatigue or otherwise fail to stabilize properly the distal movement segments, thereby subjecting them to subtle but significant changes in alignment or inefficient compensatory activity. Alternatively, it is speculated that dysfunctional reflex systems form the link between proximal and distal motor patterns. The actual consequence of proximal motor dysfunction on carpal tunnel syndrome is unknown at this time.

Discussion of cervical and scapular muscle imbalances can be found in Application Guides 10–A and 11–A, respectively. If proximal problems are identified, the clinician may reasonably consider SEMG feedback training of neck and shoulder muscles. The objective is to facilitate improved patterns of movement throughout the upper extremity kinetic chain. A more efficient proximal movement strategy may unload distal segments and decrease repetitive strain.

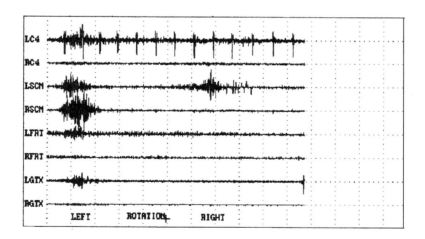

Figure 11–B–2 SEMG activity of the (**L**) left and (**R**) right (**C4**) cervical paraspinals at the level of the fourth vertebra, (**SCM**) sternomastoids, (**FRI**) wrist and finger flexors, and (**GTX**) wrist and finger extensors during left and right head rotation. Recordings were made from a patient diagnosed with chronic left carpal tunnel syndrome positioned in quiet sitting with forearms comfortably supported on chair rests. Note persistent left greater than right **C4** activity, inappropriate **SCM** co-activation during left rotation, persistent left greater than right **FRI** activity, and left **FRI** and **GTX** activity time locked to left rotation.

Training Progression for Carpal Tunnel Syndrome

- When aberrant forearm activity is produced during wrist and hand activities, refer to the Training Progression for Lateral and Medial Elbow Epicondylitis.
- When aberrant forearm activity appears linked to faulty cervical SEMG findings, refer to Application Guide 10–A:

1. Follow cervical muscle isolation and equilibration procedures recommended in Application Guide 10–A.
2. Train for forearm muscle quiescence during neck movements with forearm SEMG feedback.
3. Proceed to direct forearm training methods as indicated in Training Progression for Lateral and Medial Elbow Epicondylitis.

SUGGESTED READINGS

Grieco A, Occhipinti E, Colombini D, et al. Muscular effort and musculo-skeletal disorders in piano students: electromyographic, clinical and preventive aspects. *Ergonomics*. 1989;32:697–716.

Headley B. Is muscle failure to recover a contributing factor to the development of cumulative trauma disorder? *J Orthop Sports Phys Ther*. 1995;21:50.

Milerad E, Erickson MO, Nisell R, Kilbom A. An electromyographic study of dental work. *Ergonomics*. 1991;34:953–962.

Montes R, Bedmar M, Martin MS. EMG biofeedback of the abductor pollicis brevis in piano performance. *Biofeedback Self Regul*. 1993;18:67–77.

Peper E, Wilson V, Taylor W, Pierce A, Bender K, Tibbits V. *Repetitive Strain Injury*. Vendor monograph. Montreal, Canada: Thought Technology Ltd; 1994.

Reynolds C. Electromyographic biofeedback evaluation of a computer keyboard operator with cumulative trauma disorder. *J Hand Ther*. 1994;7:25–27.

Skubick DL, Clasby R, Donaldson CCS, Marshall WM. Carpal tunnel syndrome as an expression of muscular dysfunction in the neck. *J Occup Rehabil*. 1993;3:31–44.

Steffa ES. Lateral epicondylitis. Vendor monograph. Ft Lauderdale, FL: Verimed International; 1995.

CHAPTER 12

Low Back Dysfunction

BACKGROUND

The nature of low back pain makes it one of the more obstinate conditions in all of medicine. Clearly the persistence of pain associated with abnormal vertebral mechanics and movements is multidimensional and encompasses physical, psychosocial, cultural, environmental, and vocational domains.

Low back pain is omnipresent and pervasive in the United States. Andersson and colleagues[1] report that although the US population increased by only 7% from 1974 through 1978, disabling back injuries during that period increased by 26%. Frymoyer and coworkers[2] note that the incidence of low back pain in 1,221 men between the ages of 18 and 55 years encompassed 66.4% of their sample. In the United States alone there may be more than 2.5 million low back–injured individuals and 4.8 million low back–disabled adults.

Epidemiologic findings show that 10% to 17% of adults have at least one back pain episode each year.[3,4] Impairments related to the low back are the most frequent cause of activity limitation in people younger than age 64 years. Low back pain has ranked as high as fifth in the leading reasons for hospitalization and second only to heart disease as the basis for physician visits.[1] About 21% of all compensable work injuries involve low back pain.[5] In 1978, the Social Security Administration reported that the cost for all occupational injuries was approximately $8 bil-

lion, about one third of which were for patients with low back pain. When the associated costs for medical and surgical care are added to this expense, the enormity of the problem becomes all the more evident.

The study of epidemiologic issues underlying low back pain is fraught with methodologic difficulties. Specificity of exercise regimens, frequency and duration of treatment paradigms, and adherence to treatment instructions represent but a handful of issues requiring delineation. Cassidy and Wedge[6] surveyed the most prevalent factors associated with low back pain. These factors included increasing age (up to about 60 years of age), marked scoliosis, poor general health, lack of fitness, smoking, psychosocial problems, drug abuse, headaches, neck pain, angina pectoris, leg discomfort, and stomach pains.

Among the factors that tended not to be associated consistently with development of low back pain were gender, body build, increased lordosis, mild scoliosis, small leg length discrepancies, and psychiatric illness. Snook[7] identified that, mechanically, 37% to 49% of all industrial back injuries are associated with lifting activities and 12% to 14% are associated with bending. Closer examination of back injury trends through use of prospective or retrospective population surveys is still needed to set policy on treatment and prevention strategies. A review of interventions by the Agency for Health Care Policy and Research demonstrated that prevailing data on treatment of acute low back injury do little to justify more than provision of rest and general exercise.[8]

For the clinician eager to use surface electromyography (SEMG) as an adjunct to the treatment of low back pain symptoms, it would be prudent to recognize that despite the plethora of literature governing the biomechanics of the spine and the actions of muscles controlling it, there is little etched in stone. Only a modicum sample from the mounds of work on back muscle SEMG is addressed below. The information that follows is designed to challenge the reader to assess seriously the myriad opportunities to integrate SEMG monitoring and quantification into clinical practice.

SEMG ANALYSIS IN FREQUENCY VERSUS AMPLITUDE DOMAINS

Some controversy surrounds the essential elements of the SEMG signal and their relationship to analyses of low back pain. The integral average or RMS amplitudes derived from the SEMG signal seem to be useful for studying muscle activity during nonfatiguing conditions in patients with low back pain. Although there is considerable evidence that the magnitude of RMS SEMG diminishes with repeated contractions, the most prominent feature may be a shift or compression in the frequency domain. This observation has been supported by work from De Luca,[9] as well as from his collaborative work with other investigators,[10–13] while demonstrating accurate discrimination of patients with chronic low back pain from healthy control subjects by using frequency spectral analysis. Dolan and coworkers[14] note that when the SEMG power spectra are divided into 10 frequency bands (from 5 to 300 Hz), median frequency from erector spinae muscles at T10 and L3 decreases steadily during repeated submaximal lifting contractions. Total power and peak amplitude, however, increase. The greatest change is seen in the 5- to 30-Hz band of the SEMG power spectrum, which may provide a more meaningful linear index of erector spinae muscle fatigue. Further, in a pulling or lifting motion against a specified load, the extensor moment generated and SEMG activity recorded are a function of the lumbar posture at the time of recording, with peak extensor moment generated at 78% to 97% of full range into flexion.

Potvin and Norman[15,16] observed that during maximal and submaximal isometric trunk extensor contractions with a subject lifting inertial loads of 19 or 17 kg during 20-minute or 2-hour sessions, SEMG mean power frequency decreased by 12% at the lumbar level and 17% at the thoracic level in the 2-hour session. Decreases of 20% and 14% for these same two areas, respectively, occurred during the 20-minute session. When multiple paravertebral sites were monitored during fatiguing, intermittent isometric extension actions, the lower lumbar location showed the more consistent changes in the SEMG power spectrum, compared with findings in upper lumbar regions.[17] Collectively, these results indicate that the median frequency spectrum shifts to the lower end (lower frequency components) as a muscle fatigues, and continued efforts under this circumstance may portend muscle or ligamentous injury. However, even without spectral analysis, Robinson and coworkers[18] showed that patients with chronic low back pain produce less integrated SEMG activation from low back muscles during repeated flexion–extension loads, compared with findings in healthy subjects. If these emerging concepts remain unscathed, the possibility of using median frequency as a feedback source or guide in determining rate or intensity of effort during contextually meaningful exercise becomes inviting.

INFLUENCES OF POSTURE ON TRUNK MUSCLE ACTIVITY

For clinicians who choose to use SEMG as a monitoring device, it becomes important to examine information regarding the relationship among functional activity, SEMG, and posture as well as normalization procedures. There is little information about the trunk and body positions at which a maximal voluntary effort should be made for normalization. Fiebert and Keller[19] believe that the greatest electrical activity generated from the erector spinae occurs in extending the low back from a fully prone position. This observation may not carry over from their pain-free sample to patients with low back pain, and it has been questioned on the basis of detailed measures that suggest that there is an error factor of 75% when normalization depends on measures from one reference point.[20]

When the intricacies of interactions between loading conditions and posture are examined, many interesting observations result. All have implications for SEMG monitoring, training, and evaluation. For example, Shirado and co-workers[21] examined the relationship between trunk and neck position under different isometric loading conditions and found that the largest increase in abdominal SEMG activity during supine trunk flexion is with the neck flexed and the pelvis maintained in a posterior tilt. The greatest increase in erector spinae muscle activity is produced in prone position, also with neck flexion and pelvic stabilization. These findings indicate that neck and pelvic alignment can influence SEMG activity of trunk flexor and extensor muscles during isometric exercises. Accordingly, when using SEMG to record erector spinae or abdominal muscle activity during functional tasks or as part of a neuromuscular re-education procedure, the clinician should be aware that alignment of head, neck, and pelvis will influence the response magnitude at different trunk angles. Specifically, the operator can anticipate that the largest SEMG responses will normally occur with a maximally flexed neck and isometric posterior pelvic stabilization. This position may be optimal for decreasing lumbar lordosis and most effectively recruiting anterior or posterior trunk musculature, depending on the direction of the applied torque.

If subjects are asked to engage in lifting tasks while in a seated position, they can generate more erector spinae muscle activity during concentric contractions than under isometric conditions.[22,23] The importance of posture in extensor

torque generation was amplified further by Tan and colleagues,[24] who demonstrated in healthy subjects that more activity is seen in the lumbar erector spinae and latissimus dorsi muscles at positions of greater trunk flexion. In addition, they observed that the abdominal oblique muscles are co-activated only during 100% maximal extensor effort at each of several trunk postures. The rectus abdominis muscle fails to show activation patterns at any trunk position. Tan and associates also found that the mean maximum extension torque increases most notably at 15 and 35 degrees of trunk flexion, a finding that has implications for SEMG muscle recruitment strategies to optimize muscle activation as it relates to trunk angle and load. Their observations also raise the interesting possibility of training subjects to recruit the abdominal oblique muscles during maximal efforts into trunk extension.

MOVEMENT AND LIFTING

When Brown and coworkers[25] studied lifting loads to determine the maximum erector spinae muscle response during a squat lift, they found that the onset of this response occurred earlier in older subjects (ie, individuals aged 60–75 years), compared with onset in their younger counterparts. Scholz and colleagues[26] reported that the onset of erector spinae muscle activity is based on precise joint angles at the knee, hip, and lumbar spine at any one phase of the lifting motion. Speed of motion and load, as well as phase relationships among these joints, will affect the timing and magnitude of back muscle activity.

Toussaint and coworkers[27] exerted precision in trying to determine when a flexion–relaxation response occurs during lifting. They applied a dynamic-linked segment model to determine the momentary torques acting at the L5–S1 juncture. Markers were placed along the length of the lumbar and thoracic vertebral column, and dynamic SEMG responses were normalized to the trunk angle–dependent maximal levels. They found that dynamic lumbar SEMG activity decreased to a low level (the flexion–relaxation response) when the lumbar length increased by 25%. From this result, it is suggested that passive tissue strain provides part of the necessary extension torque. When a heavy object is lifted through the same range and under the same circumstances, however, the flexion–relaxation response occurs in the thoracic erector spinae muscles. This finding indicates that the extensor function of the lumbar portion of the vertebral column can be usurped by thoracic musculature under upper extremity loading conditions. Thus in the clinic, different loci should be monitored (and, when relevant, trained) along the vertebral column, depending on whether the task involves concurrent upper extremity efforts.

Vakos and coworkers[28] divided the squat lift (157-N crate) into four phases by using two different lumbar spine postures. They found either a trunk muscle pattern involving rectus abdominis, abdominal oblique, erector spinae, and latissimus dorsi muscles or a hip extension strategy incorporating gluteus maximus, biceps, femoris, and semitendinosus muscles. With a trunk flexion strategy, SEMG activity was greatest in these muscles during the first quarter of the movement and decreased thereafter. With an emphasis on hip extension, SEMG activity was lowest in the first quarter of the movement and highest during the next two quarters. The important point to be gleaned from this study is that different muscles are preferentially activated during different squat lift motions, and the timing for maximizing output of muscles in each differs as well.

Equally noteworthy are observations from Lavender and colleagues,[29,30] who observed that subjects develop different preparatory strategies in stopping unexpected dropped weights, but early erector spinae activation seems to characterize all of them. If subjects were asked to bend and rotate, changes in co-contraction between the erector spinae of one side and the external oblique of the other are more prominent in response to changes in the bending moment direction than in its magnitude, another observation that has profound implications for SEMG moni-

toring during lifting with use of rotatory torque exertion. Thus when recording from these muscle groups, clinicians should recognize that the moment direction created in the rotation may have a greater impact on changes in muscle activity than the actual amount of movement undertaken.

Other important parameters to consider when recording SEMG activity during dynamic movements are noting the back muscle symmetries in cardinal plane motions and asymmetries in rotational motions.[31] Ahern and coworkers[32] deciphered differences between 40 patients with low back pain and 40 healthy matched subjects on the basis of differences in the flexion–relaxation response, as well as during trunk rotation. Wolf and coworkers[33] observed that erector spinae activity detected with both surface and indwelling EMG electrodes can change dramatically as a function of movements as subtle as gentle postural sway or as obvious as cervical rotation. These factors must be considered when SEMG responses are specified during low back muscle retraining. Clinicians should consider viewing the erector spinae as one elongated dynamic chain, rather than as a discrete series of entities defined by their segmental origins and insertions. This perspective would help explain why, for example, isolated flexion of the cervical spine can cause changes in lumbar erector spinae muscle recruitment.

CLINICAL MODELS OF LOW BACK PAIN AND MUSCLE ACTIVITY

The use of SEMG in the treatment of low back pain symptoms depends, to some extent, on the orientation and belief system of the clinician. Geisser and coworkers[34] present detailed descriptions of the prevailing two models: biomechanical and reflex spasm. The former advocates that chronic back pain results from either abnormally low levels of dynamic muscle activity or muscular asymmetries during movement. These motor patterns are associated with changes in intervertebral alignment. As a result, the spine becomes unstable, and pain is mechanically induced. The reflex-spasm model purports that chronic back pain stems from physical stressors or psychophysiologic factors. As a result of either, spasms ensue. Data in support of each of the two models are equivocal. In terms of applying SEMG techniques, preferential advocacy for either model is probably superfluous. In their work, Hubbard and colleagues[35,36] have implicated hyperactivity in muscle spindles as a potential site for activation of trigger points and concomitant extrafusal muscle hyperexcitability. Indeed, deactivation of the sympathetic components, presumably innervating muscle spindles, reduces intramuscular EMG activity associated with the trigger point, along with a prolonged reduction in pain. The important issue is whether any given treatment modality can have an impact on a patient's physical or emotional behavior to enhance function and reduce pain. Inevitably, as pointed out by Arena and colleagues,[37] so many factors are summed together that a model of causation becomes ambiguous.

SEMG FEEDBACK TRAINING

The goal of the following overview is to highlight some of the SEMG observations made from patients with low back pain. However, the clinician should consult the detailed presentation by Sherman and Arena[38] for a comprehensive critique of SEMG feedback training with low back pain through 1991. A primary controversy surrounding application of SEMG monitoring of erector spinae or other trunk muscles centers around the relative level of muscle activity expected. Opinions are split as to whether SEMG activity from the low back is elevated[39-44] or unchanged[45,46] in patients with low back pain. The differences in response are attributable, in part, to methodologic considerations such as controlling for variation in arm movements, body positioning,[37] and trunk velocity. However, the issue should not necessarily revolve around whether SEMG monitoring or treatment is the sole or primary source of therapy. Asfour and coworkers[47] found that strengthening of

back musculature can be successfully undertaken in patients with chronic low back pain when SEMG is used as an adjunct to standard exercise.

Pain in low back syndromes can be related to relative magnitude of static SEMG activity, and both control subjects and patients receiving feedback can lower their SEMG response levels.[48] Patients with chronic musculoskeletal pain with higher ratings of self-dissatisfaction are more likely to respond well to SEMG feedback training, especially when the SEMG-to-pain correlates are high.[49] Well-controlled SEMG training, either in isolation or as part of a cognitive-behavioral therapy approach, leads to long-term (24-month follow-up) reductions in SEMG activity, pain severity, affective distress, and pain-related use of health care facilities, as well as to enhanced coping skills among patients with chronic low back or temporomandibular joint pain.[50] These findings suggest that elevated static SEMG activity is a reality and behavioral interventional components contribute to overall improvement. For these patients, SEMG retraining consisted primarily of using strategies to reduce activity in key muscles identified as hyperactive. Flor and colleagues[42] demonstrated that patients with pain, and not healthy subjects, show hyperreactive SEMG responses during stressful imagery. Further, these patients display a genuine deficit in their abilities to discriminate muscle tension levels. This failure is not related to physiologic changes at the site of pain, nor to lack of motivation or fatigue.[51] Such approaches work well even when the patient population is older[52] or afflicted with specific rheumatism.[53]

CONCLUSION

Patients with chronic low back pain and muscle dysfunction can be discriminated from healthy subjects by using SEMG parameters in both amplitude and frequency domains. Because chronic low back pain represents a heterogeneous set of etiologies, however, not all patients can be expected to show aberrant responses. SEMG can help delineate muscular contributions to the symptom complex. Recordings with surface electrodes also have added immensely to the understanding of spinal kinetics and trunk motor control. Finally, SEMG feedback training has been shown to contribute to positive treatment outcomes when combined with other therapies.

Perhaps the report by Geisser and coworkers[34] best summarizes the current situation regarding application of SEMG training among patients with chronic low back pain. When they studied the temporal interactions among muscle activity, physical activity, psychosocial stress, and pain, significant relationships were observed between physical activity and pain, self-reports of stress and pain, but not consistently between SEMG activity and pain. They deduced that the interrelationships are exceptionally complex, thereby re-emphasizing the immense heterogeneity in this population. This diversity is perceived as a reason for including, rather than excluding, SEMG monitoring, for only by gathering more complete profiling data can clinicians decipher the component factors for each individual.

REFERENCES

1. Andersson GBJ, Pope MH, Frymoyer JW, Nook S. Epidemiology and cost. In: Pope MH, Andersson GBJ, Frymoyer JW, Chaffin DB, eds. *Occupational Low Back Pain: Assessment, Treatment and Prevention.* St Louis, MO: Mosby; 1991;95–111.

2. Frymoyer JW, Pope MH, Costanza MC, et al. Epidemiologic studies of low back pain. *Spine.* 1980;5:419–429.

3. Cunningham LS, Kelsey JL. Epidemiology of musculoskeletal impairments and associated disability. *Am J Public Health.* 1984;74:574–579.

4. Deyo RA, Tsui-Wu Y-J. Descriptive epidemiology of low-back pain and its related medical care in the United States. *Spine.* 1987;12:264–268.

5. Antonakes JA. Claims costs of back pain. *Best's Review.* September 1981:84–87.

6. Cassidy JD, Wedge JH. The epidemiology and natural history of low back pain and spinal degeneration. In: Kirkaldy-Willis WH, ed. *Managing Low Back Pain.* 2nd ed. New York: Churchill-Livingstone; 1988:1–14.

7. Snook SH. Low back pain in industry. In: White AA, Gordon SL, eds. *Idiopathic Low Back Pain.* St Louis, MO: CV Mosby; 1982:220–239.

8. Bigos S, Bowyer O, Braen G, et al. *Acute Low Back Problems in Adults.* Rockville, MD: Agency for Health Care Policy and Research, Public Health Service, US Dept of Health and Human Services; 1994. Clinical Practice Guideline No. 14, AHCPR publication 95-0642.

9. De Luca CJ. Use of the surface EMG signal for performance evaluation of back muscles. *Muscle Nerve.* 1993;16:210–216.

10. Klein AB, Snyder-Mackler L, Roy SH, De Luca CJ. Comparison of spinal mobility and isometric trunk extensor forces with electromyographic spectral analysis in identifying low back pain. *Phys Ther.* 1991;71:445–454.

11. Roy SH, De Luca CJ, Emley M, Buijs RJC. Spectral electromyographic assessment of back muscles in patients with low back pain undergoing rehabilitation. *Spine.* 1995;20:38–48.

12. Roy SH, De Luca CJ, Snyder-Machler L, Emley MS, Crenshaw RL, Lyons JP. Fatigue, recovery, and low back pain in varsity rowers. *Med Sci Sports Exerc.* 1990;22:463–469.

13. Roy SH, De Luca CJ, Casavant DA. Lumbar muscle fatigue and chronic low back pain. *Spine.* 1989;14:992–1001.

14. Dolan P, Mannion AF, Adams MA. Fatigue of the erector spinae muscles: a quantitative assessment using "frequency banding" of the surface electromyographic signal. *Spine.* 1995;20:149–159.

15. Potvin JR, Norman RW. Quantification of erector spinae muscle fatigue during prolonged, dynamic lifting tasks. *Eur J Appl Physiol.* 1993;67:554–562.

16. DeLooze MP, Toussaint HM, van Dieen JH, Kemper HC. Joint moments and muscle activity in the lower extremities and lower back in lifting and lowering tasks. *J Biomech.* 1993;26:1067–1076.

17. Tsuboi T, Satou T, Egawsa K, Izumi Y, Miyazaki M. Spectral analysis of electromyogram in lumbar muscles: fatigue induced endurance contraction. *Eur J App Physiol.* 1994;69:361–366.

18. Robinson ME, Cassisi JE, O'Connor PD, MacMillan M. Lumbar iEMG during isotonic exercise: chronic low back pain patients versus controls. *J Spinal Disord.* 1992;5:8–15.

19. Fiebert I, Keller CD. Are "passive" extension exercises really passive? *J Orthop Sports Phys Ther.* 1994;19:111–116.

20. Mirka GA. The quantification of EMG normalization error. *Ergonomics*. 1991;34:343–452.

21. Shirado O, Ito T, Kaneda K, Strax TE. Electromyographic analysis of four techniques for isometric trunk muscle exercises. *Arch Phys Med Rehabil*. 1995; 76:225–229.

22. Dolan P, Adams MA. The relationship between EMG activity and extensor moment generation in the erector spinae muscles during bending and lifting activities. *J Biomech*. 1993;16:513–522.

23. Dolan P, Mannion AF, Adams MA. Passive tissues help the back muscles to generate extensor moments during lifting. *J Biomech*. 1994;17:1077–1085.

24. Tan JC, Parianpour M, Nordin M, Hofer H, Willems B. Isometric maximal and submaximal trunk extension at different flexed positions in standing: triaxial torque output and EMG. *Spine*. 1993;18:2480–2490.

25. Brown JM, Mills JH, Baker A. Neuromuscular control of lifting in the elderly. *Gerontology*. 1994;40:298–306.

26. Scholz JP, Millford JP, McMillan AG. Neuromuscular coordination of squat lifting, I: effect of load magnitude. *Phys Ther*. 1995;75:119–132.

27. Toussaint HM, de Winter AF, de Haas T, de Looze MP, Van Dieen JH, Kingma I. Flexion relaxation during lifting: implications for torque production by muscle activity and tissue strain at the lumbo-sacral joint. *J Biomech*. 1995;28:199–210.

28. Vakos JP, Nitz AJ, Threlkeld AJ, Shapiro R, Horn T. Electromyographic activity of selected trunk and hip muscles during a squat lift: effect of varying the lumbar posture. *Spine*. 1994;19:687–695.

29. Lavender SA, Marras WS, Miller RA. The development of response strategies in preparation for sudden loading to the torso. *Spine*. 1993;18:2097–2105.

30. Lavender SA, Tsuang YH, Anderson GB. Trunk muscle activation and cocontraction while resisting applied moments in a twisted posture. *Ergonomics*. 1993;36:1145–1157.

31. Wolf SL, Nacht M, Kelly JL. EMG feedback training during dynamic movement for low back pain patients. *Behav Ther*. 1982;13:395–406.

32. Ahern DK, Follick MJ, Council JR, Laser-Wolston N, Litchman H. Comparison of lumbar paravertebral EMG patterns in chronic low back pain patients and non-patient controls. *Pain*. 1988;34:153–160.

33. Wolf SL, Wolf LB, Segal RL. The relationship of extraneous movements to lumbar paraspinal muscle activity: implications for EMG biofeedback training applications to low back pain patients. *Biofeedback Self Regul*. 1989;14:63–74.

34. Geisser ME, Robinson ME, Richardson C. A time series analysis of the relationship between ambulatory EMG, pain, and stress in chronic low back pain. *Biofeedback Self Regul*. 1995;20:339–355.

35. Hubbard D, Burkoff G. Myofascial trigger point slow spontaneous needle EMG activity. *Spine*. 1993; 18:1803–1807.

36. McNulty W, Gevirtz R, Gerkoff G, Hubbard D. Needle electromyographic evaluation of trigger point response to a psychologic stressor. *Psychophysiology*. 1994; 31:313–316.

37. Arena JG, Sherman RA, Bruno GM, Young TR. Temporal stability of paraspinal electromyographic recordings in low back pain and non-pain subjects. *Int J Psychophysiol*. 1990;9:31–37.

38. Sherman RA, Arena JG. Biofeedback for assessment and treatment of low back pain. In: Basmajian JV, Nyberg R, eds. *Rational Manual Therapies*. Baltimore: Williams & Wilkins; 1993;177–198.

39. Ahern DK, Follick MJ, Council JR, Laser-Wolston N. Reliability of lumbar paravertebral EMG assessment in chronic low back pain. *Arch Phys Med Rehabil*. 1986;67:762–765.

40. Arena JG, Sherman RA, Bruno GM, Young TR. Electromyographic recordings of low back pain subjects and non-pain controls in six different positions: effect of pain levels. *Pain*. 1991;45:23–28.

41. Biedermann HJ, Inglis J, Monga TN, Shanks GL. Differential treatment responses on somatic pain indicators after EMG biofeedback training in back pain patients. *Int J Psychosom*. 1989;36:53–57.

42. Flor H, Birbaumer N, Schugens MM, Lutzengerger W. Symptom-specific psychophysiological responses in chronic pain patients. *Psychophysiology*. 1992;29:452–460.

43. Sihvonen T, Partanen J, Hanninen O, Soimakallio S. Electric behavior of low back muscles during lumbar pelvic rhythm in low back pain patients and healthy controls. *Arch Phys Med Rehabil*. 1991;72:1080–1087.

44. Wolf SL, Basmajian JV, Russe TC, Kutner M. Normative data on low back mobility and activity levels. *Am J Phys Med*. 1979;58:217–229.

45. Cohen MJ, Swanson GA, Naliboff BD, Schandler SL, McArthur DL. Comparison of electromyographic response patterns during posture and stress tasks in chronic low back pain patterns and control. *J Psychosom Res*. 1986;30:135–141.

46. Nouwen A, van Akkerveeken PF, Versloot JM. Patterns of muscular activity during movement in patients with chronic low-back pain. *Spine*. 1987;12:777–782.

47. Asfour SS, Kahlil TM, Waly SM, Goldberg ML, Rosomoff HL. Biofeedback in back muscle strengthening. *Spine*. 1990;15:510–513.

48. Large RG, Lamb AM. Electromyographic (EMG) feedback in chronic musculoskeletal pain: a controlled trial. *Pain*. 1983;17:167–177.

49. Large RG. Prediction of treatment response in pain patients: the illness self-concept repertory grid and EMG feedback. *Pain*. 1985;21:279–287.

50. Flor H, Birbaumer N. Comparison of the efficacy of electromyographic biofeedback, cognitive-behavior therapy, and conservative medical interventions in the treatment of chronic musculoskeletal pain. *J Consult Clin Psychol*. 1993;61:653–658.

51. Flor H, Schugens MM, Birbaumer N. Discrimination of muscle tension in chronic pain patients and healthy controls. *Biofeedback Self Regul*. 1992;17:165–177.

52. Middaugh SJ, Woods SE, Kee WG, Harden RN, Peters JR. Biofeedback-assisted relaxation training for the aging chronic pain patient. *Biofeedback Self Regul*. 1991;167:361–377.

53. Flor H, Haag G, Turk DC. Long-term efficacy of EMG biofeedback for chronic rheumatic back pain. *Pain*. 1986;27:195–202.

SEMG Program for Low Back Dysfunction

Refer to the discussion in Chapter 12 for a review of intervention approaches. The suggestions that follow are derived from those resources. Descriptions and operational definitions are provided to clarify optional practice patterns.

CANDIDATES

Implement for patients
- with chronic low back pain and in whom muscle dysfunction is suspected
- who may present with known history of
  1. motor vehicle accident
  2. work or domestic injury
  3. athletic trauma
  4. insidious symptom onset

Candidates should relate a sense of aberrant guarding or spasm, or clinical examination findings should reveal
- faulty posture
- palpable hypertonicity
- trigger points
- imbalances in muscle flexibility and strength

EVALUATION OBJECTIVES

- Assess the effects of posture and dynamic movement on lumbar muscle activity.
- Identify aberrant patterns of muscle activity about the low back and pelvic girdle, potentially contributing to musculoskeletal pain:

1. myalgia due to excessive levels or duration of muscle tension
2. imbalanced muscle activity that potentially results in soft tissue or joint dysfunction

FEEDBACK TRAINING OBJECTIVES

- Reduce excessive or imbalanced muscle tension.
- Mediate or resolve underlying lumbar mechanical dysfunction.
- Retain and generalize improved motor control to functional contexts.
- Resolve or reduce functional limitations and disability.

RECORDING SITES

- Judge the utility of each recording site on the basis of history and physical examination results.
- Include muscles that
  1. underlie the pain distribution
  2. potentially refer symptoms or are mechanically related to patient's area of complaint
  3. reproduce patient's symptoms when stretched, resisted, or palpated
- Consult Chapter 14 in the companion book, *Introduction to Surface Electromyography,* for specific electrode placement considerations.

- Confirm optimal sites from the following list by observation and palpation during isometric contraction:
  1. paraspinal group (latissimus, erector spinae, quadratus lumborum):
     - lower lumbar
     - middle lumbar
     - upper lumbar
     - lower thoracic
  2. rectus abdominis
  3. oblique abdominals
  4. hip flexors
  5. gluteus maximus
  6. hamstrings

EVALUATION PROCEDURES

- Select procedures that correspond to exacerbating and alleviating factors revealed by history and clinical examination.
- Refer to Chapter 2 for detailed discussion of evaluation methods.
- Perform at least five repetitions of each movement task to assess response consistency. Many more repetitions may be needed to assess SEMG responses with reproduction of symptoms.
- Select relevant procedures from the following:
  1. psychophysiologic stress profile
  2. postural analysis
  3. lumbar active range of motion (AROM). Implement the following with the patient's neck, upper trunk, and arms relaxed:
     - forward-bending. Examine eccentric trunk lowering, maintenance of full flexion, and concentric trunk return to neutral, each phase about 3 seconds (or about 9 seconds total). Consider repeating the same motion with a voluntary isometric contraction of gluteal muscle to assess effects on lumbar paraspinal muscle responses.
     - backward-bending
     - side-bending

     - rotation
     Repeat provocative flexion–extension movements with the patient in non–weight-bearing positions.
  4. functional activity analysis:
     - bending, stooping for activities of daily living
     - lifting from floor to table height with progressive loads
     - holding and carrying objects of progressive weight and volume
     - other home, work, sports-specific activities known to exacerbate or alleviate symptoms
  5. analysis of coordinated muscle activity patterns. Consider lumbar paraspinal, gluteal, and hamstring function. Also consider lumbar paraspinal, rectus abdominis, oblique abdominal, and hip flexor activity. Examine SEMG patterns during AROM, functional tasks, and relevant maneuvers listed below:
     - hip hiking
     - squat and arise from squat
     - prone active trunk extension
     - prone active and resisted hip extension
     - supine bridging: unilateral or bilateral
     - side-lying hip abduction
     - unilateral stance
     - gait

ASSESSMENT

- Refer to Chapter 2 for detailed discussion of SEMG assessment.
- Refer to Chapter 14 in the companion book for representative SEMG tracings of normal function.
- Select SEMG assessment parameters from the following:
  1. Amplitude and variance of each channel during baseline. Activity during resting baseline should be stable and relatively quiescent. Postural muscles tend to show low-level activity with the patient in weight-bearing positions (typically,

about 2–10 μV RMS). Use a standard bathroom scale under each of the patient's feet to ensure equal lower extremity weight bearing.

2. Amplitude, variance of each channel during contraction efforts. For comparisons across nonhomologous muscles, magnitudes may be expressed as a:

   –percentage of maximal volitional isometric contraction (%MVIC) amplitude by using standard manual muscle tests (test activity amplitude/MVIC amplitude × 100)

   –percentage of some submaximal contraction with a standardized force intensity, trunk angle, and body posture

3. Left/right paraspinal peak amplitude symmetry for forward-bending movements. Satisfactory symmetry is operationally defined as left/right scores within 35% as calculated [(higher value – lower value)/higher value] × 100. This assumes an absence of gross scoliosis or lateral trunk shift.

4. Quiescence of lumbar paraspinal activity in full flexion, the flexion–relaxation response, as a normal phenomenon (Figures 12–A–1 and 12–A–2A). Forward-bending is accomplished by spinal flexion combined with hip flexion. When a patient initiates this movement, lumbar motion predominates and paraspinal activity increases. However, lumbar activity diminishes as slack in posterior structures is taken up with increasing intervertebral flexion. A decrease in lumbar activity is usually seen between 40 and 60 degrees of gross trunk flexion, although individuals vary in both absolute levels of intervertebral mobility and lumbar:hip AROM rhythm. Forward-bending continues with a proportionately greater hip flexion contribution. Lumbar paraspinal activity declines to minimal values as full lumbar flexion is approached. An aberrant absence of a flexion–relaxation response is characterized by persistent SEMG activity through a normal AROM excursion. If for any reason the patient is severely restricted in mobility, the flexion–relaxation response cannot be reliably assessed. Simply, the presence, partial presence, or absence of the flexion–relaxation response can be reported.

5. Lumbar paraspinal concentric:eccentric ratio greater than about 2.0 as normal during trunk flexion AROM. The concentric:eccentric ratio is calculated as the peak amplitude during return from forward-bending (concentric), divided by the peak amplitude during forward-bending trunk descent (eccentric). That is, it is normal for peak paraspinal muscle activity to be substantially greater while the patient raises his or her trunk than when he or she lowers it (Figure 12–A–1). A concentric:eccentric ratio of less than about 1.8 potentially reflects aberrant paraspinal muscle activity (Figure 12–A–2A). The ratio becomes depressed because the concentric peak amplitude is diminished and the eccentric peak amplitude is increased with chronic dysfunction syndromes.

6. Lumbar paraspinal quiescence in standing backward-bending. An extension moment is produced as the trunk is backward bent. Hence, activity of the erector spinae muscles is expected to be minimal in a healthy subject. Abdominal muscle activity is correspondingly increased (Figure 12–A–3).

7. Asymmetric paraspinal muscle activity during trunk side-bending and rotation movements. Reciprocally symmetric patterns should be observed for left/right reciprocal movements (Figure 12–A–4). Assuming AROM excursion and velocity are monitored and equivalent, reciprocal asymmetry greater than 35% is operationally considered an aberrant

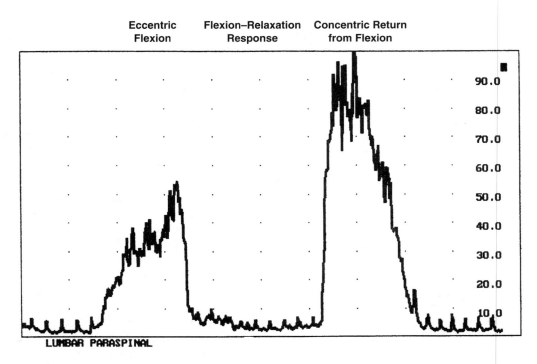

Figure 12–A–1 SEMG activity of the left lumbar paraspinals from a healthy subject. The first peak corresponds to initiation of trunk flexion from neutral standing. Flexion continues to its endpoint and is maintained during the trough between peaks. The second peak corresponds to return from flexion to neutral standing. The flexion–relaxation response is illustrated, as is the relationship between eccentric and concentric lumbar paraspinal activity.

finding. Predominance of activity from one side throughout reciprocal movement is an aberrant finding (Figure 12–A–2B), as are similar levels of left/right co-contraction within a single side unilateral movement (Figure 12–A–5A). Moderate co-contraction by itself during side-bending and rotation is not exclusively associated with low back pain. Similar levels of left/right activation may be seen in subjects without pain or disability. This is not to say that those individuals have optimal spinal function; they typically show some level of impaired intervertebral mobility on physical examination. Co-contraction tends to give way to reciprocal activation patterns in those persons after

stretching or manual mobilization. Findings in the sagittal flexion–extension plane are more discriminative between subjects who are healthy versus those with chronic dysfunction. Side-bending and rotation maneuvers are therefore of subsidiary interest.

8. Reciprocal paraspinal activity during walking. The paraspinal muscles contralateral to the stance leg are expected to be active with each step, with reciprocal symmetry across steps. Co-contraction or reciprocal asymmetry greater than 35% is considered an aberrant finding.

9. Return to baseline amplitude after activation. This is applicable to any recording site and task. Qualitatively, recovery

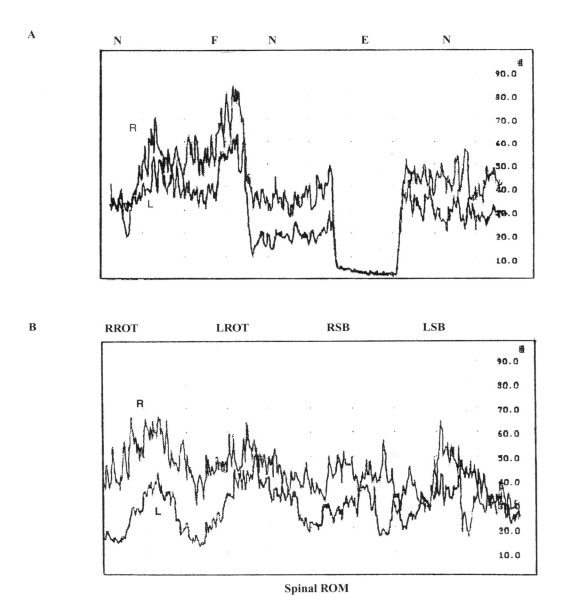

Figure 12–A–2 SEMG activity of the (**L**) left and (**R**) right lumbar paraspinal muscles during trunk range of motion recorded from a patient with chronic bilateral low back pain and disability. (**A**) Activity during (**N**) neutral standing, standing trunk flexion (**F**), return to neutral, standing trunk extension (**E**), and return to neutral. Baseline activity is elevated. Activity during flexion is asymmetric and lacks a flexion–relaxation response (despite that gross trunk motion is completed to a normal range). In addition, the concentric:eccentric peak activity ratio is depressed during trunk flexion and return to neutral. Signals achieve a stable quiescence only during true extension. (**B**) Activity during right and left trunk rotation (**RROT, LROT**) and right and left side bending (**RSB, LSB**). Rather than generating a normal left/right reciprocal pattern for reciprocal motion, signals show continual right greater than left co-activation.

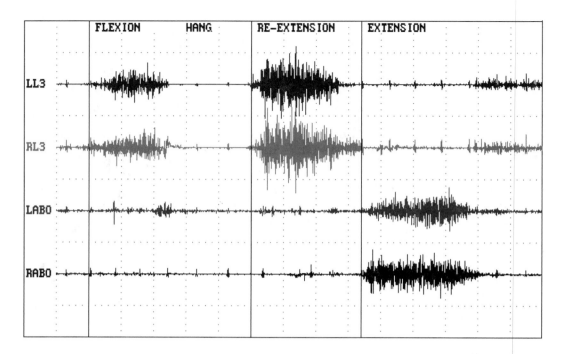

Figure 12–A–3 SEMG activity of the (**L**) left and (**R**) right (**L3**) lumbar paraspinal muscles at about the level of the third lumbar vertebra and (**ABO**) oblique abdominal muscles. Unremarkable signals from a healthy subject are shown during performance of standing trunk flexion, maintenance of flexion, return to neutral standing (re-extension), and true extension in standing. A flexion–relaxation response is present, concentric lumbar paraspinal muscle activity substantially exceeds eccentric activity, and paraspinal muscle activity is minimal in standing extension, whereas abdominal muscles are recruited. *Source:* Reprinted from JR Cram and GS Kasman, *Introduction to Surface Electromyography,* © 1997, Aspen Publishers.

can be stated as prompt and complete versus elevated and delayed. Satisfactory baseline recovery is quantitatively defined (with a smoothing time constant of 0.1 second or less) as a return to an SEMG amplitude within two standard deviations of the original baseline mean, within 3 seconds of movement cessation, and maintenance within that amplitude range for at least 30 seconds or until the next movement is initiated. Recovery can be characterized by the latency to achieve this criterion. More simply, the amplitude (expressed as percentage of baseline) observed 1 to 3 seconds after movement termination can be reported.

10. Symmetrically proportionate left/right lumbar paraspinal, abdominal, gluteal, and hamstring muscle activity during test activities. In terms of timing, the normal activation sequence for forward-bending is lumbar paraspinals-gluteus maximus-hamstrings-gastrocnemius/soleus (Figure 12–A–6), with the reverse sequence observed on return to neutral standing from flexion. Imbalances can be seen with chronic low back pain. An example is shown in Figure 12–A–7, and variations are discussed in the following section. When comparing the timing symmetry of synergist action, observe for changes in the recruitment order of muscles from one side to the

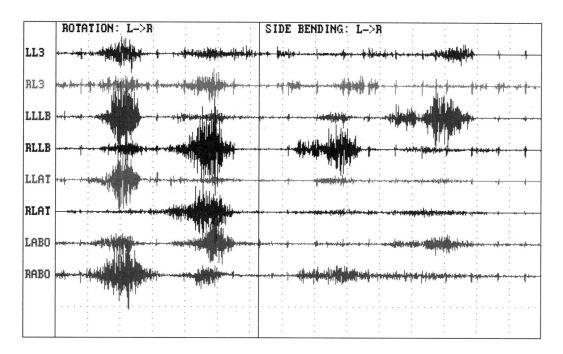

Figure 12–A–4 SEMG activity of the (**L**) left and (**R**) right (**L3**) lumbar paraspinal muscles at about the level of the third lumbar vertebra, (**LLB**) far lateral lumbar sites, as well as (**LAT**) latissimus and (**ABO**) oblique abdominal muscles. Unremarkable signals from a healthy subject are shown during performance of trunk rotation and side-bending. Left-to-right activity tends to reciprocate across reciprocal left-to-right motions. *Source:* Reprinted from JR Cram and GS Kasman, *Introduction to Surface Electromyography,* © 1997, Aspen Publishers.

other. For most clinical purposes, timing issues can be observed with rectified line tracings with a smoothing time constant of 0.1 second or less, SEMG sampling at 100 Hz or faster, frequency bandwidth filter low cutoff of 25 Hz or less, and a high resolution display with variable sweep speed. A graphic printout is useful for documentation of subtle timing differences. Documentation can be quantified with calculations of average slope, time to peak activity, or time to some percentage of MVIC activity that is clinically meaningful. Onset time can be reported simply as the latency to achieve a microvolt value equivalent to two standard deviations above the baseline mean. Duration may be noted as the amount of time between onset and baseline recovery as defined above.

11. Change in activity levels for a particular muscle and task across treatment sessions. To document this parameter a normalization procedure is preferred. A reliable maximal manual muscle test effort or a standardized submaximal contraction is required as a reference. The average amplitude during the test task is divided by that day's reference contraction amplitude, and the quotient is multiplied by 100.

COMMON PATIENT PRESENTATIONS

Lumbar Paraspinal Dysfunction

Lumbar paraspinal SEMG activity can be elevated or asymmetric in static postures in some patients with chronic low back pain (Figure

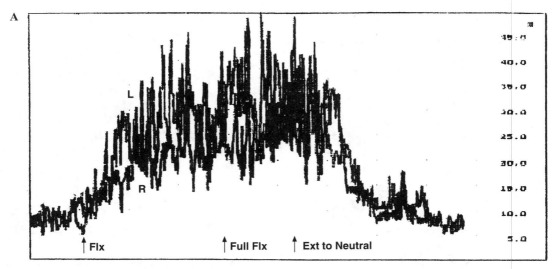

LUMBAR PARASPINALS

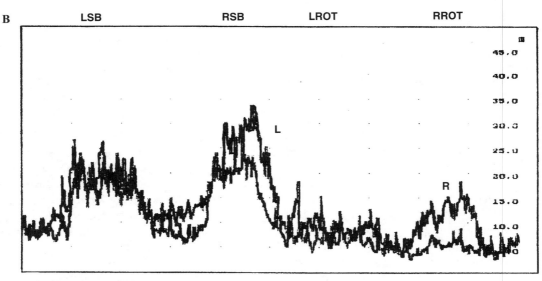

LUMBAR PARASPINALS

Figure 12–A–5 SEMG activity of the (**L**) left and (**R**) right lumbar paraspinal muscles during trunk range of motion recorded from a patient with 3-year history of bilateral, left greater than right low back pain and disability. (**A**) Activity during standing trunk (**Flx**) flexion, maintenance of (**Full flx**) full flexion, and (**Ext**) extension return to neutral standing. Baseline activity is somewhat elevated, and there is an absence of a flexion–relaxation response, along with left greater than right asymmetry and a diminished concentric:eccentric peak activity ratio. Signals are rather erratic looking throughout the sweep. (**B**) Activity during left and right side-bending (**LSB**, **RSB**) and rotation (**LROT**, **RROT**). Signals show co-activation and lack of orderly reciprocation.

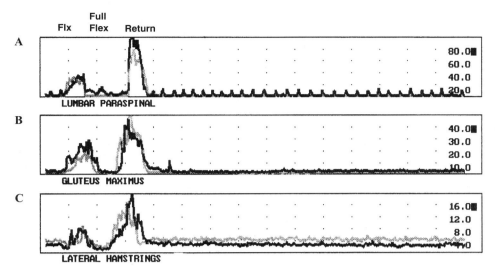

Figure 12–A–6 SEMG activity of the left (black) and right (gray) (**A**) lumbar paraspinal, (**B**) gluteus maximus, and (**C**) lateral hamstrings, showing normal relationships between muscle sites during standing trunk flexion, maintenance of full flexion, and return to neutral standing.

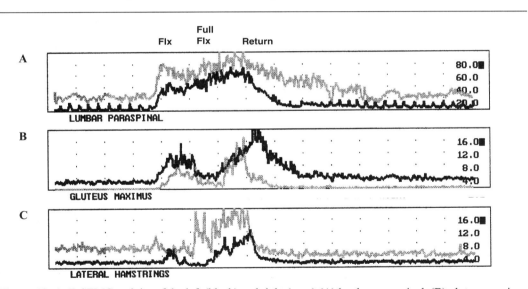

Figure 12–A–7 SEMG activity of the left (black) and right (gray) (**A**) lumbar paraspinal, (**B**) gluteus maximus, and (**C**) lateral hamstrings during standing trunk flexion, maintenance of full flexion, and return to neutral standing. Signals were recorded from a patient with chronic right low back pain, apparent right greater than left lumbar paraspinal muscle hypertrophy, and mild left lateral trunk shift. Supine straight leg raising in this patient was limited by hamstring tightness, at about 50 degrees on the right and 60 degrees on the left. Weight bearing was roughly equivalent through each lower extremity, ensured with a scale under each foot. Note right greater than left lumbar paraspinal activity (as well as absence of a flexion–relaxation response, diminished concentric:eccentric peak ratio, and delayed right baseline recovery), right less than left gluteal activity, and right greater than left hamstring activity. Recruitment/decruitment timing of gluteal and hamstring signals are also grossly asymmetric.

12–A–8). Other patients show unremarkable amplitudes in sitting or standing position, and display aberrant patterns only during movement. During forward-bending AROM, these include left/right asymmetries, absence of a flexion–relaxation response, and a depressed concentric:eccentric ratio. Further, the left and right sides can be seen to co-activate during side-bending and rotation.

Dysfunctional patterns of muscle activity at the low back are almost always associated with intervertebral dysfunction of one type or another. Sometimes SEMG activity is unequivocally aberrant, but more reflective of, than causal to, the underlying mechanical issue. For example, impingement of soft tissues by an osteophyte or herniated disk could result in reflexively elevated muscle tone. The activity of the paraspinal muscles could also be altered by working against hypomobile capsular and ligamentous structures. Thus SEMG assessment can be used to objectify muscle impairments, but not

all patients with identifiable deficits require SEMG feedback training.

Left/right paraspinal asymmetries are a common finding during postural and movement assessments. Paraspinal SEMG activity will be asymmetric with a lateral curvature that has developed with skeletal maturation. The extent to which a scoliosis represents a functional or treatable issue depends on the degree of curvature, the particular patient, and the clinician's intervention philosophy. The practitioner is not expected to restore muscle symmetry in the presence of longstanding scoliosis. Lateral trunk shifts associated with disk injury are a different matter. Some patients show marked lateral shifts that persist after spinal surgery. These shifts can also remain for a protracted period after nonsurgical intervention for presumed disk disease. Lateral shifts are associated with paraspinal and abdominal muscle asymmetry and can usually be addressed with manual therapies, exercise, education, and SEMG feedback.

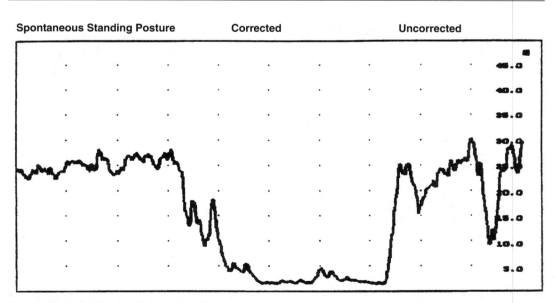

Figure 12–A–8 SEMG activity of the bilateral lumbar paraspinal muscle groups recorded from a patient with posturally related, cumulative standing back pain. Effects of the patient's spontaneous standing, corrected, and uncorrected postures are illustrated. Posture was corrected by volitionally lifting the sternum, which had the effect of slightly shifting the center of pressure posteriorly, increasing the lumbar lordosis, changing the pelvic inclination and hip extension angles, and producing a dramatic change in lumbar muscle activity.

Volitional motor control of the low back is less fine than that of cephalic and extremity musculature. The mechanical and functional demands placed on the low back also differ compared with other body regions. SEMG feedback progressions for the low back therefore emphasize different treatment techniques than advocated in other applications in this book. Postural training, functional body mechanics instruction, and therapeutic exercises with SEMG feedback are accented for the low back. Little emphasis is placed on static manipulation of SEMG signals in sitting position. Relaxation-based approaches are useful when psychophysiologic stress responses and profound guarding behaviors are identified. Otherwise, posture and movement training are the key elements.

Training Progression for Lumbar Paraspinal Dysfunction

- Refer to Chapters 3 and 4 for detailed discussion of SEMG display setups and feedback structure.
- Refer to Chapter 5 for detailed discussion of SEMG training techniques. As skill develops, generally
  1. Shape desired responses up or down.
  2. Incorporate multijoint control.
  3. Add distractions.
  4. Randomize training activities.
  5. Withdraw continuous audio/visual feedback.
- Utilize this training sequence to address focal lumbar paraspinal hyperactivity and asymmetry. Consult the following training progressions to incorporate muscles of the pelvic girdle together with the lumbar paraspinal muscles.
- Select relevant SEMG feedback training tasks from the following:
  1. isolation of target muscle activity. Use arching of the back with an anterior pelvic tilt, partial range forward-bending, side-bending, and rotation to illustrate paraspinal muscle function.

2. postural retraining with SEMG feedback
3. deactivation training
4. left/right equilibration training
5. prescription of therapeutic home exercises with SEMG feedback. Consider especially use with
   –passive prone press-ups
   –knee to chest stretches
   –spinal stabilization exercises
6. body mechanics instruction with SEMG feedback
7. functional activity performance with SEMG feedback. Select ambulation; sit-to-stand transfers; lifting; carrying; squatting; other work, home, and recreational activities that exacerbate symptoms or are performed frequently.

Lumbar Dysfunction with Gluteal Hypoactivity

A common clinical belief is that the gluteus maximus tends to become hypoactive in patients with low back pain with chronic lumbar hyperactivity. The frequency with which this imbalance actually occurs is unknown. Whether gluteal hypoactivity is caused by neurophysiologic inhibition versus altered lumbar–pelvic rhythm and gluteal atrophy—both of which have been suggested—also is unclear. Clinicians might be tempted to compare nonnormalized SEMG amplitudes of lumbar paraspinal versus gluteal muscles. However, differing amounts of subcutaneous adipose and muscle geometry exist at lumbar and gluteal sites. Gluteal readings almost always produce lower microvolt scores than lumbar paraspinal recordings. A minimal gluteal signal during forward-bending may reflect insufficient gluteal recruitment, or simply high-site impedance. Conversion to %MVIC is required to make a clinical judgment, although no quantitative standard is currently available. If the gluteus maximus generates a robust microvolt score during prone manual muscle test (or with standing hip extension/abduction/lateral rotation) and apparently minimal activity during forward-bending, the muscle is probably not recruiting to a great degree during forward-bending. Gluteal hypoactivity is presumed to shift a greater proportion of the mechanical load to the spine and associated soft tissues. SEMG feedback work emphasizes gluteal uptraining. Often, as gluteal recruitment is increased, lumbar paraspinal muscle activity decreases (Figure 12–A–9).

Training Progression for Lumbar Dysfunction with Gluteal Hypoactivity

- Refer to Chapters 3 and 4 for detailed discussion of SEMG display setups and feedback structure.
- Refer to Chapters 5 and 6 for detailed discussion of SEMG feedback training and techniques.

- As skill develops, generally
  1. Shape desired responses up or down.
  2. Incorporate multijoint control.
  3. Add distractions.
  4. Randomize training activities.
  5. Withdraw continuous audio/visual feedback.
- Also consult previous and following training progressions in this Application Guide to incorporate lumbar paraspinal, hamstring, and abdominal muscles.
- Select relevant SEMG feedback training tasks from the following:
  1. isolation of target muscle activity:
     –Use a gluteal isometric buttocks squeeze to isolate gluteus maximus.
     –If isolation of the gluteus maximus from the lumbar paraspinal muscles is difficult, display an additional SEMG

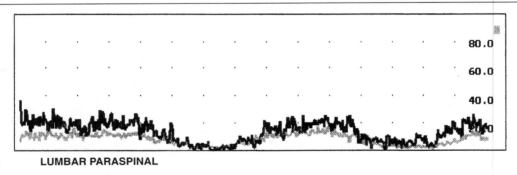

LUMBAR PARASPINAL

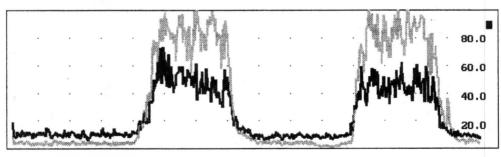

GLUTEUS MAXIMUS

Figure 12–A–9 SEMG activity of the left (black) and right (gray) lumbar paraspinal muscles and gluteus maximus during static standing in spontaneous postural alignment with and without a gluteal isometric squeeze. Activity was recorded from a patient with a 5-year history of left greater than right low back pain and disability. Paraspinal activity inversely varied with gluteal recruitment. There was no visible change in postural alignment. Gluteal uptraining over an 8-week course was accompanied by spontaneously increased gluteal activity and decreased lumbar paraspinal activity during standing and other functional tasks.

channel for co-contracting paraspinal muscles.

–Use a visual threshold or auditory function to cue minimal recruitment of lumbar muscles while maximizing the gluteal signal.

2. threshold-based uptraining. Continue with gluteal isometrics.

3. promotion of correct muscle synergies and related coordination patterns of gluteus and paraspinal muscles:

–Display both gluteal and paraspinal activity.

–Instruct the patient to observe effects of gluteal muscle activation on paraspinal activity during initiation of forward-bending or hip extension AROM.

–Progressively uptrain gluteal recruitment relative to paraspinal activity.

4. generalization to progressively dynamic movement. Perform gluteal squeeze before

–sit-to-stand, stand-to-sit
–squat
–step-ups
–lifting

Progress by increasing

–movement excursion
–movement velocity
–lifting load

5. body mechanics instruction and functional activity performance with SEMG feedback

-Use other relevant work, home, sports-specific activities.

–Increase gluteal activation during functional activities that provoke symptoms or are frequently performed.

6. therapeutic exercises with SEMG feedback. Uptrain gluteal responses, relatively downtrain lumbar paraspinal, hamstrings (see below); consider including

–prone over bolster, hip extension with bent or straight knee

–hip extension with bent or straight knee from hands-and-knees position

–hip extension/abduction/lateral rotation from hands-and-knees position

–hip extension/abduction/lateral rotation in standing position

–anterior-posterior weight shifting in stride, taking one step

–stair stepper machine

7. home exercise program emphasizing exercises that show favorable responses

8. SEMG-triggered neuromuscular electrical stimulation. Consider use of this training technique to promote gluteal muscle activation.

Lumbar Dysfunction with Gluteal Hypoactivity and Hamstring Hyperactivity

In effect, this syndrome is an extension of the previous one. The hamstrings appear hyperactive in certain patients with lumbar hyperactivity of the lumbar paraspinal muscles and hypoactivity of the gluteus maximus. Passive length of the hamstrings is also usually decreased during straight leg raising (operationally defined as less than 70 degrees of leg elevation in supine position). Patients with a relatively posteriorly tilted pelvis and diminished lower lumbar lordosis appear to display the pattern most often. Hamstring SEMG activity during forward bending tends to be of great amplitude and erratic looking. As is the case for lumbar:gluteal assessment, nonnormalized comparisons between muscle sites are confounded by differences in site impedance and muscle geometry. Quantitative SEMG standards for comparing across hamstring, gluteus maximus, and lumbar paraspinal amplitudes are not currently available. SEMG assessments must be integrated with physical examination findings and changes in symptom behavior, or be restricted to left/right symmetry comparisons for homologous muscle pairs.

Asymmetries in hamstring function tend to be linked to corresponding asymmetries along the hip–spine kinetic chain. For example, greater activity at a right hamstring recording site may be associated with right gluteal hypoactivity and right paraspinal hyperactivity (Figure 12–A–7). In patients with both lumbar and hip flexion hypomobility, the hamstrings may fire immediately as trunk forward-bending is initiated. During the return to neutral trunk position, the hamstrings may maintain high-level activity for a prolonged duration. It is assumed that decreased passive extensibility renders the hamstring length–tension relationship as less efficient, contributes to increased motor unit recruitment, and increases pathomechanical loading of the spine through the pelvis. Training is performed exactly as in the previously described treatment progressions, with the addition of hamstring stretching. Gluteal muscle activation also can result in diminution of hamstring active responses. A caution is warranted for patients after laminectomy with adhesions of the perineural connective tissue. These patients should be mobilized under the supervision of a physician or therapist specifically trained to do so.

Training Progression for Lumbar Dysfunction with Gluteal Hypoactivity and Hamstring Hyperactivity

- Refer to Chapters 3 and 4 for detailed discussion of SEMG display setups and feedback structure.
- Refer to Chapters 5 and 6 for detailed discussion of SEMG training techniques.
- As skill develops, generally
  1. Shape desired responses up or down.
  2. Incorporate multijoint control.
  3. Add distractions.
  4. Randomize training activities.
  5. Withdraw continuous audio/visual feedback.
- Refer to training progressions for Lumbar Dysfunction and Gluteal Hypoactivity for an integrated treatment approach.
- Select relevant SEMG feedback training tasks from the following:
  1. isolation of target muscle activity. Use hamstring isometric contractions in a lengthened position.

2. therapeutic exercises with SEMG feedback. Focus on hamstring stretching (Figure 5–24).
3. gluteal uptraining with concomitant hamstring downtraining during initiation of forward-bending.
4. integration of hamstring downtraining and gluteal uptraining during functional activities that reproduce symptoms or are frequently performed.

Faulty Trunk Stabilization

Many muscles work together to control pelvic inclination and spinal position. It seems reasonable that faulty coordination patterns among the muscles, in conjunction with structural deformities and dysfunction of periarticular connective tissues, could act to destabilize intervertebral segments. Segmental instability is associated with an aberrant path of the instantaneous center of rotation between two vertebrae. Instability can be found with spondylolisthesis or common degenerative disease. Coordinated function of the lumbar paraspinal, gluteus maximus, and hamstring muscles was discussed earlier. A few other muscles are added now for consideration.

Many clinicians believe that good abdominal tone is important for patients with low back dysfunction. One line of thinking suggests that the oblique and transverse abdominal muscles are most vital. This is based in part on the idea that these muscles wrap far posteriorly around the trunk and insert into the lumbodorsal fascia. Thus their activation might make the trunk into a more rigid cylinder. In addition, oblique abdominal muscle recruitment would take up slack in the lumbodorsal fascia and enable it to act as a strut. The vertebral column might then be mechanically unloaded to a degree. Abdominal muscle conditioning, as well as training in conjunction with lumbar stabilization exercises, might help reduce inappropriate intervertebral shear forces and spinal torques. Lumbar stabilization exercises are designed to train patients to recognize and maintain neutral spine positioning. Theoretically, these focus on multifidi and deep abdominal muscles. Actions of the multifidi may be uniquely important in supplying normal segmental stabilization. Some clinicians believe the quadratus lumborum is also noteworthy, because of both its propensity to develop trigger points and its potential role in pelvic–trunk stabilization. Unfortunately, it is difficult to be confident of isolating either the multifidi or quadratus lumborum with most standard clinical SEMG electrodes and processing setups. Finally, the iliopsoas affects pelvic inclination and lumbar lordosis. The iliopsoas also cannot be reliably isolated under clinical circumstances, but general hip flexor activity can be easily recorded.

When the paraspinal muscles show asymmetric SEMG activity, the oblique abdominal muscles usually do as well. Greater amplitude activity is often seen as contralaterally paired. For example, when the left paraspinal signal is of high amplitude relative to that of the right paraspinal signal, the right abdominal signal tends to be of high amplitude relative to that of the left abdominal signal. Exercises purported to recruit and train the oblique abdominal muscles selectively have variable effects. It seems that particular exercises produce greater oblique abdominal activity, expressed as a %MVIC, in some patients. In others, however, oblique abdominal activity remains low, and the rectus abdominis appears to be primarily recruited. Some clinicians believe that a muscle imbalance develops in which the oblique abdominal muscles are underused and weak and the rectus abdominis is preferentially recruited and strong. Because no single exercise seems always to be effective in promoting oblique abdominal recruitment, it is recommended that both sites be monitored, and several exercise techniques be considered, in each patient.

Hip flexor SEMG activity seems to be greater during functional movements of the hips and trunk in certain patients with low back dysfunction. These persons tend to show tightness of the iliopsoas on physical examination and excellent strength on manual muscle test. Postural analysis reveals that they stand with a relatively anterior-tilted pelvis and increased lumbar lordosis. SEMG feedback can be used with these patients as a relaxation adjunct to stretching exercise. If physical examination reveals weak hip flexors and conditioning exercises are indicated, uptraining feedback can alternatively be integrated into the exercise plan.

Training Progression for Faulty Trunk Stabilization

- Refer to Chapters 3 and 4 for detailed discussion of SEMG display setups and feedback structure.
- Refer to Chapter 5 for detailed discussion of SEMG training techniques.
- As skill develops, generally
  1. Shape desired responses up or down.
  2. Incorporate multijoint control.
  3. Add distractions.
  4. Randomize training activities.
  5. Withdraw continuous audio/visual feedback.
- Select relevant SEMG feedback training tasks from the following:
  1. isolation of target muscle activity:
     - Use a gross posterior pelvic tilt or partial sit-up for abdominal muscles in general.
     - For oblique abdominal muscles, have the patient retract the navel and use a slight posterior pelvic tilt motion. Accomplish this maneuver by instructing the patient to "suck in your navel gently and make your belly into a bowl shape or hollow."
     - Use hip flexion to recruit hip flexors.
     - Because there is no reliable technique to isolate the quadratus lumborum for surface recordings, try use of lateral paraspinal electrode placements and hip hiking. Recognize, however, that multiple muscles will be activated, the other participatory muscles have much

larger dorsal surface dimensions, and cross-talk is inevitable. Placement of electrodes just lateral to lower lumbar spinous processes may detect activity from multifidi muscles. However, with conventional-sized/configured electrodes, activity from adjacent muscles will likely be detected as well.

2. therapeutic exercises with SEMG feedback. Consider specifically:

–abdominal conditioning. Preferential activation of oblique abdominal muscles relative to rectus abdominis muscle can be achieved, but effective exercises vary across individuals. Assess the effects of partial sit-ups—pure trunk flexion versus diagonal flexion; hooklying abdominal hollow with reciprocal bent knee leg raise; hooklying abdominal hollow with reciprocal leg extension; hooklying abdominal hollow with contralateral, reciprocating arm, and leg extension; supine bilateral hip flexion with pelvic thrust—lifting soles of feet up toward ceiling;

side-lying trunk lifts with lower extremity stabilization

–hip flexor stretching as indicated. Try stretching with relaxation feedback in half-kneeling, half-hooklying position with the involved leg over the side of a bench or prone on a table with adjustable platform, raising the involved lower extremity up into hip extension with the other lower extremity over the side and pelvis stabilized

–trunk stabilization exercises. Maintain neutral spine by using abdominal and lumbar muscle co-contraction as indicated. Consider possibilities, such as hooklying abdominal sequence as described above; bridging—bilateral, single leg, maintenance of bridge with small footsteps; hands-and-knees position with reciprocal hip extension; hands-and-knees position with reciprocal, contralateral shoulder flexion and hip extension; lifting of box from floor to table height; gymnastic ball exercises

SUGGESTED READINGS

Biedermann HJ, Shanks GL, Forrest WJ, Inglis J. Power spectrum analyses of electromyographic activity: discriminators in the differential assessment of patients with chronic low back pain. *Spine*. 1991;16:1179–1184.

Cram JR, ed. *Clinical EMG for Surface Recordings*. Vol 2. Nevada City, CA: Clinical Resources; 1990.

Donaldson S, Romney D, Donaldson M, Skubick D. Randomized study of the application of single motor unit biofeedback training to chronic low back pain. *J Occup Rehabil*. 1994;4:23–37.

Fiebert I, Keller CD. Are "passive" extension exercises really passive? *J Orthop Sports Phys Ther*. 1994;19:111–116.

Flor H, Turk DC, Birbaumer N. Assessment of stress-related psychophysiological reactions in chronic back pain patients. *J Consult Clin Psychol*. 1985;53:354–364.

Geisser ME, Robinson ME, Richardson C. A time series analysis of the relationship between ambulatory EMG, pain, and stress in chronic low back pain. *Biofeedback Self Regul*. 1995;20:339–355.

Lofland KR, Mumby PB, Cassisi JE, Palumbo NL, Camic PM. Assessment of lumbar EMG during static and dynamic activity in pain-free normals: implications for muscle scanning protocols. *Biofeedback Self Regul*. 1995;20:3–18.

Roy SH, De Luca CJ, Emley M, Buijs RJC. Spectral electromyographic assessment of back muscles in patients with low back pain undergoing rehabilitation. *Spine*. 1995;20:38–48.

Sherman RA, Arena JG. Biofeedback for assessment and treatment of low back pain. In: Basmajian JV, Nyberg R, eds. *Rational Manual Therapies*. Baltimore: Williams & Wilkins; 1993;177–198.

Shirado O, Ito T, Kaneda K, Strax TE. Flexion-relaxation phenomenon in the back muscles. *Am J Phys Med*. 1995;74:139–143.

Sihvonen T, Partanen J, Hanninen O, Soimakallio S. Electric behavior of low back muscles during lumbar pelvic rhythm in low back pain patients and healthy controls. *Arch Phys Med Rehabil*. 1991;72:1080–1087.

Triano JJ, Schultz AB. Correlation of objective measure of trunk motion and muscle function with low-back disability ratings. *Spine.* 1987;12:561–565.

Vakos JP, Nitz AJ, Threlkeld AJ, Shapiro R, Horn T. Electromyographic activity of selected trunk and hip muscles during a squat lift: effect of varying the lumbar posture. *Spine.* 1994;19:687–695.

CHAPTER 13

Hip Dysfunction

BACKGROUND

Muscles about the hip joint have been studied through electromyographic analyses for more than 50 years. A review of the many sources cited by Basmajian and De Luca[1] predominantly confirms the functions that have been described for hip muscles by anatomists. To record surface electromyography (SEMG) activity, those muscles most readily accessible are the sartorius, gluteus maximus, gluteus medius, adductor mass, and tensor fasciae latae. In this regard, the sartorius has been designated a surrogate muscle for monitoring the function of hip flexion when the iliacus or psoas muscle cannot be readily approached.[2] The gluteus medius is acknowledged as an important muscle for maintaining pelvic stability during single-limb stance and assisting in hip extension, whereas the gluteus maximus functions as a preeminent extensor muscle of the hip joint. Those muscles performing rotatory motions about the hip are difficult to access with SEMG. The lateral rotation muscles are covered by the gluteus mass, and most of medial rotation must be relegated to that action subserved by portions of the nondescript adductor muscle group. The tensor fasciae latae is a flexor, abductor, and medial rotator of the hip joint; its importance in abnormalities of the hip or knee joints has often gone unheralded. Although the hip adductors have received little attention for their role at the hip joint in patients with musculoskeletal disorders, clinicians should note that augmenting activity from this muscle group in weight-bearing conditions improves recruitment of the vastus medialis oblique more than the vastus lateralis[3] but not during straight leg raising.[4]

What is of importance to clinicians who apply SEMG to hip muscles is a clear understanding of the interrelationship between these muscles and their relative contributions to normal and pathologic movement. This understanding forms the cornerstone for development and application of treatment strategies with the use of SEMG as an adjunct to manual therapy and an informational base for the patient to modify movement efforts within the context of functional restitution. The literature is remarkably sparse in these regards. Most studies are purely kinesiologic and offer little insight into how SEMG observations can be integrated into treatment plans for patients with musculoskeletal pathology.

EFFECTS OF LOAD AND SPECIFIC MOVEMENTS

Compelling data exist to support the well-known biomechanical principle that isometric torque generation and concomitant EMG activity decrease at shorter muscle lengths. Murray and Sepic[5] demonstrated this phenomenon for the gluteus medius, and this finding was confirmed and expanded by Olson and coworkers.[6] The dispersing of forces through the hip was correlated with reduced EMG output from either gluteus medius during stance when carrying loads were distributed bilaterally rather than unilaterally.[7] When gluteus medius SEMG activity was adjusted for the hip joint angle (a proxy for muscle length) at which it was recorded, the muscle was less active during ipsilateral load-carrying conditions, compared with contralaterally held loads of greater than 3% of body weight.[8] These observations become important when examining patients who have hip pain or have undergone total hip replacement. Long and colleagues[9] showed that intramuscular EMG activity from gluteus maximus and gluteus medius was reduced in some patients with osteoarthritis during ambulation before total hip replacement. Aberrant tonic activity was also produced in some patients by the tensor fasciae latae, rectus femoris, and adductor longus muscles throughout the gait cycle. After total hip replacement, force through the affected hip remained significantly lower, compared with findings in the contralateral joint or data obtained from individuals with normal hip joints. In addition, a subgroup of patients showed postoperative development of abnormal EMG activity, and revision of the noncemented hip arthroplasties was necessary. Therefore distribution of the carrying load combined with SEMG monitoring of hip muscles may represent an example of integrating a kinesiologic observation with a bona fide treatment. By training patients to recruit their gluteus medius in a timely fashion during loading of the extremities, the potential for facilitating integrity of the replaced hip joint is augmented.

On the other hand, SEMG assessment may not necessarily support the contentions of some clinicians. For example, after monitoring the gluteus medius with SEMG, Neumann and associates[10] were unable to support the notion of stretch weakness at the hip joint set forth by Kendall and McCreary.[11] When corrected for side-specific differences in maximal isometric torque–hip abduction angle curves, this observation was still preserved.[12] Specifically, right hip abductor weakness could not be attributed to persistent lengthening of these muscles due to standing postures in right-handed people.

There is little doubt that the iliopsoas is a prime mover for hip flexion. The depth of this muscle makes accurate recording with SEMG improbable. Binder and coworkers[13] described a technique to record from the origin of the sartorius muscle at the base of the anterior superior iliac spine to monitor and promote hip flexion in patients who had suffered a stroke. The application of this SEMG procedure to patients with musculoskeletal disorders affecting the initiation of the swing phase of gait awaits exploration. When use of indwelling recording electrodes is possible, however, the individual dynamics of the iliacus and psoas major muscles can be readily appreciated, as noted by Andersson and coworkers.[14] They found that both muscles can be co-activated during the generation of hip flexion torques, but the iliacus could be selectively recruited to stabilize the pelvis during contralateral hip extension in the standing position. The psoas was differentially activated in sitting with a straight back and in contralateral limb loading with the vertebral column stabilized. Relative contributions from each muscle during execution of sit-ups vary on the basis of range of motion and leg position. Collectively, these findings suggest that each muscle has task-specific activation patterns, and that these patterns are predicated on demands for stability or movement at the lumbar spine, pelvis, or hip. In this regard, clinicians should be cautious in attempting to replicate these findings using SEMG recording techniques, because the iliacus sits on the floor of the femoral triangle, and the origin of the psoas major is relatively deep to the skin surface when approached posteriorly.

There may be specific circumstances under which clinicians might use SEMG to evaluate treatment techniques for patients with hip muscle weaknesses. For example, Doorenbosch and colleagues[15] determined that the kinematics and, by deduction, the torque generated about the hip are greater in sit-to-stand activity with the trunk fully flexed than in a natural sit-to-stand transfer among healthy individuals. The implication of this finding is that posterior muscles acting about the hip should be expected to generate greater activity if the patient is engaged in forward trunk flexion during sit-to-stand training. The increasing of flexion at the hip joint can also be expected to shorten the rectus femoris as a hip flexor and reduce its output at the knee joint.[16]

Another unique muscle group requiring exploration is the medial hamstrings. These muscles contract concentrically during sit-to-stand maneuvers in children with spastic diplegia and with relatively little impedance imposed from hip flexion contractures.[17] The net effect of this activity is to aid in hip extension. This observation raises the interesting possibility of monitoring medial hamstrings to facilitate hip extension among patients with traumatic musculoskeletal injuries, who have difficulty engaging their gluteus maximus or for whom substantial subcutaneous fat dissipates signals emanating from the gluteus maximus.

Muscles can also be monitored during walking and running. DeVita[18] makes a compelling argument for rethinking the cyclic phase of recording and evaluating SEMG activity during ambulation. Larger joint torques are recorded at the swing-to-stance transition at the hip and knee for walking and running than at the stance-to-swing interval. Further, SEMG activity is lower at the latter interval. Accordingly, it is suggested that because the transition from stance to swing does not seem to be as critical a point in the gait cycle, it should be used as the beginning and ending of the cycle, whereas the more relevant transition of swing-to-stance phase should occur in the middle of the analysis.

For patients who wear knee braces during running activities, Osternig and Robertson[19] have demonstrated differences in SEMG from different muscles acting about the hip in 67% to 83% of braced versus nonbraced comparisons. These findings demonstrate that neuromotor strategies can be altered about the hip in efforts to ambulate more effectively when knee orthoses are worn, and this change can be detected electromyographically.

The influence on neuromotor control exerted from hip muscles also has been demonstrated by Brooke and associates.[20] They showed that during bicycling activity, rotary motions at the ipsilateral or contralateral hip inhibited H reflexes. These reflexes are recorded electromyographically, usually in the triceps surae, and represent the excitability state of the muscle's spinal cord motoneuron pool in response to a standardized and constant posterior tibial nerve electrical stimulation. Somatosensory receptor discharge resulting from rotatory movements at either hip may therefore induce an inhibition on ankle extension. This finding dramatically shows an effect of proximal joint motion patterns on peripheral joint behavior. The clinical relevance relates to the SEMG monitoring of hip muscles during functional activities such as bicycling. Output from lower extremity muscles can vary during the cycle phase, and each phase can have an impact on ankle muscle activity, which the clinician might monitor with SEMG.

HIP MUSCLE COMPARTMENTALIZATION

Muscle compartmentalization, called partitioning by some,[21] may prove to be another important concept in SEMG and hip dysfunction. The notion is that individual muscles may have discrete cytoarchitectural and nerve innervation patterns, leading to the possibility for discrete task-specific behaviors within the same muscle. In this regard, Soderberg and Dostal[22] observed that the gluteus medius may actually have three distinct portions, each of which can make a unique contribution to movement components of hip extension and abduction. In addition, the tensor fasciae latae has been differentiated on the basis of intramuscular EMG and anatomic study by Pare and coworkers.[23] The anteromedial portion of the tensor fasciae latae contributes to hip flexion, whereas the posterolateral fibers produce hip abduction and medial rotation. Activity levels of the two portions of this muscle vary widely during performance of functional activities, and each may selectively atrophy or hypertrophy. These findings point to a need for heightened awareness by clinicians as to where electrodes are placed with respect to training objectives.

CONCLUSION

Electromyography has been used primarily for kinesiologic study of hip function. Investigations have generally supported long-held beliefs as to the roles of specific muscles in regulating motion about the hip, with implications for control of the trunk and lower extremity during functional tasks. There is a paucity of clinical literature relating hip muscle activity to commonly diagnosed musculoskeletal problems. Neverthe-less, it seems inevitable that patterns of muscle activity would be altered with chronic pain, restricted mobility, and deconditioning. Electromyography may be reasonably used to evaluate the effects of lower extremity orthoses, gait activity, and performance of other physical activities in patients with known musculoskeletal pathology. The use of SEMG feedback training may contribute to postoperative rehabilitation outcomes by fostering gains in strength and functional motor control. Nonoperative patients may benefit by neuromuscular re-education and, consequently, more efficient dispersion of forces through the hip complex.

REFERENCES

1. Basmajian JV, De Luca CJ. *Muscles Alive: Their Functions Revealed by Electromyography*. 5th ed. Baltimore: Williams & Wilkins; 1985.

2. Wolf SL, Binder-Macleod SA. EMG biofeedback applications to the hemiplegic patient: changes in lower extremity neuromuscular and functional status. *Phys Ther*. 1983;63:1404–1413.

3. Hodges PW, Richardson CA. The influence of isometric hip adduction on quadriceps femoris activity. *Scand J Rehabil Med*. 1993;25:57–62.

4. Karst GM, Jewett PD. Electromyographic analysis of exercises proposed for differential activation of medial and lateral quadriceps femoris muscle components. *Phys Ther*. 1993;73:286–295.

5. Murray MP, Sepic SB. Maximum isometric torque of the hip abductor muscle. *Phys Ther*. 1968;48:1327–1335.

6. Olson VL, Smidt GL, Johnson RC. The maximum torque generated by the eccentric, isometric, and concentric contractions of the hip abductor muscles. *Phys Ther*. 1972;52:149–157.

7. Neumann DA, Cook TM, Sholty RL, Sobush DC. An electromyographic analysis of hip abductor muscle activity when subjects are carrying loads in one or both hands. *Phys Ther*. 1992;72:207–217.

8. Neumann DA, Hase AD. An electromyographic analysis of the hip abductors during load carriage: implications for hip joint protection. *J Orthop Sports Phys Ther*. 1994;19:296–304.

9. Long WT, Dorr LD, Healy B, Perry J. Functional recovery of noncemented total hip arthroplasty. *Clin Orthop*. 1993;288:73–77.

10. Neumann DA, Soderberg GL, Cook TM. Electromyographic analysis of hip abductor musculature in healthy right-handed persons. *Phys Ther*. 1989;69:431–440.

11. Kendall FP, McCreary EK. *Muscle Testing and Function*. 3rd ed. Baltimore: Williams & Wilkins; 1983.

12. Neumann DA, Soderberg GL, Cook TM. Comparison of maximal isometric hip abduction muscle torques between hip sides. *Phys Ther*. 1988;68:496–502.

13. Binder SA, Moll CB, Wolf SL. Evaluation of EMG biofeedback as an adjunct to therapeutic exercise in treating the lower extremities of hemiplegic patients. *Phys Ther*. 1981;61:886–894.

14. Andersson E, Oddsson L, Grundstrom H, Thorstensson A. The role of psoas and iliacus muscles in stability and movement of the lumbar spine, pelvis and hip. *Scand J Med Sci Sports*. 1995;5:10–16.

15. Doorenbosch CA, Harlaar J, Roebroeck ME, Lankhorst GL. Two strategies of transferring from sit-to-stand; the activation of monoarticular and biarticular muscles. *J Biomech*. 1994;27:1299–1307.

16. Hasler EM, Denoth J, Stacoff A, Herzog W. Influence of hip and knee joint angles on excitation of knee extensor muscles. *Electromyogr Clin Neurophysiol*. 1994;34:355–361.

17. Hoffinger SA, Rab GT, Abou-Ghaida H. Hamstrings I cerebral palsy crouch gait. *J Pediatr Orthop*. 1993;13:722–726.

18. DeVita P. The selection of a standard convention for analyzing gait data based on the analysis of relevant biomechanical factors. *J Biomech*. 1994;27:501–508.

19. Osternig LR, Robertson RN. Effects of prophylactic knee bracing on lower extremity joint position and muscle activation during running. *Am J Sports Med*. 1993;21:733–737.

20. Brooke JD, Misiaszek JE, Cheng J. Locomotor-like rotation of either hip or knee inhibits soleus H reflexes in humans. *Somatosens Mot Res*. 1993;10:357–364.

21. English AW, Wolf SL, Segal RL. Compartmentalization of muscles and their motor nuclei: the partitioning hypothesis. *Phys Ther*. 1993;73:857–867.

22. Soderberg GL, Dostal WF. Electromyographic study of three parts of the gluteus medius muscle during functional activities. *Phys Ther*. 1978;58:691–696.

23. Pare EB, Stern JT, Schwartz JM. Functional differentiation within the tensor fasciae latae. *J Bone Joint Surg Am*. 1981;63:1457–1471.

SEMG Program for Hip Dysfunction

Refer to the discussion in Chapter 13 for a review of intervention approaches. The suggestions that follow are derived from those resources. Descriptions and operational definitions are provided to clarify optional practice patterns.

CANDIDATES

Implement for patients
- with chronic pain and in whom hip muscle dysfunction is suspected
- who present with a diagnosis of
  1. chronic hamstring muscle origin tendinitis
  2. trochanteric bursitis
  3. iliotibial band friction syndrome
  4. degenerative joint disease

Physical examination should reveal
- faulty pelvic–lower extremity structural alignment
- palpable hypertonicity
- trigger points
- imbalances in muscle flexibility and strength

EVALUATION OBJECTIVES

- Assess effects of postural alignment on hip muscle activity.
- Identify aberrant patterns of dynamic muscle activity about the pelvic girdle, potentially contributing to musculoskeletal pain:

1. myalgia due to excessive levels or duration of muscle tension
2. imbalanced muscle activity that potentially results in soft tissue or joint dysfunction

FEEDBACK TRAINING OBJECTIVES

- Improve postural alignment.
- Reduce excessive or imbalanced muscle tension.
- Retain and generalize improved motor control to functional contexts.
- Resolve or reduce functional limitations and disability.

RECORDING SITES

- Judge the utility of each recording site on the basis of history and physical examination results.
- Include muscles that
  1. underlie the pain distribution
  2. potentially refer symptoms or are mechanically related to the patient's area of complaint
  3. reproduce patient's symptoms when stretched, resisted, or palpated
- Consult the companion book, *Introduction to Surface Electromyography*, for specific electrode placement considerations.
- Confirm optimal sites from the following

list by observation and palpation during isometric contraction:

1. gluteus maximus
2. gluteus medius
3. tensor fasciae latae
4. hip flexors
5. hip adductors
6. hamstrings

EVALUATION PROCEDURES

- Select procedures that correspond to exacerbating and alleviating factors revealed by history and clinical examination.
- Refer to Chapter 2 for detailed discussion of evaluation methods.
- Perform at least five repetitions of each movement task to assess response consistency. Many more repetitions may be needed to assess SEMG responses with reproduction of symptoms.
- Select relevant procedures from the following:
  1. postural analysis. Examine relationships throughout the lower extremity kinematic chain; assess effects of temporarily altering foot pronation and hip rotation angle with the patient in a standing position.
  2. hip active range of motion (AROM). Test in open versus closed kinematic chains; examine concentric versus eccentric movement phases (use a standard bathroom scale under each foot to ensure equal lower extremity weight bearing during closed chain movement), as relevant:
     –flexion
     –extension
     –abduction
     –adduction
     –medial rotation
     –lateral rotation
  3. isometric contractions:
     –maximal effort

     –progressively graded submaximal efforts
  4. dynamic contractions at progressive intensities. Emphasize movement planes that were provocative of symptoms or accompanied by faulty SEMG patterns during no. 2 above.
  5. dynamic contractions at progressive velocities. Emphasize movement planes that were provocative of symptoms or accompanied by faulty SEMG patterns during no. 2 above.
  6. analysis of coordinated muscle activity patterns. Consider hamstrings and gluteus maximus, tensor fasciae latae and gluteus medius, and others as indicated; test with AROM and the following tasks as indicated:
     –prone active hip extension: knee bent versus straight
     –step-up, step-down
     –unilateral stance
     –bilateral partial squat
     –unilateral partial squat
     –lunge
     –gait
     –jumping, hopping, cross-cutting
  7. functional activity analysis. Use other home, work, sports-specific activities known to exacerbate or alleviate symptoms.

ASSESSMENT

- Refer to Chapter 2 for detailed discussion of SEMG assessment.
- Refer to Chapter 14 in the companion book for representative SEMG tracings of normal function.
  1. Amplitude, variance, recruitment, and decruitment timing of each channel during contraction efforts. Recruitment and decruitment should be prompt and smooth, to and from a stable baseline. Activity during standing baseline should be stable and of relatively low amplitude (typically about 2–15 μV RMS).

2. Relationship of salient SEMG events to particular range of motion arcs. Observe for consistent amplitude elevations or depressions during a painful portion of the AROM arc.

3. Left/right peak amplitude symmetry for bilateral and unilateral reciprocal movements. Satisfactory symmetry is operationally defined as left/right scores within 35% as calculated [(higher value − lower value)/higher value] × 100. Symmetry assessment assumes a symmetric AROM excursion and velocity. The tonic amplitude should also be roughly symmetric between repeated task trials.

4. Symmetrically proportionate left/right gluteus maximus/hamstring and gluteus medius/tensor fasciae latae activity during test activities. For comparisons across nonhomologous muscles, amplitudes may be expressed as a:

   –percentage of maximal volitional isometric contraction (%MVIC) amplitude by using standard manual muscle tests (test activity amplitude/MVIC amplitude × 100)

   –percentage of some submaximal contraction with a standardized force intensity, joint angle, and body posture. Normalized gluteus maximus:hamstring and gluteus medius:tensor fascia latae ratios can then be constructed if desired.

5. Left/right timing symmetry for symmetric movements: coincident recruitment, peak, and decruitment patterns during bilateral symmetric tasks (eg, partial squat). Timing relationships should be roughly symmetric for repetitious reciprocal tasks (eg, walking [see Pare and coworkers[1] and Perry[2] for detailed gait analysis]). Observe timing differences with rectified line tracings with a smoothing time constant of 0.1 second or less, SEMG sampling at 100 Hz or faster, frequency bandwidth filter low cutoff of 25 Hz or less, and a high resolution display with variable sweep speed. A graphic printout is useful for documentation of subtle timing differences. Documentation can be quantified with calculations of average slope, time to peak activity, or time to some percentage of MVIC activity that is clinically meaningful. Onset time can be reported simply as the latency to achieve a microvolt value equivalent to two standard deviations above the baseline mean. Duration may be noted as the amount of time between onset and baseline recovery (amplitude recovery within two standard deviations of the baseline mean).

6. Change in activity levels for a particular muscle and task across treatment sessions. To document this parameter a normalization procedure is preferred. A reliable maximal manual muscle test effort or a standardized submaximal contraction is required as a reference. Average amplitude during the test task is divided by that day's reference contraction amplitude, and the quotient is multiplied by 100.

COMMON PATIENT PRESENTATIONS

Recurrent Hamstring Origin Tendinitis with Hamstring Hyperactivity and Gluteal Hypoactivity

Patients with this disorder have chronic aching rest pain over the ischial tuberosity. Sharp pain tends to be provoked with sports activities involving robust or ballistic hamstring contractions from a stretched position. Sports examples include volleyball, skating, uphill running, hiking, climbing, and any activity that includes sprinting. Physical examination is usually notable for marked hamstring shortness on a straight leg raise and weak gluteus maximus on manual muscle test. Many repetitions of a provocative functional activity can be required to reproduce symptoms. Maximally resisted hip extension and resisted knee flexion may reproduce symptoms if the patient is acutely flared.

Although patterns of structural alignment, flexibility, and strength may be similar for both lower extremities, usually only one side is symptomatic. Physical impairments tend to be more pronounced on the symptomatic side, and hamstring SEMG activity tends to be hyperactive (Figure 13–A–1). Moreover, SEMG activity recorded from the gluteus maximus on the symptomatic side tends to be hypoactive relative to activity from the asymptomatic side. Thus there appears to be a hamstring–gluteus maximus muscle imbalance in supporting hip extension. It is hypothesized that the hamstrings become habitually overused, and the gluteus maximus becomes underused, poorly recruited, and deconditioned. No quantitative SEMG standards for hamstring:gluteus maximus comparisons are currently available. However, left/right asymmetries for each muscle recording site can be calculated. Asymmetric normalized hamstring: gluteus maximus activity ratios can also be found in individuals.

Training Progression for Recurrent Hamstring Tendinitis with Hamstring Hyperactivity and Gluteal Hypoactivity

- Refer to Chapters 3 and 4 for detailed discussion of SEMG display setups and feedback structure.
- Refer to Chapters 5 and 6 for detailed discussion of SEMG feedback training techniques.
- As skill develops, generally
  1. Shape desired responses up or down.
  2. Incorporate multijoint control.
  3. Add distractions.
  4. Randomize training activities.
  5. Withdraw continuous audio/visual feedback.
- Select relevant SEMG feedback training tasks from the following:
  1. isolation of target muscle activity.
     –Use gently resisted isometric knee flexion with the patient in prone or sit-

ting position, or gentle standing knee flexion, for hamstrings.
     –Isolate gluteus maximus with an isometric squeeze. Isolation of the gluteus maximus may be extremely difficult for the patient at the start of progression. That is, the patient may not be able to activate the gluteus maximus without also recruiting the hamstrings (Figure 13–A–2). Experiment with different hip and knee flexion angles in non–weight bearing to find the best position. As isolation skill develops, transition the patient to weight-bearing postures.
  2. deactivation training for the hamstrings
  3. uptraining of gluteus maximus relative to hamstrings during AROM. Consider use of display thresholds for each; include
     –open chain hip extension with gluteal squeeze
     –unilateral stance
     –taking one step forward and backward on the involved side, level gait, ramps
     –sit-to-stand, stand-to-sit
     –front step-ups/step-downs, lateral step-ups/step-downs
     –stair-stepper
     –lunges
  4. generalization to progressively dynamic movement. Progressively increase
     –AROM excursion
     –movement velocity
     –addition of extrinsic loads
  5. functional activity performance with SEMG feedback. Continue gluteal–hamstring training during exacerbating work or sports-specific tasks.
  6. prescription of therapeutic home exercises with SEMG feedback
     –hamstring relaxation during stretching
     –isolated gluteal uptraining. Experiment as above, and prescribe successful maneuvers for home practice.
  7. motor copy training. Use the symptomatic side of the gluteal maximus to pattern-match the asymptomatic side.

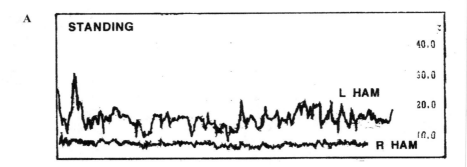

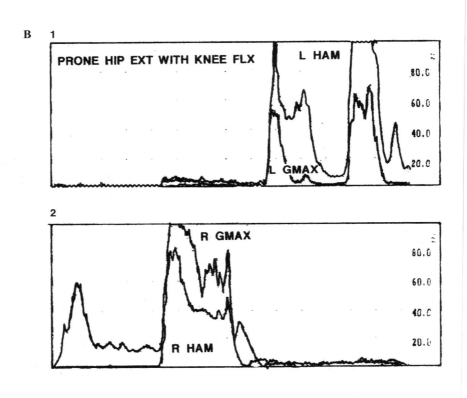

Figure 13–A–1 SEMG activity of the (**L**) left and (**R**) right medial hamstring (**HAM**) and (**GMAX**) gluteus maximus, recorded from a patient with left ischial tuberosity pain that was chronically reproduced with running, uphill biking, volleyball, lunging, in-line skating, and cross-country skiing. (**A**) Activity during static standing with equal lower extremity weight bearing. (**B**) Activity during prone hip (**EXT**) extension with knee (**FLX**) flexion on the (**1**) left and (**2**) right through a symmetric range of motion arc. Note the tendency for left greater than right hamstring activity and left less than right gluteal activity.

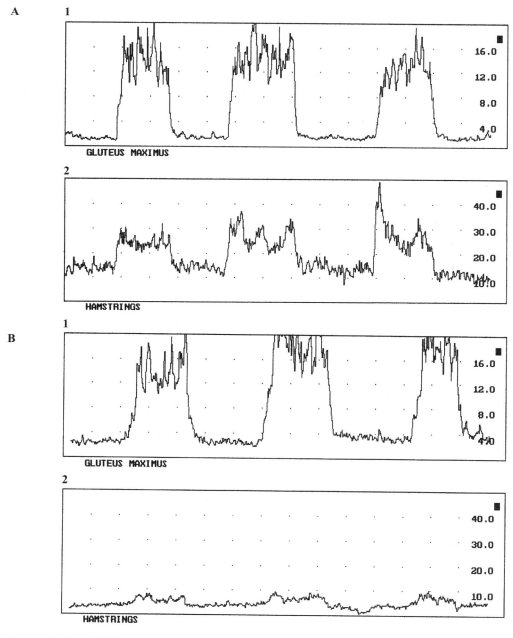

Figure 13–A–2 SEMG activity of the gluteus maximus and lateral hamstrings during attempted isolation of gluteal recruitment recorded from a patient with chronic buttock pain linked to athletic activity. (**A**) Activity at the start of SEMG feedback training. The patient is unable to recruit (**A1**) gluteus maximus without also increasing (**A2**) hamstring activity. (**B**) Activity after 4 weeks of weekly feedback training, home hamstring stretching, and gluteal muscle uptraining exercises. The patient can now recruit (**B1**) gluteus maximus in an isolated manner without co-activation of (**B2**) hamstring activity. Symptoms resolve as skills for increased gluteal activation are transferred to sport tasks.

8. SEMG-triggered neuromuscular electrical stimulation. Consider use of this training technique for the gluteus maximus muscle during the above-listed procedures.

- Integrate SEMG feedback training into a comprehensive approach to patient management. Consider the need for
    1. adjunctive physical agents and manual therapies
    2. comprehensive lower extremity conditioning
    3. shoe orthotics
    4. guided return to sport and technique modification by a trained coach

Lateral Hip Pain with Tensor Fasciae Latae Hyperactivity and Gluteus Medius Hypoactivity

Patients with this syndrome have pain over the lateral or anterolateral portion of the hip. Dysesthetic burning pain and soreness tend to be produced and progressively increased with weight-bearing activity. The problem occurs in trained athletes, as well as in persons engaging regularly in recreational walking and running. Elite bicyclists and runners may complain of an associated friction syndrome at the iliotibial band insertion. The syndrome seems to be most common in women with a wide pelvic brim who have suddenly started exercising or increased their exercise level. When there is a flare-up of pain, simple tasks such as arising from a squat or sitting position can be exacerbating.

Physical examination tends to be notable for marked tightness of the iliotibial band as well as weak gluteus medius on manual muscle test. During unilateral stance tasks, excessive lateral hip drop, hip medial rotation, genu valgum, and foot pronation may be observed. Symptoms can sometimes be reproduced by manual muscle test of the tensor fasciae latae. In most cases, many repetitions of a provocative functional task are required to reproduce symptoms.

Patterns of structural alignment, flexibility, and strength may be similar for both lower extremities, but usually only one side is symptomatic. Physical impairments tend to be more pronounced on the symptomatic side, and SEMG activity from the tensor fasciae latae is often hyperactive. Moreover, SEMG activity recorded from the gluteus medius on the symptomatic side tends to be hypoactive relative to the activity on the asymptomatic side (Figures 13–A–3 and 13–A–4). Thus there appears to be a tensor fasciae latae–gluteus medius muscle imbalance. It is hypothesized that the tensor fasciae latae (especially the posterolateral fibers) becomes habitually overused to stabilize the hip during stance. The gluteus medius becomes underused, poorly recruited, and deconditioned. It is conceivable that a similar progression takes place in many patients with degenerative hip disease. The progression of muscle imbalance and arthritis may ultimately necessitate arthroplasty. Slower postoperative rehabilitation may follow in persons with longstanding muscle imbalance.

Training Progression for Lateral Hip Pain with Tensor Fasciae Latae Hyperactivity and Gluteus Medius Hypoactivity

- Refer to Chapters 3 and 4 for detailed discussion of SEMG display setups and feedback structure.
- Refer to Chapters 5 and 6 for detailed discussion of SEMG feedback training techniques.
- As skill develops, generally
    1. Shape desired responses up or down.
    2. Incorporate multijoint control.
    3. Add distractions.
    4. Randomize training activities.
    5. Withdraw continuous audio/visual feedback.
- Select relevant SEMG feedback training tasks from the following:
    1. isolation of target muscle activity. Use standing hip flexion/abduction/medial rotation combined with knee extension to recruit the tensor fascia latae muscle. Isolating gluteus medius from the tensor fasciae latae may be extremely difficult

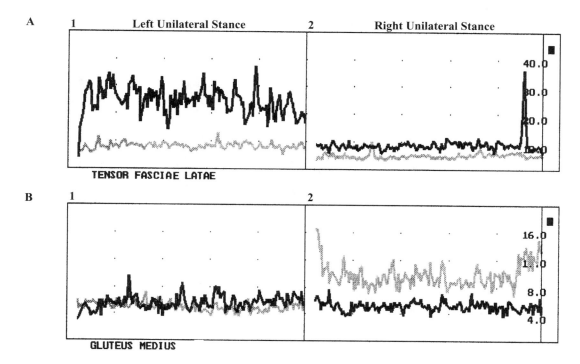

Figure 13–A–3 SEMG activity of the left (black) and right (gray) tensor fascia latae and gluteus medius during unilateral stance in a modified functional climbing position (with toe touch weight bearing with the contralateral limb) of the (**A1, B1**) left or (**A2, B2**) right lower extremity. Signals were recorded from an elite alpine climber during an acute flare-up of chronic left lateral hip pain. There is a tendency for reciprocally greater tensor fascia latae activity and lower gluteus medius activity on the left compared with the right side.

for the patient at the start of the progression. That is, the patient may not be able to activate the gluteus medius without also recruiting the tensor fasciae latae (Figure 13–A–5). Prone hip abduction in lateral hip rotation tends to be most successful for isolating activity of the gluteal muscle from that of the tensor fasciae latae. Posterior fibers of the gluteus medius can also be isolated with standing abduction/extension/lateral rotation.

2. uptraining of gluteus medius relative to tensor fasciae latae. Include display thresholds for each muscle; consider including
   –prone hip abduction, starting training

with lateral hip rotation and progressing to neutral rotation
–side-lying hip abduction/extension with slight lateral rotation
–unilateral stance
–bilateral and unilateral partial squats
–sit-to-stand, stand-to-sit
–taking one step forward and backward on the involved side, level gait, ramps
–front step-ups/step-downs, lateral step-ups/step-downs
–stair-stepper

3. generalization to progressively dynamic movement. Progressively increase
   –AROM excursion
   –movement velocity
   –addition of extrinsic loads

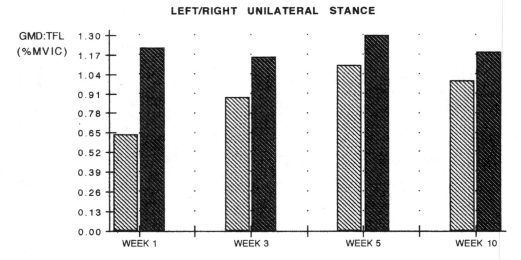

Figure 13–A–4 Ratios of SEMG activity of (**GMD**) gluteus medius to (**TFL**) tensor fasciae latae muscles during unilateral stance with weight bearing on left or right hip. Each signal was normalized to a percentage of maximal volitional isometric contraction (%MVIC) amplitude before ratio construction. Recordings were derived from a novice climber 9 weeks after a long alpine ascent and accompanied by left dysesthetic lateral hip pain. Regular clinic visits were discontinued at week 5 with follow up at week 10. *Source:* Copyright © 1997, G Kasman.

4. functional activity performance with SEMG feedback. Continue gluteal–tensor fasciae latae training during exacerbating home, work, and sports-specific tasks.

5. prescription of therapeutic home exercises with SEMG feedback
   –tensor fasciae latae relaxation during iliotibial band stretching
   –isolated gluteal uptraining. Experiment as above, and prescribe successful maneuvers for home practice.

6. motor copy training. Use the symptomatic side of the gluteus medius to pattern-match the asymptomatic side.

7. SEMG-triggered neuromuscular electrical stimulation. Consider use of this training technique for the gluteus me-

dius during the above-listed procedures.

• Integrate SEMG feedback training into a comprehensive approach to patient management. Consider the need for
1. adjunctive physical agents and manual treatments
2. comprehensive lower extremity conditioning
3. shoe orthotics
4. guided return to athletic activity

• Be aware that this tends to be one of the most difficult muscle imbalances to alter with SEMG training. SEMG-triggered neuromuscular electrical stimulation, soft tissue mobilization along the iliotibial band, and diligent home exercise compliance are helpful adjuncts.

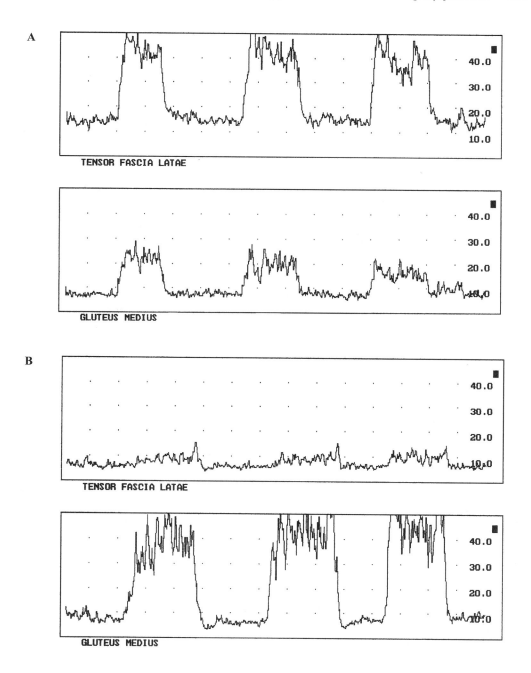

A

TENSOR FASCIA LATAE

GLUTEUS MEDIUS

B

TENSOR FASCIA LATAE

GLUTEUS MEDIUS

Figure 13–A–5 SEMG activity of the tensor fasciae latae and gluteus medius muscles during attempted isolation of gluteal recruitment recorded from a patient with chronic lateral hip pain linked to athletic activity. (**A**) Activity at start of EMG feedback training. The patient is unable to recruit gluteus medius without also increasing tensor fasciae latae activity. (**B**) Activity after 4 weeks of weekly feedback training and home exercise. The patient can now recruit the gluteus medius in an isolated manner. Symptoms resolve as skills for increased gluteal activation are transferred to sport tasks.

REFERENCES

1. Pare EB, Stern JT, Schwartz JM. Functional differentiation within the tensor fasciae latae. *J Bone Joint Surg Am.* 1981;63:1457–1471.

2. Perry J. *Gait Analysis.* Thorofare, NJ: Slack; 1992.

SUGGESTED READINGS

Long WT, Dorr LD, Healy B, Perry J. Functional recovery of noncemented total hip arthroplasty. *Clin Orthop.* 1993;288:73–77.

Lyons K, Perry J, Gronley JK, Barnes L, Antonelli D. Timing and relative intensity of hip extensor and abductor muscle action during level and stair ambulation. *Phys Ther.* 1983;63:1597–1605.

Neumann DA, Cook TM, Sholty RL, Sobush DC. An electromyographic analysis of hip abductor muscle activity when subjects are carrying loads in one or both hands. *Phys Ther.* 1992;72:207–217.

CHAPTER 14

Knee Dysfunction

BACKGROUND

Control of the knee is an integral part of human locomotion and other functional activities. The knee complex is composed of the tibiofemoral, patellofemoral, and superior tibiofibular joints. Large forces are transmitted through the knee, with stability being provided by the shapes of the joint surfaces and key ligamentous structures (Figure 14–1). Stability is also gained by the dynamic action of muscles that cross the tibiofemoral and patellofemoral joints. These muscles additionally generate mobility, and their function interacts with that of the articular connective tissues to control the biomechanics of the joint complex.

Kinesiologic electromyographic studies of knee musculature have been conducted since the 1940s.[1] Muscles of the knee that are accessible for surface electromyography (SEMG) recordings include the rectus femoris, vastus medialis (VM), and vastus lateralis (VL) components of the quadriceps, hamstrings—consisting of the lateral biceps femoris and medial semimembranosus/semitendinosus group—and gastrocnemius. Rarely, the tensor fasciae latae can be selected for recording on the basis of its action at the knee through the iliotibial band and the relationship of the iliotibial band to the lateral retinaculum of the knee.[2] The sartorious, gracilis, adductor longus, adductor magnus, adductor brevis, and gluteal muscles contribute less directly to knee function. They generally are not related to knee pathology evaluated with SEMG, although they bring about balanced muscle function throughout the lower extremity kinetic chain.

Elaborate synergistic and antagonistic relationships exist among all these muscles. For example, the VM and VL function synergistically to produce knee extension in the sagittal plane, but act antagonistically on the patella in the frontal plane. With the exception of the vastus muscles, each muscle's action crosses either the hip or ankle in addition to the knee. The ankle, knee, and hip form a closed kinetic chain when the foot is weight bearing on the ground; movement at one joint produces or constrains motion at the other joints. Ground reaction forces generated during stance are transmitted throughout the kinetic chain and met by the coordinated action of the uniarticular and biarticular musculature. When the lower extremity is engaged in the swing phase of gait, muscles acting on the knee must again contract in a manner that coordinates with hip and ankle control. Thus motor programs must be implemented that regulate flexion-extension of the knee in a way that reconciles control of all joints of the lower extremity kinetic chain.

The largest volume of clinical descriptions involving SEMG relates to the patellofemoral joint. SEMG has been used to investigate presumed motor control imbalances between the VM and VL in patients with patellofemoral pain. Exercises purported to have selective training

CLINICAL APPLICATIONS IN SURFACE ELECTROMYOGRAPHY

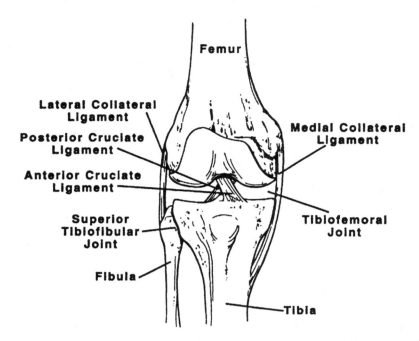

Figure 14–1 Anterior view of bones and major ligaments of the right knee, excluding the patellofemoral joint. *Source:* Reprinted with permission from JP Tomberlin and HD Saunders, Vol 2. *Extremities, Evaluation, Treatment, and Prevention of Musculoskeletal Disorders*, 3rd ed, p 218, © 1994, The Saunders Group, Inc.

effects on the VM have also been examined with SEMG. Finally, SEMG feedback training has been used in attempts to facilitate motor learning and rehabilitation in this population. Application of SEMG to patellofemoral dysfunction has emerged as a popular topic in educational programs, and several controversies exist in the literature.

Most of this chapter focuses in depth on SEMG and the patellofemoral pain syndrome (PFPS). However, injuries and postsurgical rehabilitation of the anterior cruciate ligament (ACL) will also be discussed as a common concern in dysfunction of the knee.

ANTERIOR CRUCIATE LIGAMENT AND GENERAL POSTSURGICAL KNEE REHABILITATION

The ACL runs from the anterior intercondylar area of the tibial plateau in a posterior, lateral,

and superior direction in the intercondylar notch to the medial part of the lateral femoral condyle[3] (see Figure 14–1). This alignment acts to limit anterior translation and rotation of the tibia relative to the femur. The ACL also functions with the posterior cruciate ligament and other structures to control the complex rolling–gliding arthrokinematics of the tibia and femur during flexion–extension.[4] Injury to the ACL is caused by application of valgus force with the knee flexed and the leg laterally rotated in stance, associated also with trauma to the medial collateral ligament and potentially to the medial meniscus.[5,6] Isolated ACL injuries occur with the leg in medial rotation and knee hyperextension, and other less common mechanisms have been reported.[7–11] Tears of this ligament lead to intrinsic knee instability and significant disability. SEMG has been used as a component of both nonsurgical and postsurgical rehabilitative efforts.

Several investigators have reported altered EMG activity in subjects with ACL deficiencies.[12–14] Sinkjaer and Arendt-Nielsen[15] investigated patterns of SEMG activity from semimembranosus/semitendinosus, biceps femoris, medial gastrocnemius, VM, and VL during treadmill walking. Compared with findings in matched control subjects, men and women with arthroscopically verified complete ACL ruptures (10–12 months after injury) tended toward earlier onset time and prolonged duration at all muscle sites during the normalized gait cycle. The trend was most pronounced with biceps femoris and medial gastrocnemius muscle activity. Subjects with ACL ruptures were then divided into two groups on the basis of knee stability and functional assessment. Evaluation revealed that subjects with good stability displayed significantly earlier and prolonged medial gastrocnemius muscle activity than subjects with poor stability. Finally, the investigators used SEMG feedback to train two subjects with poor functional stability to recruit the medial gastrocnemius earlier in stance. The subjects achieved greater recruitment of this muscle during early stance, apparently by using a slight manipulation of foot position, and improved their functional assessment scores over a 15-week rehabilitation period.

Co-activation training of the hamstrings with the quadriceps has also been advocated for rehabilitation in patients with deficiencies of ACL.[16] Healthy subjects naturally co-activate the hamstrings during active knee extension.[17,18] It is assumed that hamstring co-activation assists the ACL in limiting anterior translation of the tibia relative to the femur and in apt distribution of articular forces. Decreased mechanical strain of the ACL has been suggested or reported during hamstrings and quadriceps co-activation.[19,20] Gryzlo and associates[21] used fine wire EMG to study activation patterns of the vastus medialis oblique (VMO), VL, rectus femoris, biceps femoris, and semimembranosus muscles in healthy subjects during several common rehabilitative exercises. They concluded that certain variations of short arc knee extension exercises

with deliberate hamstring co-contraction, as well as isometric knee co-contraction exercises, resulted in adequate hamstring/quadriceps co-activation whereas the squat maneuver had an insufficient effect. The investigators suggested that therapists who design rehabilitation programs for ACL take these findings into account during exercise prescription. Another approach, as yet untested, would be to use SEMG feedback to uptrain hamstrings/quadriceps co-activation during functional sports training and activities of daily living.

Ciccotti and colleagues[13] examined non-injured individuals, subjects who had rehabilitated after bone–patella–bone autograft reconstruction, and subjects who had completed nonsurgical rehabilitation. The investigators noted increases in fine wire EMG activity from several muscles during a series of functional tasks in the nonsurgical rehabilitation group. The surgical reconstruction group tended to show more normal EMG patterns. Thus the nonsurgical rehabilitation group continued to use altered patterns of motor control to support functional lower extremity movements. The investigators interpreted these as compensatory motor control patterns that were not required in subjects who underwent surgical repair. A coordinated quadricep–hamstring response was supported, and protective mechanical effects subserved by the actions of the VL, biceps femoris, and tibialis anterior were proposed. It was suggested that these muscle actions counter untoward medial tibial rotation moments that occur as the knee is extended. Attention to rehabilitation of the VL, biceps femoris, and tibialis anterior was therefore encouraged. Although not addressed by the investigators, SEMG feedback could be integrated with functional retraining to enhance such muscle responses.

Draper[22] and Draper and Ballard[23] chose another tack with patients who underwent surgical ACL repairs. They believed that postsurgical quadriceps dysfunction might be a limiting factor for early rehabilitation. Draper[22] reported that patients receiving quadriceps SEMG feedback after surgery as an adjunct to exercise demonstrate faster recovery of knee extensor peak torque than patients training with exercise alone. Draper and Ballard[23] then compared a group performing postsurgical quadriceps rehabilitation exercises with SEMG feedback to a group training with the same exercise protocol but with adjunctive neuromuscular electrical stimulation (NMES) instead of SEMG. The exercise group receiving SEMG feedback demonstrated greater knee extensor peak torque (expressed as a percentage of the torque from the nonoperative limb) than shown in the exercise group receiving NMES. Generalization of the results of these studies may be limited by the relative level of aggressiveness of the rehabilitation protocols and type of NMES used.[24] Nevertheless, Draper and Ballard suggested that SEMG training can serve as a vehicle for motor learning in the early postoperative period, especially for patients training with less therapist supervision at home. Subjects may learn to increase neural drive to the quadriceps and overcome inhibitory processes occurring in response to pain and edema.[25–30]

It therefore seems reasonable to use SEMG feedback to teach patients to maximize quadriceps recruitment during postoperative ACL exercise prescription. The feedback may help patients quickly learn proper exercise technique and then transfer motor skills to independent practice. Persistent difficulties with postoperative quadriceps recruitment can be confirmed by comparing SEMG activity on the involved versus uninvolved sides. A course of SEMG training, either in the clinic or with an inexpensive home trainer, can be prescribed for patients who are lagging in improvement relative to expected clinical pathways. The feedback device can be quickly set up and integrated with a protocol rehabilitation program. Patients can maximize display output by using protocol exercises and functional activities. Therapists may choose to go on to hamstring/quadriceps co-activation training or medial gastrocnemius gait training for ACL patients with poor outcomes or unrepaired instabilities.

Early reports on surgical techniques that are now outdated also noted apparent quadriceps in-

hibition after meniscectomy.[31–34] SEMG feedback training of the quadriceps was offered as a means of counteracting this effect and promoting improved muscle function after meniscectomy by arthrotomy.[35] Less morbidity is associated with current surgical interventions, and it seems unlikely that SEMG feedback will be a critical adjunct for many patients. However, use of SEMG feedback is appropriate for patients who are progressing slowly relative to expected clinical pathways with persistent quadriceps weakness. The case is similar for patients who show difficulty recovering quadriceps function after total knee replacement. For example, at one medical center, patients who undergo total knee replacement are expected to achieve certain exercise and functional milestones each postoperative day during the hospital stay. On average, active terminal knee extension and straight leg raising are performed without therapist assistance by day 3 after surgery. This is associated with progression in ambulation and transfer abilities in preparation for hospital discharge. Patients who do not meet functional discharge criteria by day 4 or 5 tend to show persistent problems with quadriceps strength during terminal knee extension and straight leg raising exercises. Anecdotally, use of SEMG feedback or SEMG-triggered NMES with patients whose progress falls below pathway expectations seems to help restore quadriceps activity and function to expected levels, or to reduce length of stay below the time that might have been anticipated based on the early course. Patients continue to train with an identical rehabilitation protocol, but with the use of SEMG feedback or SEMG-triggered NMES as an adjunct. Application Guide 14–A summarizes SEMG methods for therapists to consider in working with ACL and general postsurgical knee patients.

PATELLOFEMORAL PAIN SYNDROME

PFPS is chronic anterior knee pain related to the patellofemoral articulation. This syndrome can be associated with inflammation, patellar dislocation, patellar subluxation, chondromalacia patella, hypertrophied infrapatellar fat pad, plica syndrome, quadriceps tendinitis, and patellar tendinitis.[36,37] The syndrome tends to be linked with increased pain on ascending or descending stairs, squatting, kneeling, prolonged sitting, and general activity.[38] PFPS is one of the more commonly encountered knee problems in athletic populations.[39–42]

Contributory causes of PFPS include the following:

- excessive Q angle (the acute angle formed by the intersection of a line from the anterior superior iliac spine to the center of the patella with a line from the center of the patella to the tibial tubercle)[43–45]
- passive and active structural factors such as excessive foot pronation, genu recurvatum, patella alta, excessive tibial torsion, genu varum/valgum deformities, femoral anteversion or excessive medial rotation, and lateral displacement of the tibial tubercle[38,41,46–48]
- trochlear groove dysplasia[41,49]
- tight lateral retinaculum or iliotibial band (or both)[2,50,51]
- tight gastrocnemius, hamstring, and rectus femoris muscles[52,53]
- weakness or faulty motor control of the distal VM muscle[37,41,45]

Pain is presumably generated from nociceptors in the synovium, subchondral bone, and retinaculum.[45,49,54]

Anatomy and Biomechanics

The quadriceps femoris muscle acts in a concentric fashion to extend the knee and in an eccentric manner to decelerate knee flexion. The four components of the quadriceps—the VM, VL, vastus intermedius, and rectus femoris—act together to produce a knee extension moment. Each component generates tension with a particular magnitude and direction. The components insert commonly to the patella (Figure 14–2), a sesamoid bone that imparts mechanical

advantage to the extensor mechanism by increasing the lever arm through which the quadriceps acts.[55] The resultant force vector tends to displace the patella laterally as knee extension forces are created,[53,56] and this effect is in part attributable to the line of pull of the VL.[57] Lateral displacement of the patella is resisted by congruency of the lateral aspect of the patella with the lateral femoral condyle,[41,53] medial retinaculum,[45] medial patellofemoral and patellotibial ligaments,[45,47] and distal portion of the VM termed the VMO.[53,57,58]

A patellofemoral joint reaction force is generated during knee extension. This force creates compressive loads at approximately half the body weight during ambulation, approximately three times body weight during stair climbing, and approximately seven times body weight during squat activity.[55,59] Normal contact areas

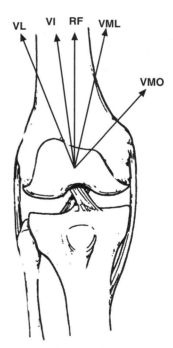

Figure 14–2 Approximate action lines of the components of the quadriceps: vastus lateralis (VL), vastus intermedius (VI), rectus femoris (RF), vastus medialis longus (VML), and vastus medialis oblique (VMO).

of the patella and trochlear groove vary as a function of range of motion in a defined manner.[56,60–62] When there is proper balance of muscle tension and passive restraints acting on the patella, it tracks along the femoral trochlear groove in a way that compressive loading from the patellofemoral joint reaction force is optimally dissipated at the articular surfaces. Pathomechanical situations arise in which abnormally located, excessively compressive loads and lateral displacement are imparted to the patella, leading to acute and cumulative trauma.[49,53,59,63]

Role of the VM

Contrary to early descriptions, the VM is active throughout knee extension range of motion.[1,64,65] Along with the rest of the quadriceps, the VM is most active at terminal range during active knee extension in sitting and at the nadir of a closed chain squat, with more activity displayed during the concentric than in the eccentric phase.[1,66] In contrast to the phasic action of the rectus femoris, and to a lesser extent to that of the VL, the VM is tonically active during rapid flexion–extension movements of the knee.[67]

On the basis of anatomic, physiologic, and mechanical criteria,[57,58,68] as well as of innervation and perhaps morphologic characteristics,[69] the VM can be functionally classified into two distinct portions. The proximal component, or vastus medialis longus, acts with a fiber orientation of 15 to 18 degrees medially from the longitudinal femoral axis, mechanically contributes to knee extension, and may share a common spinal and peripheral innervation with that of the vastus intermedius. The VMO is so named for its oblique fiber orientation of 40 to 60 degrees.[53,57] Fibers of the VMO originate from the adductor magnus tendon, medial intermuscular septum, and adductor longus tendon.[58,69] These fibers insert onto the patella and medial retinaculum, and superficially onto the rectus femoris tendon. The spinal and peripheral innervations of the VMO

are distinct from that of the vastus medialis longus.[69] It is likely that the VMO does not contribute directly to knee extension torque and its activity is not required to effect the "screw home" mechanism of the knee at terminal extension.[57] Rather, the VMO provides dynamic medial stabilization of the patella and is believed to be of primary importance in resisting lateral patellar displacement.[47,57]

The fibers of the VL attach to the patella at an angle between 12 and 15 degrees and, unlike the rectus femoris, vastus intermedius, or vastus medialis longus, are capable of direct lateral displacement of the patella.[57] Thus these four muscles act synergistically to extend the knee, and the unique role of the VMO is to function as an antagonist to the lateral force of the VL. By balancing patellar tracking, the VMO increases the mechanical efficiency of the VL as a knee extensor.[57] The capacities of VL and VMO to produce frontal plane forces are determined by their respective insertion locations on the patella, angles of fiber insertion, cross-sectional dimensions, morphologic characteristics, and properties relating to active neuromuscular recruitment. In addition to the anatomic differences discussed above, the cross-sectional area of the VL exceeds that of the VM and a moderately greater proportion of type II fibers is found in the VL compared with that in the VM.[70] It is obvious that a complex interplay of dynamic and passive factors contributes to balanced patellar tracking.

The quadriceps components, specifically including the VM, are reflexively inhibited by pain and joint effusion,[25,71] the effects perhaps being greater at terminal extension.[29] Spencer and colleagues[27] showed that the VM is inhibited after a saline injection of 20 to 30 mL into the knee joint space, whereas an injection of 50 to 60 mL is required to reach the threshold for reflex inhibition for the VL and rectus femoris. Some clinicians have suggested that the VMO atrophies first and is last to be rehabilitated.[49] Others[57] have argued that the prominence of the VMO is more apparent because of its thinner fascial covering and fiber obliquity, and that

VMO atrophy simply reflects generalized quadriceps muscle weakness.

SEMG in Discrimination of VMO:VL Function

SEMG seems to be an attractive tool for clinicians in identifying VMO insufficiency. Without a practical way of isolating the force contributions of VMO and VL, and with a lack of a simple, reliable means of assessing patellofemoral kinematics, SEMG adds a unique dimension of information to the evaluation process. Recording with SEMG allows for relatively quick, low-cost assessment and collection of objective data regarding muscle function. If PFPS is truly a multifactorial problem, and if VMO insufficiency can be confidently ruled in or out for particular patients by analysis with SEMG, treatment might be directed to meet the peculiar needs of each patient. Insufficiency of the VMO could be a contributory factor for some patients and not others. Patients who have PFPS with VMO insufficiency might need to work on VMO strengthening or improved motor control timing. Other patients might demonstrate normal VMO function but presumably faulty lower extremity kinetic chain mechanics and passive tightness. In an era of cost containment, SEMG assessment might help to assign the greatest resource value to each patient.

Results of early work with both surface and intramuscular electrodes established that VM and VL EMG activity tends to be relatively balanced in timing and magnitude during knee extension in healthy subjects.[1,29,64,72,73] Results of other studies specifically targeting the VMO and VL were similar, without a clear tendency of one muscle's recruitment to exceed the other during routine quadriceps contraction.[21,65,74–81] Taken together, these investigations argue for similar VMO and VL EMG patterns as the norm. The investigators used a variety of recording techniques and quantification methods. Isometric, concentric, and eccentric quadriceps contractions were tested throughout joint range of motion, and both open and closed kinetic chain conditions were included.

Another methodologic approach has been to generate a mathematical ratio of VMO and VL EMG activity. This method has intuitive appeal as a basis for standardized patient and exercise comparisons, and it has been adopted by a number of investigators. Integrated or root-mean-square SEMG amplitude scores have been used most commonly to produce VMO:VL ratios.

Several groups have published results for healthy subjects. Souza and Gross[82] reported normalized VMO:VL SEMG amplitude ratios during 25% of maximal volitional effort isometric knee extension in sitting, stair ascent, and stair descent. SEMG ratios for VMO:VL function were 0.96 ± 0.17, 1.15 ± 0.36, and 1.18 ± 0.22, respectively, or 1.10 ± 0.27 overall across the three conditions. Cuddeford and associates[83] studied stationary bike, single leg quarter squat, step-up, isometric quadriceps setting, straight leg raising, and short arc knee extension exercises by using normalized VMO:VL activity ratios. SEMG ratios ranged from 0.71 ± 0.52 (straight leg raising) to 1.19 ± 0.44 (bike) and averaged 1.15 ± 0.42 across closed chain exercises and 0.77 ± 0.41 across open chain exercises. Karst and Jewett[68] used normalized data to calculate VMO:VL ratios ranging from approximately 0.8 ± 0.23 to 1.0 ± 0.08 during maximal effort quadriceps setting and several submaximal variations of quadriceps setting plus straight leg raising. Kasman and colleagues[84] generated normalized VMO:VL activity ratios from subjects positioned in recumbent sitting as a function of isometric contraction intensity. There was a significant trend for VMO:VL ratios to increase as contraction intensity decreased, with ratio values ranging from 0.84 ± 0.19 to 1.22 ± 0.49. SEMG activity ratios for VMO and VL derived from nonnormalized data have been reported at a similar range,[85–87] somewhat higher,[88,89] or somewhat lower.[82] Normalized amplitude comparisons generated from fine wire EMG recordings during a large number of knee extension exercises produced VMO:VL ratios ranging from 1.0 to 1.3.[90] Thus results of study with both surface and intramuscular electrodes have proved to be broadly consistent for healthy subjects across diverse conditions, especially when normalization procedures have been included.

A number of investigators have attempted to discriminate between patients with PFPS and healthy subjects by using SEMG methods (Table 14–1). Of the 11 studies reviewed, results of 9 revealed differences in SEMG activity between these two groups[76,78,82,88,91–95]; results of the other two[96,97] failed to show any differences. In 10 of the studies, VM or VMO and VL activity was specifically compared with that of VL. In 6 of those 10, selective VM or VMO versus VL effects of PFPS were revealed,[76,82,88,93–95] whereas in four,[78,92,96,97] no selective differences were identified. Results of an additional study[98]—not included in Table 14–1 but discussed later—documented responsiveness of VMO:VL ratios to a rehabilitation training program that was associated with patient improvement. These contrasting results may be due to different criteria for subject inclusion, as well as to differences in tested activities, SEMG measurement techniques, and data management.

In five of the studies, SEMG activity was evaluated during seated isometric contractions,[76,78,82,88,92] and in one of those,[82] step-up and step-down procedures were also used. Seated isokinetic knee extension was tested in another study,[93] treadmill running was studied in another report,[97] and seated patellar tendon reflex latencies were investigated in the other three studies.[94–96] It may be that VMO and VL activity patterns are differentially affected by subtle but significant effects of joint angle, contraction type (isometric, concentric, or eccentric), contraction intensity, and open versus closed kinetic chains.[82,84,86,86,89] In some of the studies, SEMG activity from the symptomatic knee was compared with that in the asymptomatic knee within the same patient.[78,82,91,93] In other cases, data recorded from healthy subjects were used for comparison against those of the affected knees of patients.[76,82,88,92,94–97] Two groups found that SEMG

VMO:VL activity of each knee of unilaterally symptomatic patients was similar to each other but different from that in knees of healthy subjects.[82,95] Hence sole use of the contralateral side for comparison in unilaterally symptomatic patients with PFPS may be inadequate.

PFPS may take in a heterogeneous patient population. At the outset of this section on PFPS, it was stated that many different factors are believed to contribute to the disorder. For example, greater Q angles are often found with this syndrome.[44] Larger Q angles in PFPS patients are associated with smaller VMO:VL activity ratios.[9] Because the Q angle affects VMO:VL activity ratios and because Q angles vary with gender,[43] it may be important to gender match experimental groups. Gender effects have been suggested in experimental SEMG recordings of quadriceps components.[74] Further, age is a predictor of PFPS rehabilitation outcome and it may be important to match or stratify patients on this parameter.[99] It also seems unlikely that patients with recurrent subluxations or frank chondromalacia would test the same as patients with hypomobility problems. Many of the investigators accepted PFPS subjects with a variety of clinical diagnoses or provided nonspecific clinical descriptions of their samples. Perhaps some subpopulations with this syndrome show altered VMO and VL activity and others do not. Finally, normalization of SEMG amplitude scores is an accepted practice to reduce data variance.[100,101] As alluded to above, such procedures may be useful in studying VMO and VL activity. Yet several of the investigators did not normalize their data for comparisons across recording sites and between subjects, and the normalization procedures used by others are potentially confounding.[82,97] Souza and Gross[82] provide a compelling argument that if the relative activities of VMO and VL are aberrant in the same way for the normalizing reference contraction as they are for the test activity, true differences between patients with PFPS and healthy subjects would be obscured.

The VMO:VL ratiometric approach may not be straightforward for a few more reasons. It can be speculated that the SEMG activity ratio has different biomechanical implications in different cases. Perhaps PFPS subjects should be trained to a greater VMO:VL ratio value to compensate with dynamic muscle control for deficient structural elements. That is, patients potentially require a greater VMO:VL ratio than that required by healthy subjects to achieve the same patellofemoral tracking efficiency (Figure 14–3A). The activity of each muscle is typically expressed as a percentage of maximal voluntary isometric contraction (%MVIC) for normalization before ratio calculation. A 5% MVIC VMO:5% MVIC VL ratio may not have the same effect on dissipation of the patellofemoral joint reaction force as a 50% MVIC VMO:50% MVIC VL ratio, despite that both ratios are computed as 1.0 (Figure 14–3B). These models would account for many of the experimental findings discussed above. Patients with PFPS would be characterized as showing depressed activity of the VMO in relation to the VL, or producing nonspecific changes in the intensity of quadriceps recruitment, depending on the patient and task type. In a patient with active pain and effusion, the VMO might be more inhibited, and a lower VMO:VL ratio would result. Decreases in both VMO and VL activity would be seen with maximal effort contraction in the presence of quadriceps atrophy. This would occur because of neurophysiologic factors and loss of cross-sectional volume. However, greater nonspecific SEMG activity could be produced at submaximal loads to compensate for inefficient excitation–contraction coupling. Thus a depressed VMO:VL ratio would indicate muscle imbalance, but a ratio approximating 1.0 would not in and of itself rule out muscle insufficiency.

Multiple investigators have commented on patellofemoral dysfunction from the perspective of faulty timing and neuromuscular control.[67,94,102] Their view is one of motor control imbalance through a functional range of motion arc rather than through simple strength or SEMG peak amplitude differences. Indeed, peak SEMG activity from the VMO and VL is limited to about 5% of maximum while a patient arises

from a partial squat,[80] making it unlikely that weakness is the pivotal factor in producing patellofemoral dysfunction during this motion. To the extent that the VMO and VL are antagonistic to each other for medial–lateral dynamic control of the patella and ultimately synergistic to the other quadriceps components for efficient biomechanical function of the knee, their recruitment levels must be appropriately timed to each other and to the other quadriceps components for any given functional task. Studies that limit testing to peak SEMG amplitude comparisons during isometric contractions may be insensitive to timing issues.

Karst and Willet[96] did not detect any onset timing differences of VMO and VL in PFPS patients and healthy subjects after tendon tap, nor after initiation of concentric knee extension in sitting, or a concentric step-up task. However, Voight and Wieder[94] and Witvrouw and associates[95] identified altered VMO and VL reflex latency patterns in response to patellar tendon tap in PFPS. Decrements in VMO/VL onset timing related to PFPS during voluntary contraction also have been reported.[103] In none of these studies was there an attempt to track motor function throughout a functional range of motion arc. Souza and Gross[82] did find differences between PFPS patients and healthy control subjects in peak VMO:VL activity extracted during functional concentric and eccentric stepping tasks. MacIntyre and Robertson,[97] using an SEMG ensemble averaging technique throughout the gait cycle, could not demonstrate any changes in VM and VL function between PFPS patients and controls during treadmill running.

Perhaps the most thorough EMG study that addresses timing and function was reported by Powers and colleagues.[79] Intramuscular fine wire electrodes were used to record EMG activity from the VMO, vastus medialis longus, VL, and vastus intermedius during free-speed–level walking, fast-level walking, stair ascent, stair descent, ramp ascent, and ramp descent. No differences in activity onset, nor cessation, were detected among the muscles for either PFPS patients or healthy control subjects. In addition,

Table 14–1 SEMG Discrimination of Subjects with Patellofemoral Pain Syndrome

Study	Subject Groups	SEMG Sites	SEMG Measure	Tested Activities
Mariano & Caruso, 1979[76]	Preoperative unilateral patellar subluxation Healthy controls	VMO, VL	Visual inspection of peak-to-peak amplitude	Seated concentric knee extension
Moller et al, 1986[78]	Unilateral patellar instability Unilateral idiopathic chondromalacia Asymptomatic knees of same subjects	VMO, VL	Zero crossings	Maximal effort isometric seated knee extension at 0, 15, 30, 45, 60, and 90 degrees
Doxey & Eisenman, 1987[91]	Unilateral PFPS Asymptomatic knees of same subjects	Distal aspect of quadriceps, medial–lateral	Integral average, submaximal testing normalized to seated 100% MVIC	Seated isometric extension—maximal and submaximal with 0.56 kg and 2.72 kg lower extremity loads at 0 and 40 degrees
Petschnig et al, 1991[93]	Unilateral unspecified knee pain, injury Asymptomatic knees of same subjects	Distal aspect of VM, VL	Ordinal ranking of amplitudes and activity patterns	Seated concentric knee extension from 90 to 20 degrees, at a constant velocity of 10 degrees/second
Souza & Gross, 1991[82]	Symptomatic knees of subjects with unilateral PFPS Asymptomatic knees of same subjects with PFPS Healthy controls	VMO, VL	Integral average, normalized to seated 100% MVIC, VMO:VL ratios	Seated knee extension at 25% MVIC torque level, 10 inch step-up, 10 inch step-down
Voight & Wieder, 1991[94]	PFPS Healthy controls	VMO, VL	VMO, VL response latencies	Seated patellar tendon reflex elicitation

Results	Comments
Decreased VMO activity relative to VL in subjects with subluxation, compared with control subjects, especially in terminal extension range.	Restoration of normal SEMG patterns after surgery. No quantification or statistical testing. Small subject number.
No differences between VMO and VL activity counts in symptomatic versus asymptomatic knees.	Investigators suggest a trend toward deceased activity from VMO and VL in both PFPS groups relative to asymptomatic knees at 45 degrees.
Significantly decreased maximal activity, but significantly greater submaximal activity under all tested conditions, from symptomatic compared with asymptomatic knees.	Investigators suggest symptomatic knees displayed decreased maximal activity due to pain-induced inhibition and increased submaximal activity due to decreased limb efficiency.
Decreased peak torque and SEMG activity from injured compared with uninjured knees. No significant SEMG activity differences between VMO and VL. Significant differences in VMO activity as a function of joint angle and VL as a function of joint angle from injured versus uninjured sides.	Investigators suggest a trend of VMO dominance in terminal range of uninjured knees that is reversed in injured knees. Statistical methods and interpretation are difficult to understand, and relationship between conclusions and data is not clear.
No significant differences between PFPS symptomatic knees, asymptomatic knees, and control knees in VMO:VL activity ratios with use of normalized data. With use of nonnormalized data, significantly lower VMO:VL activity ratios for both knees of unilateral PFPS subjects compared with findings in control subjects.	Investigators proposed that significant differences between groups might have been masked by normalization (ie, if VMO:VL ratios were aberrant during 100% MVIC normalizing contraction and during test contractions in a similar way, between-group differences would be obscured).
Significantly shorter VMO, compared with VL, response latencies in healthy subjects. Significantly shorter VL, compared with VMO, response latencies in PFPS subjects. Significantly shorter VL response latencies in PFPS subjects compared with controls; no between group differences in VMO latencies.	Investigators believe their results argue against VMO inhibition in PFPS patients, noting reversal in VMO/VL firing order was caused by a decrease in VL latency in PFPS subjects. They suggest changes in motor control timing may be a critical factor in PFPS.

continues

Table 14–1 continued

Study	Subject Groups	EMG Sites	EMG Measure	Tested Activities
Boucher et al, 1992[88]	PFPS Healthy controls	VMO, VML, VL	Integral amplitude VMO:VL ratios	100% MVIC seated knee extension at 15, 30, and 90 degrees
Grabiner et al, 1992[92]	Symptomatic knees of subjects with unilateral and bilateral PFPS Healthy controls	VMO, VL	Integral average, normalized to seated 50% MVIC; normalized peak force, peak rate of force change	Seated knee extension: ~ 3 second ramp 0%–100% MVIC Constant 20%, 80% MVIC Immediate step 0%–100% MVIC
MacIntyre & Robertson, 1992[97]	Recreational runners with PFPS Healthy recreational runners	RF, VM, VL motor points	Ensemble–averaged, linear envelope amplitude, normalized as % maximal value of stride cycle	Treadmill running at 80% of normal speed and 12 km/hour
Karst & Willet, 1995[96]	Symptomatic knees of subjects with unilateral and bilateral PFPS Healthy controls	VMO, VL	VMO, VL onset latency differences	Seated patellar tendon reflex elicitation, seated voluntary knee extension, 8 cm lateral step-up
Witvrouw et al, 1996[95]	Symptomatic and asymptomatic knees of subjects with unilateral/bilateral PFPS Healthy controls	VMO, VL	VMO, VL response latencies and latency differences	Seated patellar tendon reflex elicitation

Results	*Comments*
No significant differences across primary subject groups. Isolation of subjects with Q angles > 22 degrees revealed decreased VMO:VL versus findings in controls at 15 degrees knee extension. No significant VML effects.	Investigators suggested caution with terminal range exercises. Mechanical factors may start PFPS. Neuromuscular dysfunction may have an additive effect in chronic or severe cases. Results support differential function of VMO and VML.
Decreased PFPS group peak ramp and step force. Decreased PFPS group peak rate of force change during step contractions. Decreased VMO and VL SEMG amplitudes during step contractions in PFPS versus control group. No selective VMO or VL intergroup differences.	SEMG data during ramp contractions collected at peak force. Averaged SEMG data during constant force contractions. SEMG data during step condition collected at force initiation. Investigators speculate that findings may represent disuse atrophy or inhibition of high threshold motor units in PFPS.
No significant differences in activity between subjects with PFPS and healthy runners over the stride cycle.	Normalization method may have been suboptimal; no significant differences using nonnormalized data.
No significant effects between subject groups in VMO/VL onset timing differences during any test conditions.	Investigators propose that reflex latencies are not suitable for clinical PFPS assessment and that clinical SEMG devices are largely inadequate to assess subtle timing phenomena.
Significantly shorter VMO, compared with VL, response latencies in healthy subjects. Response sequence reversed in both symptomatic and asymptomatic PFPS knees.	General agreement with Voight and Wieder, 1991. Also suggested that changes in VL are the critical factor and that PFPS can be thought of in terms of muscle balance and neuromotor control.

Abbreviations: PFPS, patellofemoral pain syndrome; %MVIC, percentage of maximal volitional isometric contraction; RF, rectus femoris muscle; SEMG, surface electromyograph; VL, vastus lateralis muscle; VM, vastus medialis muscle; VML, vastus medialis longus muscle; VMO, vastus medialis oblique muscle.

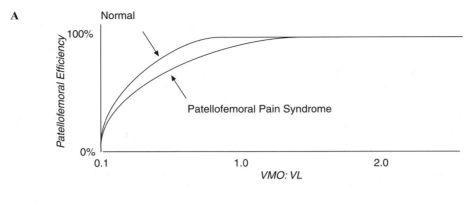

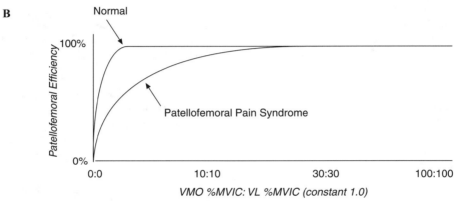

Figure 14–3 Speculative effects of vastus medialis oblique (VMO) and vastus lateralis (VL) on mechanical efficiency of the patellofemoral joint. (**A**) Potential changes in the relationship between normalized VMO:VL SEMG ratios and patellofemoral efficiency in normal and dysfunctional conditions. (**B**) Absolute SEMG activity levels of VMO and VL—each expressed as a percentage of maximum voluntary isometric contraction (%MVIC)—vary. The VMO:VL ratio, however, remains constant at 1.0. Patients with patellofemoral dysfunction are represented as less efficient than healthy subjects at an equivalent %MVIC intensity, until a certain intensity is reached. Patients might gain efficiency by either increasing the VMO:VL ratio (**A**) or raising both VMO and VL activity levels to a greater intensity (**B**).

there were no selective differences in VMO and VL mean intensities, each respectively normalized to seated maximal effort contractions. However, the vastus muscles of patients with PFPS subjects demonstrated generally decreased mean intensities, compared with findings in healthy subjects, during the level walking and ramp tasks. There was also a general delay in onset of vastus muscle activity in the PFPS group during fast-level walking and ramp descent, as well as a later cessation during stair descent. Thus selec-

tive VMO:VL effects in PFPS patients were not supported, although nonspecific trends among the vastus muscles were observed.

A number of methodologic issues and implications were discussed in an expert panel commentary that followed this report.[104] A point of consensus among panel members was that patients with PFPS probably represent a heterogeneous population. Because of practical considerations, Powers and associates[79] did not attempt to discriminate among different types of patients with this syndrome. The same point has been raised regarding earlier investigations, and the development of a valid and reliable classification system is needed to resolve conflicting study results.

Another plausible explanation for selective VMO:VL effects is that the fatigue resistance of the VMO might be lower than that of the VL in PFPS patients. Runners with PFPS do not differ from healthy control subjects in isokinetic strength, but they do vary in isokinetic endurance parameters.[44] Large numbers of task repetitions have, for the most part, not been studied with SEMG and PFPS subjects. Fatigability can be assessed by analyzing the frequency spectrum of the SEMG signal. In brief, the frequency spectrum shifts toward lower values as fatigue is produced.[1] There are no selective differences in frequency analyses from VMO and VL recordings after repeated isometric contractions or terminal knee extension exercises in healthy subjects.[105] However, this issue has yet to be studied in PFPS patients and in none of the previously reviewed investigations was there an attempt to monitor the effects of sustained or repeated contractions to a fatigue point.

The authors have observed numerous PFPS cases wherein SEMG VMO:VL activity has seemed depressed in magnitude (Figure 14–4). Open chain testing has been included, but emphasis has been primarily on the closed chain. Closed chain tasks more appropriately reflect functional limitations in PFPS patients. Activities have included unilateral weight acceptance during gait, step-ups, step-downs, leg press exercise, partial squats, and lunge steps. At times, similar VMO and VL peak magnitudes have been observed, but the recruitment timing of the VMO has appeared altered relative to that of the VL through a functional range of motion arc. Sometimes such changes are observed only during closed chain tasks, with relatively unremarkable activity during open chain tasks (Figure 14–5). Other patients show changes in magnitude or timing relationships only during the eccentric phase of closed chain maneuvers and particularly through range of motion arcs that correlate

to subjective pain reports (Figure 14–6). Recommendations for SEMG assessment of PFPS patients are summarized in Application Guide 14–B. Not all patients with this syndrome require SEMG evaluation.

Effects of Specific Exercises on VMO and VL Activity

Rehabilitative exercises have long been proposed for PFPS.[37,45] Investigators using surface and intramuscular EMG have sought to identify particular positions or exercises that selectively enhance components of the quadriceps, and the VM or VMO in particular. Early reports indicated that selective VM recruitment during knee extension could be facilitated by foot and ankle movements or tibial rotation in some persons, although no clear trend was identified across subjects and studies.[1,106–108]

A subsequent body of work has emerged that, with few exceptions, has failed to identify any exercise that selectively enhances the VM or VMO in a statistically significant way. Results of systematic studies have not supported tibial rotation maneuvers in healthy subjects,[36,65,90] nor effects of ankle and foot position during quadriceps contraction in healthy subjects or patients with PFPS.[90] Also, there is no evidence for selective VMO recruitment during quadriceps setting at various joint angles in either healthy subjects[65,90] or patients with PFPS,[77,90] nor during straight leg raising in healthy subjects or patients with knee pathology.[21,68,109–111] In fact, normalized peak activity from both VM and VL muscles is lower during maximally resisted straight leg raising than during maximal effort quadriceps setting.[110,111] Conscious combination of quadriceps setting with straight leg raising does not seem to make a difference.[68] A sustained training program with quadriceps setting produces general increases in SEMG activity, but it has no selective effects.[77] Conjoint lateral hip rotation with straight leg raising also does not increase VM, VMO:VL, or VMO:VML function, compared with standard straight leg raising.[1,68,81] Maximal hip lateral rotation is infe-

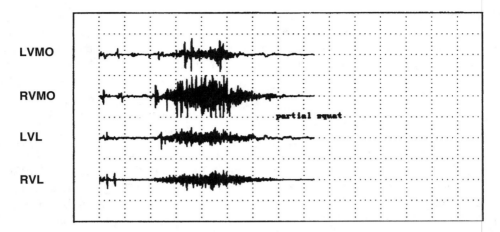

Figure 14–4 SEMG activity of the (**L**) left and (**R**) right (**VMO**) vastus medialis oblique and (**VL**) vastus lateralis during a bilateral symmetric partial squat. Signals were recorded from a patient with chronic left patellofemoral pain syndrome. Lower extremity alignment and weight bearing were symmetric throughout the procedure.

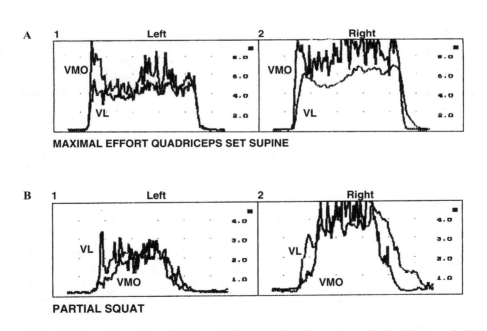

Figure 14–5 SEMG activity of the (**L**) left and (**R**) right (**VMO**) vastus medialis oblique and (**VL**) vastus lateralis, recorded from a patient with chronic bilateral patellofemoral pain syndrome after bilateral lateral release surgery. (**A**) Activity for (**1**) left VMO and VL and (**2**) right VMO and VL during open chain (supine) isometric quadriceps set at 0 degrees of knee flexion. (**B**) Activity for (**1**) left VMO and VL and (**2**) right VMO and VL during bilateral symmetric partial squat. Note the change in relative VMO and VL timing relationships from open to closed chain conditions.

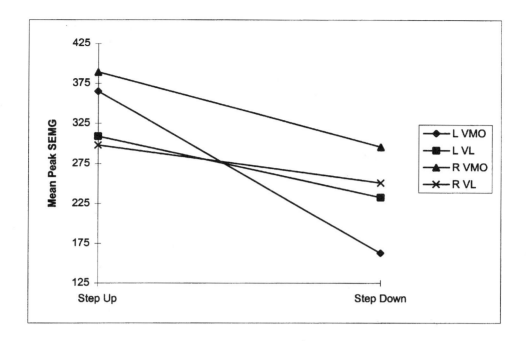

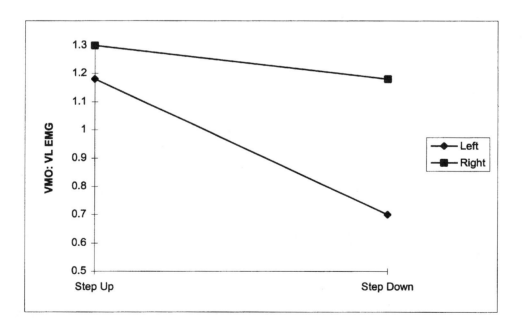

Figure 14–6 SEMG activity of the (**VMO**) vastus medialis oblique and (**VL**) vastus lateralis during step-up (concentric) and step-down (eccentric) maneuvers recorded frpm a patient with chronic left patellofemoral pain syndrome. Note the change in relative VMO and VL activity patterns from concentric to eccentric conditions.

rior to hip medial rotation positioning when terminal knee extension exercises are performed.[90] With healthy subjects, standard terminal knee extension exercises do not produce significant differences in fatigue-related SEMG frequency data between VMO and VL muscles,[105] do not improve patellar alignment as assessed by radiographic studies,[112] nor do they selectively affect VMO or VL intramuscular EMG amplitudes.[21,90] Addition of hamstring co-activation to short arc knee extension does not selectively change VMO or VL amplitudes in healthy subjects.[21]

Rehabilitative programs for PFPS that incorporate quadriceps setting, straight leg raising, and terminal knee extension exercises have been heavily promoted and seem to be associated with improvement for patients.[45,49,52,53,113,114] Despite this positive trend, there is no evidence that these exercises selectively enhance the function of the VMO relative to the VL. The rationale for use of quadriceps setting (in full extension), straight leg raising, and terminal knee extension exercises has been that the patellofemoral joint reaction force is relatively low, and that the exercises are well tolerated by patients.[37,61,81] Results of early studies also showed that greater levels of quadriceps recruitment are produced at the terminal range of active knee extension.[39,72,86,95] This latter effect is probably due to decreased mechanical efficiency of the extensor mechanism in the terminal range.[64] As stated earlier, there is no enhancement of VMO activity relative to that of the VL as the knee approaches full extension. It is generally agreed that although these exercise methods are useful in producing gains in general quadriceps strength, they are unlikely to affect VMO:VL balance.[36,68,77,90,105,112]

Grabiner and colleagues[115] have reviewed this apparent lack of selective EMG effect with common knee exercises. They have speculated that there might be some threshold level of VMO function required for satisfactory patellofemoral tracking. Atrophy might decrease the force-generating ability of all quadriceps components, including the VMO. According to this line of thinking, exercise results in general quadriceps recruitment and strength gain, which bring the VMO above its threshold level. There are reports of nonselective alterations in VMO and VL EMG activity in knees of patients with PFPS versus knees of healthy subjects that lend support to this view.[78,92]

Selective effects on SEMG amplitude VMO:VL ratios were, however, demonstrated by Sczepanski and associates[89] with isokinetic exercise in healthy subjects. A higher VMO:VL ratio was noted with concentric contractions at 120 degrees per second, compared with eccentric contractions at 120 degrees per second, or concentric contractions at 60 degrees per second. These investigators also found a significantly greater VMO:VL ratio for the 60- to 85-degree arc of motion than the 35- to 60-degree arc, which in turn yielded a greater VMO:VL ratio than the 10- to 35-degree arc. The investigators concluded that arc of motion, as well as contraction type combined with angular velocity, were important parameters to consider.

The exercises discussed so far focus on work in the open kinetic chain. The use of closed chain rehabilitation has been strongly advocated for PFPS.[37,116] McConnell[102,117,118] believes it is appropriate to correct patellofemoral arthrokinematics with taping techniques and thus enable patients to tolerate functional closed chain activities. She postulates that this method improves the length–tension relationship of the VMO and, along with similar comments by Shelton and Thigpen,[37] emphasizes that the problem of VMO retraining can be thought of in terms of motor skill acquisition, learning, and functional task performance. Higher VM:VL or VMO:VL activity has been reported with SEMG during certain closed chain tasks, compared with findings with traditional open chain exercises.[82,83,85,119] This trend is consistent with the author's recommendations, favoring unilateral stance, step-up, squat, lunges, and leg press. The effect is not apparent, though, in two reports with the use of fine wire intramuscular electrodes with both closed and open chain exercises.[21,90] As an aside, the SEMG activity of the

VM is facilitated (and that of the medial gastrocnemius, semimembranosus, and rectus femoris is inhibited) when graded hip extension contractions are added to knee extension efforts in an open chain.[120] Hip extension is naturally combined with knee extension in the closed chain, and perhaps there is a facilitory effect on the monoarticular extensors and the VM in particular.

Another area of uncertainty relates to the effect of adductor activity on VMO function. Because fibers of the VMO take origin from the adductor tendons and disruption of these attachments has been identified in patients with recurrent patellar dislocations,[58,69] clinical use of hip adduction exercises has been proposed by several investigators.[3,36,58,74,80,102] Wheatley and Jahnke[108] recorded with surface electrodes and noted increased VM activity with adductor activation. Hanten and Schulties[36] used intramuscular electrodes to show that normalized VMO activity was significantly greater than VL activity during non–weight-bearing maximal effort hip adduction. They tested adduction resistance applied to the distal aspect of the thigh, without a directed knee extension effort and without measuring knee extension torque. Grabiner and coworkers[121] also used intramuscular recordings and tested the effect of hip adduction on non–weight-bearing isometric knee extensor contractions at several intensities. Normalized VMO and VL activity levels were not changed by the addition of 50% maximum isometric hip adductor force to the knee extensor efforts. Andriacchi and associates[122] found that addition of graded abduction moments to a knee flexion moment produced changes in VM and VL intramuscular EMG activity at some knee joint angles. Although not directly compared, alterations in VM and VL activity in their report seem to follow parallel trends, without an apparent differential effect.

Using surface recordings, Karst and Jewett[68] did not find a facilitative influence of concomitant adductor contraction on VMO:VL or VMO:vastus medialis longus activity. They supplied 5% body weight adduction resistance with a pulley apparatus affixed to the distal aspect of the leg. Adductor contraction was added to quadriceps setting plus straight leg raising with 5% body weight ankle cuff load. There was no effect of adductor contraction when compared to quadriceps setting/straight leg raising alone, nor with maximal effort quadriceps setting alone.

Finally, Hodges and Richardson[85] studied VMO:VL SEMG activity in both weight-bearing and non–weight-bearing conditions with addition of 15%, 50%, and maximal hip adductor force to knee extension. Their weight-bearing position consisted of maintenance of 60 degrees of knee extension and 60 degrees of hip extension in a squat position. The non–weight-bearing position involved the same joint angles in supine without external load applied to the leg. There was no attempt to control for equivalent knee extensor loads. Average VMO:VL baseline activity was greater in the weight-bearing posture than in the non–weight-bearing position. Increased VMO:VL ratios were produced by addition of each of the adductor contractions in the weight-bearing position. However, only the maximal adductor contraction increased VMO:VL activity in the non–weight-bearing posture.

Collectively, this existing evidence runs contrary to the notion of adductor facilitation of VMO recruitment during open chain knee extension, unless perhaps very high intensity contractions are used. Improved effects may be produced with closed chain exercise. None of the investigations included PFPS patients, nor a series of conditioning exercise sessions. Both might be important variables for study.

The most effective method of exercise prescription for individual patients with VMO insufficiency may be to assess SEMG responses during trial of various movement tasks. Emphasis should be placed on SEMG evaluation of functionally relevant exercises in the closed chain. Assessed with SEMG, this is one practical aspect of exercise that supports higher VMO:VL activity with consistency.[82,83,85] Motor programming schema (see Chapter 3) for VMO and VL function will probably differ for purposeful closed chain movements versus open chain exercises. Thus exercise prescription can be viewed from the standpoint of neural adaptation and training in addition to peripheral conditioning effects.[123] This perspective is not meant to imply that open chain exercises should be excluded but, rather, that exercise prescription should include functional considerations. If certain exercises act to facilitate the VM selectively, they may be relatively idiosyncratic. Specific recommendations are listed in Application Guide 14–B.

SEMG Feedback Training

A number of investigators have promoted the use of SEMG feedback to retrain the VM or VMO.[37,98,102,106,112] SEMG feedback coupled with exercise has produced outcomes superior to those with exercise alone or exercise combined with NMES in patients with knee problems other than PFPS.[22,23,35,124] SEMG feedback from the rectus femoris has produced greater gains in knee extension torque when combined with exercise, compared with findings in exercise-only in no treatment control groups.[125]

McConnell[102,118] has suggested that VMO feedback training may be combined with patellofemoral taping. The latter treatment has become popular with many physical therapists as part of a core approach to PFPS. Although such taping techniques reduce symptomatic complaints, they do not seem to alter VMO:VL activity assessed with fine wire EMG electrodes.[90] Patellofemoral taping and SEMG feedback training may each be useful in rehabilitation, but perhaps through different mechanisms or in different subpopulations. Application of NMES to facilitate and strengthen the VMO has also been proposed by several groups,[3,114,126] and the concept of SEMG feedback combined with NMES has been suggested for knee rehabilitation programs.[23,127] Thus quadriceps SEMG feedback seems generally useful in rehabilitation, and options exist for innovative combination, of SEMG training with other therapies.

Several investigators have systematically examined the effects of SEMG feedback training from VMO and VL with reference to PFPS.

Wise and colleagues[98] trained patients diagnosed with PFPS to increase the activity of the VMO and maintain stable VL activity by using SEMG feedback. Patients used auditory and visual feedback during a progressive series of exercises. Phase I consisted of one to two orientation sessions of quadriceps setting and straight leg raising with the use of a 7.5:7.5 second work:rest cycle, as well as a supplementary home exercise program of 10 repetitions of each of these two exercises with the same timing two times per day. Phase II was implemented over two to six sessions and was similar to phase I except that patients were instructed to increase VMO activity and maintain VL activity at baseline. Terminal knee extension exercises and resistive cuff weights were then added at the therapist's discretion. Once patients became pain free, they entered phase III, during which they practiced VMO:VL training while bicycling, ambulating, and stair climbing. Total training lasted 4 to 6 weeks. Patients decreased their pain and returned to desired functional activities. Pretraining quadriceps setting VMO:VL ratios ranged from 0.38 to 0.79. Posttraining VMO:VL ratios ranged from 0.64 to 1.0. No attempt was made to normalize the SEMG data across sessions or subjects, and no formal statistical tests were reported. It is not clear whether data collection before and after training took place at equivalent contraction intensities. A control group was not included in the design.

LeVeau and Rogers[106] demonstrated that healthy subjects can be trained to increase the activity of the VM compared with that of the VL by using SEMG feedback. Subjects practiced for 30 minutes 5 days per week for 3 weeks with seated isometric contractions. For each day of training, each subject's isometric one repetition maximum load was determined, and 80% of that load was used as reference contraction for VM and VL SEMG activity levels. Each day's work consisted of 5 sets of 6 contractions, each set separated by a 30-second rest. Throughout the experiment, subjects received visual feedback when VM activity exceeded the VM training threshold, and auditory feedback when VL activity exceeded the VL threshold level. During the initial 2 weeks, subjects attempted to contract the VM to 25% or greater of that day's SEMG reference level while progressively reducing VL recruitment. Subjects had difficulty reducing VL activity without also decreasing VM activity. Hence there was little change in relative balance over the training period. During the third training week, subjects succeeded in increasing VM recruitment while maintaining VL activity below threshold level, producing a significant training effect. The investigators therefore believed that uptraining the VM was a more successful strategy than downtraining the VL.

Also using healthy subjects, Ingersoll and Knight[112] showed that VMO feedback can result in improved patellofemoral congruence. They trained one group of subjects with the Daily Adjustable Progressive Resistive Exercise technique for four sets of 20-degree terminal knee extension exercises three times per week for 3 weeks. A second group of normal subjects worked three times per week for 3 weeks with a SEMG feedback program with the use of auditory and visual cues for VMO and VL feedback. Subjects receiving feedback increased SEMG activity of the VMO while minimizing that of the VL through a progressive series of exercises, including quadriceps setting, straight leg raising, terminal knee extension, stationary bicycle, ambulation, and stair climbing. A third group of normal subjects served as untrained control subjects. SEMG data were not reported, but subjects receiving feedback demonstrated significantly more medial patellofemoral congruence angle change between pretraining and posttraining periods as assessed with the quadriceps contracted, compared with findings in the group training with terminal knee extension exercises alone. The patellar rotation angle during quadriceps contraction was changed between pretraining and posttraining periods in a more posterior direction for the feedback group compared with findings in the control group. The investigators concluded that the SEMG feedback program produced changes in VMO:VL motor behavior, favoring improved medial patellar tracking and tilt, that were not obtained in the control group or the group receiving only terminal knee exten-

sion exercises. Unfortunately, it cannot be stated with certainty whether results in the group trained with SEMG were derived from the addition of feedback or of other training tasks.

Taken together, results of these reports seem to indicate that SEMG feedback can be used to change the relationship of the VMO to the VL, with potential consequences for patellofemoral function. Carefully controlled investigations with the use of SEMG feedback training with different types of PFPS patients are needed. If, as has been suggested, a key to managing VMO insufficiency is to view the problem as one of faulty motor control rather than as pure weakness, both amplitude and timing measures should be included in experimental designs. Analysis of SEMG frequency data and large numbers of task repetitions may also be useful during assessment. Functional outcomes measurement and comparison of SEMG training to other therapies, as well as combination approaches, would be helpful to determine optimal training programs.

Limitations of SEMG Methods

Thus far, the use of VMO and VL recordings to gauge dynamic medial and lateral control of the patella has been described. Throughout the chapter, limitations of SEMG techniques as a potential source of conflict in the literature have been alluded to. The discussion will now focus on bringing together and amplifying some of those points. SEMG electrodes record the algebraic sum of muscle action potential voltages from their pick-up zones.[1] This approach neglects passive patellar restraints. Therefore the extent to which SEMG methods characterize resultant forces acting on the patella must be incomplete. To be meaningful, SEMG findings must be interpreted within the context of a complete history and relevant clinical tests.

SEMG recordings from specific portions of the quadriceps muscle may be vulnerable to signal cross-talk from nontargeted areas of the quadriceps and adjacent muscles. Cross-talk is influenced by muscle bulk dimensions, proximity to co-activated muscles, intervening tissue conductances between the skin and the target muscle as well as between co-activated muscles, electrode location, size and spacing, and other aspects of the recording and processing set-up.[1,128,129] Recordings of VL activity may be contaminated by activity from the adjacent bulk of the vastus intermedius, rectus femoris, and hamstrings during knee extension.[105] Because of the proximity of the adductor bulk and potential co-activation of the VMO and hip adductors, surface recordings of VMO activity may be subjected to signal contamination from the adductor muscles. This factor has gone uncontrolled in some studies during which the hip adductors might have been active in stabilizing weight-bearing limbs. No studies have been identified in which intramuscular recordings, which are far less susceptible to cross-talk, are compared directly with surface recordings specifically for the VMO. It is somewhat reassuring that in the existing body of literature results obtained with intramuscular electrodes are broadly consistent with findings with surface recordings under similar testing circumstances.

Although a linear or near-linear relationship between percentage of maximal SEMG activity and force output has been demonstrated under isometric nonfatiguing conditions for many muscles, the relationship may be influenced by sarcomere resting length, contraction velocity, proportionate amounts and geometric distributions of type I and II fibers, angle of insertion, fatigue, and neurophysiologic mechanisms. (See Chapter 3 in the companion book.)[130] How these factors specifically influence VMO versus VL activity detected by SEMG and their respective contributions to patellar stabilization is unknown. Investigators have advised caution in interpreting SEMG data with respect to VMO and VL functions, noting differences in muscle cross-sectional area, angle of fiber insertion, and morphologic characteristics.[115] The relationship between SEMG and force may be different for VMO and VL, and may be differentially affected by changes in contraction type, velocity, and intensity.

Because of the previously discussed issues and differences in electrical conductance,

SEMG data should be normalized in some fashion before multisite or across-subject comparison. For example, different thicknesses of subcutaneous adipose tissue and skin impedances across subjects would differentially suppress the magnitude and frequency content of each subject's surface electrical signal.[1] Within subjects, the fascia overlying the VL is approximately twice as thick as that overlying the VMO.[57] Other things being equal, this would tend to attenuate VL activity to a greater extent than VMO activity for surface recordings. Any type of normalization procedure, however, has its limitations. As was stated earlier, problems here can confound interpretation of SEMG studies of the VM and VMO in relation to the VL.[82,97]

In discussing SEMG studies of movement, it has been assumed that factors that enhance recruitment of the VMO relative to the VL lead to lasting changes in VMO:VL function if repeated in a training regimen. This may be a reasonable postulate,[68] but in much of the work to date no attempt has been made to monitor subjects over time. Caution must be used in extrapolating results of these experimental designs to patient training programs that target lasting gains in strength, motor skill, and functional activity performance.

Some clinical SEMG devices incorporate a frequency bandwidth filter with a low bandpass cutoff at 100 Hz. It is suggested that investigation of quadriceps SEMG activity be performed with equipment that has a low cutoff of about 20 to 25 Hz and that devices with a low cutoff of 100 Hz not be used. The frequency spectrum of the SEMG signal typically includes a great deal of activity below 100 Hz. Thus with a progressive left shift in power density plots during fatigue,[1] it is vitally important that bandwidth filters pass the appropriate range of frequencies during clinical work. Research findings have been reported on VMO:VL activity detected by SEMG devices with a bandpass low cutoff of 100 Hz. The magnitude of effect, if any, is unknown.

SEMG assessment and feedback training for PFPS should be performed with units that have dual channel capacity or greater. Although single channel SEMG units are less expensive and easy to operate, there is no way to monitor directly the balance of VMO and VL activities. In general, VM and VMO activity tends to parallel that of the other quadriceps components. Increased or decreased activity from a single VMO recording site does not imply that anything meaningful has happened in terms of VMO:VL balance, and selective gains in VMO function should not be assumed.[77,112]

Finally, it is recommended that SEMG feedback training to change the timing of muscle activity be executed with sampling rates of 100 Hz or faster, line tracing visual displays, and minimal display smoothing. Systems with high temporal resolution and offline software analysis are required to assess onset timing precisely. Karst and Willet[96] have emphasized that many handheld SEMG devices are wholly inadequate to detect subtle timing parameters. Thus clinicians working in the temporal domain should expect to purchase more sophisticated equipment and be able to detect only gross changes through a range of motion arc.

CONCLUSION

Knee extension is accompanied by a tendency to displace the patella laterally, which is dynamically opposed by the VMO. Imbalance of active and passive factors acting on the patella can lead to faulty compressive loading, cumulative trauma, and PFPS. It is likely that not all patients with PFPS have VMO insufficiency as a primary cause. The literature suggests substantial intersubject variability in terms of structural alignment and passive flexibility, quadriceps recruitment, and successful training regimens. Intramuscular as well as surface EMG have been used successfully in kinesiologic studies of the quadriceps as a unit and the actions of its component parts. The SEMG activity of the VMO has been qualified and quantified relative to that of the VL. Analysis of SEMG activity has been used to distinguish PFPS patients from healthy control subjects. Additional study is required to discern assessment procedures with optimal sensitivity and specificity. No open chain exercise has been shown conclusively to facilitate the VMO in a selective manner. There have been favorable outcomes with knee extension and hip adduction maneuvers in the closed chain. SEMG feedback training has been used successfully to train the quadriceps in general and the VMO relative to the VL in particular. Training with SEMG feedback should be performed in patients with identifiable SEMG deficits, as opposed to applying a blanket PFPS protocol to all. Feedback training ought to be regarded as an adjunctive component of a comprehensive rehabilitation program.

REFERENCES

1. Basmajian JV, De Luca CJ. *Muscles Alive: Their Functions Revealed by Electromyography*. Baltimore, MD: Williams & Wilkins; 1985.

2. Puniello MS. Iliotibial band tightness and medial patellar glide in patients with patellofemoral dysfunction. *J Orthop Sports Phys Ther*. 1993;17:144–148.

3. Arnocyzky SP. Anatomy of the anterior cruciate ligament. *Clin Orthop*. 1983;172:19–25.

4. Kapandji IA. *The Physiology of the Joints, Vol 2 Lower Limb*. Edinburgh, Scotland: Churchill Livingstone; 1970.

5. O'Donoghue D. Treatment of acute ligamentous injuries to the knee. *Orthop Clin North Am*. 1973;4:617–624.

6. O'Donoghue D. Surgical treatment of injuries to the knee. *Clin Orthop*. 1960;18:11–17.

7. Feagan J, Abbott H. The isolated tear of the anterior cruciate ligament. *J Bone Joint Surg Am*. 1972;54:1340–1347.

8. Losse GM. Anterior cruciate ligament injuries in downhill skiing: evaluation, surgical treatment, and rehabilitation. *Top Acute Care Trauma Rehabil*. 1988;3:41–72.

9. McMaster J, Weinert C, Scranton P. Diagnosis and management of isolated anterior cruciate ligament tears. *J Trauma*. 1974;14:230–242.

10. Pickett J, Altizer T. Injuries to the ligaments of the knee. *Clin Orthop*. 1971;76:27–34.

11. Wang JB, Rubin RM, Marshall JL. A mechanism of isolated anterior cruciate ligament rupture. *J Bone Joint Surg Am.* 1975;57:411–413.

12. Branch TP, Hunter R, Donath M. Dynamic EMG analysis of anterior cruciate deficient legs with and without bracing during cutting. *Am J Sports Med.* 1989;17:35–41.

13. Ciccotti MG, Kerlan RK, Perry J, Pink M. An electromyographic analysis of the knee during functional activities, II: the anterior cruciate ligament-deficient and -reconstructed profiles. *Am J Sports Med.* 1994;22:651–658.

14. Tibone, JE, Antich TJ, Fanton GS, Moynes DR, Perry J. Functional analysis of anterior cruciate ligament instability. *Am J Sports Med.* 1986;14:276–283.

15. Sinkjaer T, Arendt-Nielsen L. Knee stability and muscle coordination in patients with anterior cruciate ligament injuries: an electromyographic approach. *J Electromyogr Kinesiol.* 1991;1:209–217.

16. Seto JL, Brewster CE, Lombardo SJ, Tibone JE. Rehabilitation of the knee after anterior cruciate ligament reconstruction. *J Orthop Sports Phys Ther.* 1989;11:8–18.

17. Baratta R, Solomonow M, Zhoue BH, Letson E, Chuinard R, D'Ambrosia R. Muscular coactivation: the role of the antagonist musculature in maintaining knee joint stability. *Am J Sports Med.* 1988;16:113–122.

18. Draganich LF, Jaeger RJ, Krajl AR. Coactivation of the hamstrings and quadriceps during extension of the knee. *J Bone Joint Surg Am.* 1989;71:1071–1081.

19. Kain CC, McCarthy JA, Arms SW, et al. An in vivo analysis of the effect of transcutaneous electrical stimulation of the quadriceps and hamstring on anterior cruciate ligament deformation. *Am J Sports Med.* 1988;16:147–152.

20. Renstrom P, Arms SW, Stanwyck TS, Johnson RJ, Pope MH. Strain within the anterior cruciate ligament during hamstring and quadriceps activity. *Am J Sports Med.* 1986;14:83–87.

21. Gryzlo SM, Patek RM, Pink M, Parry J. Electromyographic analysis of knee rehabilitation exercises. *J Orthop Sports Phys Ther.* 1994;20:36–43.

22. Draper V. Electromyographic biofeedback and recovery of quadriceps femoris muscle function following anterior cruciate ligament reconstruction. *Phys Ther.* 1990;9:11–17.

23. Draper B, Ballard L. Electrical stimulation versus electromyographic biofeedback in the recovery of quadriceps femoris muscle function following anterior cruciate ligament surgery. *Phys Ther.* 1991;71:455–463.

24. Snyder-Mackler L. Commentary. *Phys Ther.* 1991;71:461–463.

25. de Andre J, Grant C, Dixon A. Joint distension and reflex inhibition in the knee. *J Bone Joint Surg Am.* 1965;47:313–322.

26. Fahrer H, Rentsch HU, Gerber NJ, Beyeler CH, Heiss CW, Grunig B. Knee effusion and reflex inhibition of the quadriceps. *J Bone Joint Surg Br.* 1988;70:635–638.

27. Spencer J, Hayes K, Alexander I. Knee joint effusion and quadriceps reflex inhibition in man. *Arch Phys Med Rehabil.* 1984;65:171–177.

28. Stokes M, Young A. The contribution of reflex inhibition to arthrogenous muscle weakness. *Clin Sci.* 1984;67:7–14.

29. Stratford P. Electromyography of the quadriceps femoris muscles in subjects with normal knees and acutely effused knees. *Phys Ther.* 1981;62:279–283.

30. Wood L, Ferrell WR, Baxendale RH. Pressures in normal and acutely distended human knee joints and effects on quadriceps maximal voluntary contractions. *Q J Exp Physiol.* 1988;73:305–314.

31. Santavirta S. Integrated electromyography of the vastus medialis muscle after meniscectomy. *Am J Sports Med.* 1979;7:40–42.

32. Shakespeare DT, Stokes M, Sherman KP, Young A. Reflex inhibition of the quadriceps after meniscectomy: lack of association with pain. *Clin Physiol.* 1985; 5:137–144.

33. Shakespeare DT, Stokes M, Sherman KP, Young A. The effect of knee flexion on quadriceps inhibition after meniscectomy. *Clin Sci.* 1983;65:64–65.

34. Young A, Stokes M, Shakespeare DT, Sherman KP. The effect of intra-articular bupivicaine on quadriceps inhibition after meniscectomy. *Med Sci Sports Exerc.* 1983;15:154–159.

35. Sprenger CK, Carlson K, Wessman HC. Application of electromyographic biofeedback following medial meniscectomy. *Phys Ther.* 1979;59:167–169.

36. Hanten WP, Schulties SS. Exercise effects on electromyographic activity of the vastus medialis oblique and vastus lateralis muscles. *Phys Ther.* 1990;70:561–565.

37. Shelton GL, Thigpen LK. Rehabilitation of patellofemoral dysfunction; a review of literature. *J Orthop Sports Phys Ther.* 1991;14:243–249.

38. Insall J. Chondromalacia patellae: patellar malalignment syndrome. *Orthop Clin North Am.* 1979;10:117–124.

39. Chesworth BM, Culham EG, Tata GE, Peat M. Validation of outcome measures in patients with patellofemoral syndrome. *J Orthop Sports Phys Ther.* 1989;11:302–308.

40. DeHaven KE, Lintner DM. Athletic injuries: comparison by age, sport, and gender. *Am J Sports Med.* 1986;14:218–224.

41. Fox TA. Dysplasia of the quadriceps mechanism: hypoplasia of the vastus medialis muscle as related to the hypermobile patella syndrome. *Surg Clin North Am.* 1975;55:199–226.

42. Kannus P, Aho H, Jarvinen M, Niittymaki S. Computerized recording of visits to an outpatient sports clinic. *Am J Sports Med.* 1987;15:79–85.

43. Horton MG, Hall TL. Quadriceps femoris muscle angle: normal values and relationships with gender and selected skeletal measures. *Phys Ther.* 1989;69:897–901.

44. Messier SP, Davis SE, Curl WW, Lowert RB, Pack RJ. Etiologic factors associated with patellofemoral pain in runners. *Med Sci Sports Exerc.* 1991;23:1008–1015.

45. Woodall W, Welsh J. A biomechanical basis for rehabilitation programs involving the patellofemoral joint. *J Orthop Sports Phys Ther.* 1990;11:535–542.

46. Buchbinder R, Naporo N, Rizzo E. The relationship of abnormal pronation to chondromalacia patellae in distance runners. *J Am Podiatr Assoc.* 1979;69:159–161.

47. Hungerford DS. Patellar subluxation and excessive lateral pressure as a cause of fibrillation. In: Pickett JC, Radin EL, eds. *Chondromalacia of the Patella.* Baltimore: Williams & Wilkins, 1983;24–42.

48. Walker HL, Schreck RC. Relationship of hyperextended gait pattern to chondromalacia patellae. *Phys Ther.* 1975;55:259–262.

49. Grana W, Kriegshauser L. Scientific basis of extensor mechanism disorders. *Clin Sports Med.* 1985;4:247–258.

50. McNichol K. Iliotibial tract friction syndrome in athletes. *Can J Appl Sports Sci.* 1981;6:76–80.

51. Noble C. Iliotibial band friction syndrome in runners. *Am J Sports Med.* 1980;8:232–234.

52. Henry J. Conservative treatment of patellofemoral subluxation. *Clin Sports Med.* 1989;8:261–277.

53. Hughston JC, Walsh WM, Puddu G. *Patellar Subluxation and Dislocation.* Philadelphia: WB Saunders Co; 1984.

54. Fulkerson JP, Tennant R, Jaivin JS, Grunnet M. Histologic evidence of retinacular nerve injury associated with patellofemoral malalignment. *Clin Orthop.* 1985;197:196–205.

55. Fulkerson J, Hungerford D. *Disorders of the Patellofemoral Joint.* 2nd ed. Baltimore, MD: Williams & Wilkins; 1990.

56. Maquet PGJ. *Biomechanics of the Knee.* New York: Springer-Verlag; 1984.

57. Lieb FJ, Perry J. Quadriceps function: an anatomical and mechanical study using amputated limbs. *J Bone Joint Surg Am.* 1968;50:1535–1548.

58. Bose K, Kanagasuntheram R, Osman MBH. Vastus medialis oblique: an anatomic and physiologic study. *Orthopedics.* 1980;3:880–883.

59. Reilly D, Martens M. Experimental analyses of the quadriceps muscle force and patellofemoral joint reaction force for various activities. *Acta Orthop Scand.* 1972;43:126–137.

60. Goodfellow J, Hungerford D, Zindel M. Patellofemoral joint mechanics and pathology, part 1, part 2. *J Bone Joint Surg Br.* 1976;58:287–299.

61. Huberti HH, Hayes WC. Patellofemoral contact pressures. *J Bone Joint Surg Am.* 1984;66:715–724.

62. Matthews LS, Sonstegard DA, Henke JA. Load bearing characteristics of the patellofemoral joint. *Acta Orthop Scand.* 1977;48:511–521.

63. Minns RJ, Birnie AJM, Abernethy PJ. A stress analysis of the patella and how it relates to patellar articular cartilage lesions. *J Biomech.* 1979;12:699–711.

64. Lieb FJ, Perry J. Quadriceps function: an electromyographic study under isometric conditions. *J Bone Joint Surg Am.* 1971;53:749–758.

65. Signorile JF, Kacisk D, Perry A, et al. The effect of knee and foot position on the electromyographic activity of the superficial quadriceps. *J Orthop Sports Phys Ther.* 1995;22:2–9.

66. Komi PV, Kaneko M, Aura O. EMG activity of the leg extensor muscles with special reference to mechanical efficiency in concentric and eccentric exercise. *Int J Sports Med.* 1987;8S:22–29.

67. Richardson C, Bullock MI. Changes in muscle activity during fast, alternating flexion–extension movements of the knees. *Scand J Rehabil Med.* 1986;18:51–58.

68. Karst GM, Jewett PD. Electromyographic analysis of exercises proposed for differential activation of medial and lateral quadriceps femoris muscle components. *Phys Ther.* 1993;73:286–295.

69. Thiranagama R. Nerve supply of the human vastus medialis muscle. *J Anat.* 1990;170:193–198.

70. Johnson MA, Polgar J, Weightman D, Appleton D. Data on the distribution of fiber types in thirty six human muscles: an autopsy study. *J Neurol Sci.* 1973;18:111–129.

71. Stokes M, Young A. Investigations of quadriceps inhibition: implications for clinical practice. *Physiotherapy.* 1984;70:425–428.

72. Basmajian JV, Harden TP, Regenos EM. Integrated actions of the four heads of the quadriceps femoris: an electromyographic study. *Anat Rec.* 1972;172:15–20.

73. Pocock GS. Electromyographic study of the quadriceps during resistive exercise. *Phys Ther.* 1963;43:422–434.

74. Brownstein BA, Lamb RL, Mangine RE. Quadriceps torque and integrated electromyography. *J Orthop Sports Phys Ther.* 1985;6:309–314.

75. Lange GW, Hintermeister RA, Schlegal T, Dillman CJ, Steadman JR. Electromyographic and kinematic analysis of graded treadmill walking and the implications for knee rehabilitation. *J Orthop Sports Phys Ther.* 1996;23:294–301.

76. Mariano P, Caruso I. An electromyographic investigation of subluxation of the patella. *J Bone Joint Surg Br.* 1979;61:169–171.

77. Moller BN, Jurik AG, Tidemand-Dalc, Krebs B, Aaris K. The quadriceps function in patellofemoral disorder: a radiographic and electromyographic study. *Arch Orthop Trauma Surg*. 1987;106:195–198.

78. Moller BN, Krebs B, Tidemand-Dal C, Krebs B, Aaris K. Isometric contractions in the patellofemoral pain syndrome. *Arch Orthop Trauma Surg*. 1986;105:24–27.

79. Powers CM, Landel R, Perry J. Timing and intensity of vastus muscle activity during functional activities in subjects with and without patellofemoral pain. *Phys Ther*. 1996;76:946–955.

80. Reynolds L, Levin TA, Mederios JM, Adler NS, Hallum A. EMG activity of the vastus medialis oblique and the vastus lateralis in their role in patellar alignment. *Am J Phys Med*. 1983;62:61–70.

81. Wild J, Franklin T, Woods W. Patellar pain and quadriceps rehabilitation: an EMG study. *Am J Sports Med*. 1982;10:12–15.

82. Souza DR, Gross MT. Comparison of vastus medialis oblique: vastus lateralis muscle integrated electromyographic ratios between healthy subjects and patients with patellofemoral pain. *Phys Ther*. 1991;71:310–320.

83. Cuddeford T, Williams AK, Medeiros JM. Electromyographic activity of the vastus medialis oblique and vastus lateralis muscles during selected exercises. *J Orthop Sports Phys Ther*. 1996; 4:10–15.

84. Kasman G, Cram J, Miller D. Electromyographic assessment of the distal vastus medialis and vastus lateralis as a function of contraction intensity. *J Orthop Sports Phys Ther*. 1994;19:72. Abstract.

85. Hodges P, Richardson C. The influence of isometric hip adduction on quadriceps femoris activity. *Scand J Rehabil Med*. 1993;25:57–62.

86. Simoneau GG, Wilk K. Electromyographic activity ratio between the vastus medialis and the vastus lateralis for four exercises. *Phys Ther*. 1993;73:S78.

87. Wilk KE, Simoneau G, McGraw J. The electromyographic activity of the quadriceps femoris vastus medialis/lateralis ratio during knee bend squats, knee extensions, and leg press exercises. *Phys Ther*. 1993;73:S80.

88. Boucher JP, King MA, Lefebvre R, Pepin A. Quadriceps femoris muscle activity in patellofemoral pain syndrome. *Am J Sports Med*. 1992;20:527–532.

89. Sczepanski TL, Gross MT, Duncan PW, Chandler JM. Effect of contraction type, angular velocity, and arc of motion on VMO:VL EMG ratio. *J Orthop Sports Phys Ther*. 1991;14:256–262.

90. Cerny K. Vastus medialis oblique/vastus lateralis muscle activity ratios for selected exercises in persons with and without patellofemoral pain syndrome. *Phys Ther*. 1995;75:672–683.

91. Doxey GE, Eisenman P. The influence of patellofemoral pain on electromyographic activity during submaximal isometric contractions. *J Orthop Sports Phys Ther*. 1987;9:211–216.

92. Grabiner MD, Koh TJ, Andrish JT. Decreased excitation of vastus medialis oblique and vastus lateralis in patellofemoral pain. *Eur J Exp Musculoskel Res*. 1992;1:33–39.

93. Petschnig R, Baron R, Engel A, Chomiak J, Ammer K. Objectivation of the effects of knee problems on vastus medialis and vastus lateralis with EMG and dynamometry. *PMR*. 1991;2:50–54.

94. Voight ML, Wieder DL. Comparative reflex response times of vastus medialis obliques and vastus lateralis in normal subjects and subjects with extensor mechanism dysfunction: an electromyographic study. *Am J Sports Med*. 1991;19:131–137.

95. Witvrouw E, Sneyers C, Lysens R, Victor J, Bellemans J. Reflex response time of vastus medialis oblique and vastus lateralis in normal subjects and in subjects with patellofemoral pain syndrome. *J Orthop Sports Phys Ther*. 1996;24:160–165.

96. Karst GM, Willet GM. Onset timing of electromyographic activity in the vastus medialis oblique and vastus lateralis muscles in subjects with and without patellofemoral pain syndrome. *Phys Ther*. 1995; 75:813–823.

97. MacIntyre DL, Robertson DG. Quadriceps muscle activity in women runners with and without patellofemoral pain syndrome. *Arch Phys Med Rehabil*. 1992;73:10–14.

98. Wise HH, Fiebert IM, Kates J. EMG biofeedback as treatment for patellofemoral pain syndrome. *J Orthop Sports Phys Ther*. 1984;6:95–103.

99. Kannus P, Niittymaki S. Which factors predict outcome in the nonoperative treatment of patellofemoral pain syndrome? A prospective follow-up study. *Med Sci Sports Exerc*. 1994;26:289–296.

100. Knutson LM, Soderberg GL, Ballantyne BT, Clarke WR. A study of various normalization procedures for within day electromyographic data. *J Electromyogr Kinesiol*. 1994;4:47–60.

101. Redfern MS. Functional muscle: effects on electromyographic output. In: Doderberg GL, ed. *Selected Topics in Surface Electromyography for Use in the Occupational Setting: Expert Perspectives*. Rockville, MD: US Dept of Health and Human Services; 1991:104–120. National Institute for Occupational Safety and Health publication no. 91-100.

102. McConnell JS. Management of patellofemoral problems. *Manual Ther*. 1996;1:60–66.

103. Perez PL, Gossman MR, Lechner D, Stepenson SX, Katholi C. Electromyographic temporal characteristics of the vastus medialis oblique and the vastus lateralis in

women with and without patellofemoral pain. In: *Proceedings of the World Confederation for Physical Therapy 13th General Meeting, Washington, DC, June 1995.* Alexandria, VA: American Physical Therapy Association; 1995. Paper no. PO-RR-0239-T.

104. Fitzgerald GK, Karst G, Malone T, Wilk K, Rothstein J. Conference. *Phys Ther.* 1997;76:956–966.

105. Grabiner MD, Koh TJ, Miller GF. Fatigue rates of vastus medialis oblique and vastus lateralis during static and dynamic knee extension. *J Orthop Res.* 1991;9:391–397.

106. LeVeau BF, Rogers C. Selective training of the vastus medialis muscle using EMG biofeedback. *Phys Ther.* 1980;60:1410–1415.

107. Tepperman PS, Mazliah J, Naumann S, Delmore T. Effect of ankle position on isometric quadriceps strengthening. *Am J Phys Med.* 1986;65:69–74.

108. Wheatley MD, Jahnke WD. Electromyographic study of the superficial thigh and hip muscles in normal individuals. *Arch Phys Med Rehabil.* 1951;32:508–515.

109. Skurja M, Perry J, Gronley J, et al. Quadriceps action in straight leg raise versus isolated knee extension. *Phys Ther.* 1980;60:582.

110. Soderberg GL, Cook TM. An electromyographic analysis of quadriceps femoris muscle setting and straight leg raising. *Phys Ther.* 1983;63:1434–1438.

111. Soderberg GL, Duesterhaus Minor S, Arnold K, et al. Electromyographic analysis of knee exercise in healthy subjects and in patients with knee pathologies. *Phys Ther.* 1987;67:1691–1696.

112. Ingersoll C, Knight K. Patellar location changes following EMG biofeedback or progressive resistance exercises. *Med Sci Sports Med.* 1991;23:1122–1127.

113. Knight KL, Martin JA, Londeree BR. EMG comparison of quadriceps femoris activity during knee extension and straight leg raises. *Am J Phys Med.* 1979;58:57–69.

114. Montgomery JB, Steadman JR. Rehabilitation of the injured knee. *Clin Sports Med.* 1985;4:333–343.

115. Grabiner MD, Koh TJ, Draganich LF. Neuromechanics of the patellofemoral joint. *Med Sci Sports Exerc.* 1994;26:10–21.

116. Stiene HA, Brosky T, Reinking MF, Nyland J, Mason MB. A comparison of closed kinetic chain and isokinetic joint isolation exercise in patients with patellofemoral dysfunction. *J Orthop Sports Phys Ther.* 1996;24:136–141.

117. McConnell JS. The management of chondromalacia patellae: a long term solution. *Austr J Physiother.* 1986;32:215–223.

118. McConnell JS. Training the vastus medialis oblique in the management of patellofemoral pain. *Proceedings of the Tenth International Conference of the WCPT, Sydney, Australia, May 1987.*

119. Duarte Cintra AI, Furlani J. Electromyographic study of quadriceps femoris in man. *Electromyogr Clin Neurophysiol.* 1981;21:539–554.

120. Yamashita N. EMG activities in mono and bi-articular thigh muscles in combined hip and knee extension. *Eur J Appl Physiol.* 1988;58:274–277.

121. Grabiner MD, Koh TJ, Von Haffen L. Effect of concomitant hip joint adduction and knee joint extension forces on quadriceps activation. *Eur J Exp Musculoskel Res.* 1992;1:155–160.

122. Andriacchi TP, Andersson GBJ, Ortengren R, Mikosz RP. A study of factors influencing muscle activity about the knee joint. *J Orthop Res.* 1984;1:266–275.

123. Sale D. Neural adaptation to strength training. In: Komi PV, ed. *Strength and Power in Sport.* Oxford, England: Blackwell Scientific Publications; 1992;249–265.

124. King AC, Ahles TA, Martin JE, White R. EMG biofeedback-controlled exercise in chronic arthritic knee pain. *Arch Phys Med Rehabil.* 1984;65:341–343.

125. Lucca JA, Recchiuti SJ. Effect of electromyographic biofeedback on an isometric strengthening program. *Phys Ther.* 1983;63:200–203.

126. Bohannon RW. Effects of electrical stimulation to the vastus medialis muscle in a patient with chronically dislocating patellae. *Phys Ther.* 1983;63:1445–1447.

127. Kasman G. Use of integrated electromyography for the assessment and treatment of musculoskeletal pain: guidelines for physical medicine practitioners. In: Cram JR, ed. *Clinical EMG for Surface Recordings.* Vol 2. Nevada City, CA: Clinical Resources; 1990:255–302.

128. De Luca CJ, Merletti R. Surface myoelectric signal cross-talk among muscles of the leg. *Electroencephalogr Clin Neurophysiol.* 1988;69:568–575.

129. Winter DA, Fuglevand AJ, Archer SE. Crosstalk in surface electromyography: theoretical and practical estimates. *J Electromyogr Kinesiol.* 1994;4:15–26.

130. Cram JR, Kasman GS. *Introduction to Surface Electromyography.* Gaithersburg, MD: Aspen Publishers; 1997.

SEMG Program for General Knee Rehabilitation

Refer to the discussion in Chapter 14 for a review of intervention approaches. The suggestions that follow are derived from those resources. Descriptions and operational definitions are provided to clarify optional practice patterns.

CANDIDATES

Implement for patients with
- apparent quadriceps weakness who are lagging in functional recovery relative to an expected clinical pathway. Quadriceps dysfunction may be of posttraumatic or postsurgical origin.
- functional limitation due to instability after ACL injury.

EVALUATION OBJECTIVES

- Identify poorly recruited quadriceps function.
- Identify potential lower extremity compensatory patterns for patients with ACL deficiencies.

FEEDBACK TRAINING OBJECTIVES

- Increase magnitude of quadriceps recruitment.
- In patients with ACL deficiencies increase hamstring/quadriceps co-activation or increase magnitude/duration of gastrocnemius, tibialis anterior recruitment during gait.

- Resolve mechanical dysfunction and pain.
- Retain and generalize improved motor control to functional contexts.
- Resolve or reduce functional limitations and disability.

RECORDING SITES

- Judge utility of each recording site on the basis of history and physical examination results.
- Consult Chapter 14 in the companion book, *Introduction to Surface Electromyography*, for specific electrode placement considerations.
- Confirm optimal sites from the following list by observation and palpation during isometric contraction:
  1. general quadriceps:
     - rectus femoris
     - VM
     - VL
  2. medial gastrocnemius
  3. lateral hamstrings
  4. medial hamstrings
  5. tibialis anterior

EVALUATION PROCEDURES

- Select procedures that correspond to findings of pain, weakness, or instability revealed by history and clinical examination.
- Refer to Chapter 2 for detailed discussion of evaluation methods.

- Perform at least five repetitions of each movement task to assess SEMG response consistency.
- Select relevant procedures from the following:
  1. seated maximal and submaximal isometric contractions. Use these contractions as a baseline for comparison with other test activities.
  2. seated full or partial arc active range of motion (AROM)
  3. seated AROM against progressively increased loads at approximately constant velocity
  4. seated AROM with fixed load at progressively greater velocities
  5. closed kinetic chain tasks:
     –Place a standard bathroom scale under each of the patient's feet to ensure equal weight bearing.
     –Examine both concentric and eccentric movement phases.
     –Include bilateral partial squat, unilateral squat, lunge, step-up, step-down as indicated.
  6. functional activity analysis of work, home, sports-specific activities
  7. repeated tests with positive findings after application of an indicated orthotic appliance

ASSESSMENT

- Refer to Chapter 2 for detailed discussion of SEMG assessment.
- Refer to Chapter 14 in the companion book for representative SEMG tracings of normal function.
- Select SEMG assessment parameters from the following:
  1. Amplitude, variance, recruitment slope, decruitment slope during contraction effort. SEMG activity should be stable and quiescent before command to contract. Recruitment and decruitment should be prompt and smooth.
  2. Left/right peak amplitude symmetry for symmetric movements. Satisfactory symmetry is operationally defined as left/right scores within 35% as calculated [(higher value – lower value)/higher value] × 100. Symmetry assessment assumes an equivalent left/right AROM excursion, velocity, and extrinsic load.
  3. Relationship of salient SEMG events to particular range of motion arcs. Observe for consistent magnitude elevations or depressions during a painful portion of the AROM arc.
  4. Proportionate lower extremity SEMG patterns across muscle sites that are symmetric from left to right. For comparisons across recording sites, magnitudes may be expressed as:
     –percentage of MVIC amplitude by using standard manual muscle tests (test activity amplitude/MVIC amplitude × 100)
     –percentage of some standardized submaximal contraction. Normalized quadriceps:hamstring or quadriceps:gastrocnemius ratios can then be constructed if desired.
  5. Symmetric left/right timing relationships among lower extremity muscles (ie, quadriceps, hamstring, gastrocnemius, tibialis anterior). When comparing the timing symmetry of synergist action, observe for changes in the recruitment order of muscles from one side to the other. For most clinical purposes, timing issues can be observed with rectified line tracings with a smoothing time constant of 0.1 second or less, SEMG sampling at 100 Hz or faster, frequency bandwidth filter low cutoff of 25 Hz or less, and a high resolution display with variable sweep speed. A graphic printout is useful for documentation of subtle timing differences. Documentation can be quantified with calculations of average slope, time to peak activity, or time to some percentage of MVIC activity that is clinically meaningful. Onset time can be reported simply as the latency to achieve a micro-

volt value equivalent to two standard deviations above the baseline mean. Duration may be noted as the amount of time between onset and baseline recovery (amplitude recovery within two standard deviations of the baseline mean).

6. Change in activity levels for a particular muscle and task across treatment sessions. To document this parameter a normalization procedure is preferred. A reliable maximal manual muscle test effort or a standardized submaximal contraction is required as a reference. For example, seated knee 45-degree isometric hold of a cuff weight (equal to 5% of body weight) applied to the ankle can be used for the quadriceps. The average amplitude during a functional task is divided by that day's reference contraction amplitude, and the quotient is multiplied by 100.

COMMON PATIENT PRESENTATIONS

Posttraumatic/Postsurgical Quadriceps Weakness

Some patients show persistent quadriceps weakness after immobilization for fracture or total knee replacement, ACL repair, and other surgical procedures. Weakness may be caused by a combination of neurophysiologic quadriceps inhibition and muscle atrophy. SEMG activity is characterized by quadriceps hypoactivity on the involved side, compared with findings on the uninvolved side. Hamstring activity may also be imbalanced with that of the quadriceps. Imbalance can be documented by either quadriceps hypoactivity in conjunction with hamstring hyperactivity on the involved side (each side expressed as a left/right percent difference) or a depressed normalized quadriceps: hamstring ratio on the involved side. Training focuses on quadriceps uptraining. Additional suggestions are provided below for patients who demonstrate inappropriate hamstring guarding, or who have ACL deficiencies.

Training Progression for Posttraumatic/Postsurgical Quadriceps Weakness

- Refer to Chapters 3 and 4 for detailed discussion of SEMG display setups and feedback structure.
- Refer to Chapters 5 and 6 for detailed discussion of SEMG feedback training techniques.
- As skill develops, generally
  1. Shape desired responses up or down.
  2. Incorporate multijoint control.
  3. Add distractions.
  4. Randomize training activities.
  5. Withdraw continuous audio/visual feedback.
- Select SEMG feedback training tasks from the following:
  1. isolation of target muscle activity. Use quadriceps setting or seated active knee extension to orient the patient to quadriceps function and the feedback display.
  2. threshold-based uptraining. Continue with maximal effort quadriceps setting at various joint angles.
  3. therapeutic exercises with SEMG feedback/generalization to progressively dynamic movement. For each training task, progress as appropriate from
     –small to large movement arcs
     –slow to fast speed
     –light to heavy resistance
     Select activities relevant to the patient's routine rehabilitation protocol from the following:
     –seated/supine terminal knee extension, full arc knee extension
     –straight leg raising
     –standing quadriceps setting
     –sit-to-stand, stand-to-sit
     –standing in stride, left/right weight shifting
     –involved side unilateral stance
     –taking of one step forward and backward with the involved side, level gait, ramps
     –stationary bike
     –bilateral partial squats

–stair-stepper

–front step-ups/step-downs, lateral step-ups/step-downs

–cross-over and braiding steps, balancing on rocker platforms and rolls

–partial squats in stride, lunge steps, jumping, hopping

4. functional activity performance with SEMG feedback. Use other relevant work and sports-specific activities that require high-intensity or high-velocity quadriceps activity.

5. motor copy training. Use the uninvolved quadriceps as a template for pattern-matching with the involved quadriceps during any of the above-listed tasks.

6. SEMG-triggered NMES. This technique is recommended for quadriceps uptraining if there are no contra-indications or precautions.

• Integrate SEMG feedback training with indicated physical agents, manual therapies, orthoses, and home exercise programs.

• Consider also the potential utility and cost-effectiveness of a home SEMG feedback trainer.

Quadriceps Weakness Combined with Pain and Hamstring Guarding

Pain and decreased extension range of motion can accompany postsurgical quadriceps weakness. Hamstring guarding may be displayed in response to therapist efforts to extend the patient's knee into a painful range. Training combines hamstring relaxation with quadriceps uptraining.

Training Progression for Quadriceps Weakness Combined with Pain and Hamstring Guarding

• Refer to Chapters 3 and 4 for detailed discussion of SEMG display setups and feedback structure.

• Refer to Chapter 5 for detailed discussion of SEMG feedback training techniques.

• As skill develops, generally
  1. Shape desired responses up or down.
  2. Incorporate multijoint control.
  3. Add distractions.
  4. Randomize training activities.
  5. Withdraw continuous audio/visual feedback.

• Select SEMG feedback training tasks from the following:
  1. isolation of target muscle activity. Use gently resisted knee flexion to orient the patient to hamstrings function and the SEMG feedback display.
  2. relaxation-based downtraining. Combine SEMG feedback with
    –verbal cues
    –supported lower extremity positioning.
    –voluntary contraction followed by relaxation.
  3. therapeutic exercises with SEMG feedback.
    –Continue hamstring muscle relaxation during passive stretch.
    –Include SEMG feedback during all routine mobilization procedures for the patient.
  4. implementation of quadriceps uptraining progression described above.

ACL-Related Knee Instability

Insufficient function of the ACL results from traumatic tearing injuries. Patients with ACL insufficiency are unable to stabilize the tibial–femoral joint properly, leading to acute knee dysfunction, progressive degenerative disease, and disability. SEMG feedback training can be used in postsurgical and nonsurgical rehabilitation programs.

Training Progression for ACL-Related Knee Instability

• Refer to Chapters 3 and 4 for detailed discussion of SEMG display setups and feedback structure.

• Refer to Chapter 5 for detailed discussion of SEMG feedback training techniques.

- As skill develops, generally
  1. Shape desired responses up or down.
  2. Incorporate multijoint control.
  3. Add distractions.
  4. Randomize training activities.
  5. Withdraw continuous audio/visual feedback.
- Select SEMG feedback training tasks from the following:

Postsurgical patients with satisfactory ligament repair:

1. Follow preceding uptraining guidelines for quadriceps weakness during the patient's routine exercise and functional activity protocol progression.
2. Consider use of dual channel SEMG feedback from the quadriceps and hamstrings.
3. Follow the patient's routine exercise protocol, training for quadriceps/hamstring co-contraction.
4. Promote deliberate co-activation of the hamstrings during knee extension tasks.

One of the following for nonsurgical patients or postsurgical patients with persistent laxity:

1. Train quadriceps/lateral hamstrings co-contraction.
2. Train quadriceps/gastrocnemius co-contraction. Focus on training increased gastrocnemius SEMG amplitude as well as earlier onset and longer duration timing during lower extremity stance with walking, running, and sport-specific maneuvers.
3. Train increased tibialis anterior activity, especially during cross-cutting or other movements that require rotation on a stance leg.

- Integrate SEMG training with indicated physical agents, manual therapies, orthoses, and home exercise programs.
- Consider the potential utility and cost-effectiveness of a home SEMG feedback trainer.

SUGGESTED READINGS

Ciccotti MG, Kerlan RK, Perry J, Pink M. An electromyographic analysis of the knee during functional activities, II: the anterior cruciate ligament-deficient and -reconstructed profiles. *Am J Sports Med*. 1994;22:651–658.

Draper V. Electromyographic biofeedback and recovery of quadriceps femoris muscle function following anterior cruciate ligament reconstruction. *Phys Ther*. 1990;9:11–17.

Draper B, Ballard L. Electrical stimulation versus electromyographic biofeedback in the recovery of quadriceps femoris muscle function following anterior cruciate ligament surgery. *Phys Ther*. 1991;71:455–463.

Gryzlo SM, Patek RM, Pink M, Parry J. Electromyographic analysis of knee rehabilitation exercises. *J Orthop Sports Phys Ther*. 1994;20:36–43.

Sinkjaer T, Arendt-Nielsen L. Knee stability and muscle coordination in patients with anterior cruciate ligament injuries: an electromyographic approach. *J Electromyogr Kinesiol*. 1991;1:209–217.

SEMG Program for PFPS

Refer to the discussion in Chapter 14 for a review of intervention approaches. The suggestions that follow are derived from those resources. Descriptions and operational definitions are provided to clarify optional practice patterns.

Consult Application Guide 13–A for associated problems with the proximal lower extremity.

CANDIDATES

Implement for patients
- with PFPS with marked quadriceps atrophy, history of subluxation/dislocation, or apparent patellofemoral tracking problems assessed radiographically.
- with PFPS who have not responded to other conservative measures within 4 to 6 weeks.
- who have undergone knee surgery and have secondary PFPS.

EVALUATION OBJECTIVES

- Identify generally depressed quadriceps activity.
- Identify poorly coordinated quadriceps function, specifically decreased or ill-timed VMO recruitment relative to VL.

FEEDBACK TRAINING OBJECTIVES

- Generally increase quadriceps recruitment.

- Restore normal patterns of muscle synergy. Increase magnitude, improve timing of VMO recruitment relative to VL.
- Resolve mechanical dysfunction and pain.
- Retain and generalize improved motor control to functional contexts.
- Resolve or reduce functional limitations and disability.

RECORDING SITES

- Judge utility of each recording site on the basis of history and clinical examination results. Consult Chapter 14 in the companion book, *Introduction to Surface Electromyography*, for specific electrode placement considerations.
- Confirm optimal sites from the following list by observation and palpation during patient's execution of isometric contraction:
  1. VMO
  2. VL
- Consider additional sites, such as the hamstrings, tensor fasciae latae, or gluteals, if PFPS is accompanied by hip muscle weakness or tightness.
- Consult Application Guide 13–A for additional recommendations.

EVALUATION PROCEDURES

- Select procedures that correspond to exacerbating and alleviating factors revealed in the history and clinical examination.

- Refer to Chapter 2 for detailed discussion of evaluation methods.
- Perform at least five repetitions of each task movement to assess response consistency. Many more repetitions may be needed to assess SEMG responses with reproduction of symptoms.
- Select relevant procedures from the following:
  1. seated maximal and submaximal isometric contractions
  2. seated active range of motion (AROM):
     –repeated trials at progressively increased loads
     –repeated trials at progressively greater velocities
  3. closed kinetic chain tasks:
     –Place a standard bathroom scale under each of the patient's feet to ensure equal weight bearing.
     –Examine both concentric and eccentric movement phases.
     –Include bilateral partial squat, unilateral squat, lunge, step-up, step-down.
  4. functional activity analysis of work, home, sports-specific activities that exacerbate symptoms or are performed frequently

ASSESSMENT

- Refer to Chapter 2 for detailed discussion of SEMG assessment.
- Refer to Chapter 14 in the companion book for representative SEMG tracings of normal function.
- Select SEMG assessment parameters from the following:
  1. Amplitude, variance, recruitment slope, decruitment slope of each channel during contraction efforts. SEMG activity should be stable and quiescent before command to contract. Recruitment and decruitment should be prompt and smooth.
  2. Relationship of salient SEMG events to particular range of motion arcs. Observe for consistent magnitude elevations or depressions during a painful portion of the AROM arc.
  3. Left/right peak amplitude symmetry for VMO and VL recordings, respectively. That is, left and right side of each muscle site should function symmetrically. Satisfactory symmetry is operationally defined as left/right scores within 35% as calculated [(higher side value − lower side value)/higher side value] × 100. Symmetry assessment assumes an equivalent left/right AROM excursion, velocity, and extrinsic load. It may be that just VMO activity is depressed on the involved side or that both VMO and VL intensities are altered.
  4. Nonnormalized VMO:VL peak amplitude ratios. Divide the VMO peak amplitude by the VL peak amplitude during a test task to produce an activity ratio. The left side VMO:VL ratio should be approximately symmetric to the right side ratio.
  5. Normalized VMO:VL ratios. Activity from each recording site should be normalized for comparison with a population standard. To construct a normalized VMO:VL ratio, perform the following:
     –Express the activity of each muscle site as a percentage of MVIC amplitude for each respective muscle by using standard manual muscle tests (test activity amplitude/MVIC amplitude × 100). Maximally resisted isometric seated knee extension at about 45 degrees serves well as a reference contraction for VMO and VL conjointly.
     –Divide the normalized VMO percent score by the normalized VL percent score. Normalized VMO:VL activity ratios should approximate 1.0. Values less than 0.6 are potentially aberrant.
  6. VMO:VL timing. Timing analyses require raw or rectified line tracing graph-

ics display with a smoothing time constant of 0.1 second or less, SEMG sampling at 100 Hz or faster, frequency bandwidth filter low cutoff of 25 Hz or less, and a high resolution display with variable sweep speed. A graphic printout is useful for documentation of subtle timing differences. Documentation can be quantified with calculations of average slope, time to peak activity, or time to some percentage of MVIC activity that is clinically meaningful. Onset time can be reported as the latency to achieve a microvolt value equivalent to two standard deviations above the baseline mean. Duration may be noted as the amount of time between onset and baseline recovery (amplitude recovery within two standard deviations of the baseline mean). Assessment tends to be easiest with VMO- and VL-rectified line tracings overlaid in the same field. Expect coincident tracking of VMO and VL display channels from the same limb through an AROM arc. With use of current commercially available SEMG devices, any difference in recruitment, peak, or decruitment timing that is visibly apparent is potentially significant.

COMMON PATIENT PRESENTATIONS

VMO and VL Hypoactivity

Some patients with unilateral PFPS show asymmetrically depressed activity from the involved side VMO and VL during maximal effort contractions (Figure 14–B–1). Submaximal contractions are also accompanied often by nonselective hypoactivity, although this finding may be variable and sometimes reversed. In these patients, however, VMO and VL activity patterns always follow the same course; there is no evidence of a selective change of VMO function. A generalized quadriceps impairment is presumed to contribute to patellofemoral dysfunction. Such a pattern may be most common with pa-

tients who have withdrawn from normal physical activity, or who are recovering strength or mobility after a period of immobilization.

Training Progression for VMO and VL Hypoactivity

These patients tend to progress with a carefully graded exercise program. If desired, SEMG feedback can be combined with exercise for general quadriceps muscle uptraining (see Application Guide 14–A).

VMO:VL Imbalance

Imbalance of the VMO:VL relationship can be characterized with SEMG in several ways. Patients with unilateral complaints may show decreased VMO activity on the involved side with relative left/right symmetry (or a lesser amount of asymmetry) for the VL (see Figures 14–4 through 14–6). This difference can also be represented by an asymmetrically depressed nonnormalized or normalized VMO:VL ratio. Persons with asymmetric SEMG patterns often seem to have asymmetric patterns of lower extremity alignment and flexibility. The involved side may be observed with greater femoral anteversion, hip medial rotation, iliotibial band tightness, Q angle, or foot pronation.

Symmetry assessment with SEMG is less revealing in patients with bilateral PFPS. Moreover, some patients show bilateral deficits in alignment and flexibility, but complain only of unilateral symptoms. Thus SEMG activity in some patients with unilateral PFPS may be similar when recorded from each limb but different from that displayed by healthy subjects. Calculation of normalized VMO:VL activity ratios and comparison with an approximate 1.0 standard is probably the best documentation method currently available in these circumstances. Activity ratios and timing phenomena should be monitored through functional movements. Problematic range of motion arcs and tasks vary across individuals. Patients with recurrent dislocation or marked hypomobility following surgery or

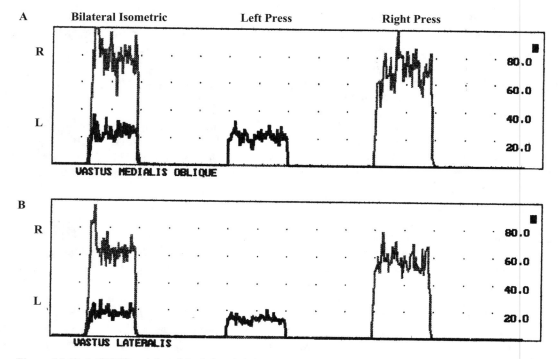

Figure 14–B–1 SEMG activity of the left and right (**A**) vastus medialis oblique and (**B**) vastus lateralis recorded from a postsurgical patient with chronic left PFPS pain syndrome. The first set of peaks corresponds to bilateral maximal effort isometric quadriceps setting with the patient in the supine position. The second and third set of peaks correspond to an equivalent submaximal unilateral leg press task performed on the left and right, respectively. Activity at both recording sites appears proportionately diminished on the left compared with the right.

immobilization tend to show the most aberrant SEMG patterns. However, activity can be altered in patients with subtle disease. In a manner analogous to the assessment of patients with low back or shoulder girdle dysfunction, the potential role of muscular imbalance probably varies in different subpopulations. The clinician should not expect to find evidence of VMO insufficiency in all, or perhaps even most, patients with nonspecific complaints of anterior knee pain. SEMG feedback training is indicated when aberrant muscle activity patterns are substantiated during assessment. Patellofemoral tracking dysfunction and muscle imbalance are then suspected syndrome components. Training focuses on VMO uptraining.

Training Progression for VMO:VL Imbalance

- Refer to Chapters 3 and 4 for detailed discussion of SEMG display setups and feedback structure.
- Refer to Chapters 5 and 6 for detailed discussion of SEMG feedback training techniques.
- As skill develops, generally
  1. Shape greater VMO responses.
  2. Incorporate multijoint control.
  3. Add distractions.
  4. Randomize training activities.
  5. Withdraw continuous audio/visual feedback.

- Select relevant SEMG feedback training tasks from the following:
  1. isolation of target muscle activity:
     –Use seated quadriceps setting and knee extension to demonstrate VMO and VL contributions to knee function. There is no simple maneuver to isolate the VMO from the VL; explain their balancing contribution to control of the patella to the patient.
     –Display both VMO and VL tracings throughout training.
  2. threshold-based uptraining for VMO:
     –Set a threshold for the VMO and one for the VL at levels consistently reached during comfortable, quadriceps setting trials at about 15% to 25% of maximal effort.
     –Instruct the patient to try to increase VMO activity above the VMO threshold and to maintain VL activity below the VL threshold.
     –To free the patient to focus visually on the VMO, use an auditory function as an alarm if VL activity exceeds its threshold. Alternatively, set an auditory reward to sound if the baseline VMO:VL ratio is exceeded.
  3. therapeutic exercises with SEMG feedback. Use the following to facilitate VMO activity:
     –Have the patient perform partial squats combined with hip adductor squeeze by using a semirigid pad between his or her thighs.
     –Consider that with standard commercial electrode configurations and signal processing it is not possible to rule out cross-talk from adductor muscles as contributing to the appearance of increased VMO activity.
     –Experiment with different foot pronation/supination and hip medial/lateral rotation positions during training tasks. Individual responses may be noted, but there are no known suc-

cessful training effects for most persons.
  4. generalization to progressively dynamic movement. For each task, progress VMO:VL training as appropriate from
     –small to large movement arcs
     –slow to fast speed
     –light to heavy resistance
     Select activities that can be performed without exacerbating symptoms:
     –standing quadriceps setting
     –standing in stride, left/right weight shifting
     –involved side unilateral stance
     –taking of one step forward and backward on the involved side, level gait, ramps
     –stationary bike
     –bilateral partial squats
     –sit-to-stand, stand-to-sit
     –stair-stepper
     –front step-ups/step-downs, lateral step-ups/step-downs
     –cross-over and braiding steps, balancing on rocker platforms and rolls
     –partial squats in stride, lunge steps, jumping, hopping, cross-cutting
  5. functional activity performance with SEMG feedback. Use other relevant work and sports-specific activities. Continue training with other movements required to meet the patient's functional activity goals.
  6. motor copy training. Use an uninvolved side VMO as a template for pattern matching with the involved side VMO during any of the above-listed tasks.
  7. SEMG-triggered NMES.
     –Apply this technique to the VMO during any of the above-listed tasks.
     –This procedure is recommended for VMO uptraining if there are no contraindications or precautions (Figure 14–B–2).
     –Set the triggering SEMG threshold so that it is exceeded with the initiation of movement.

A

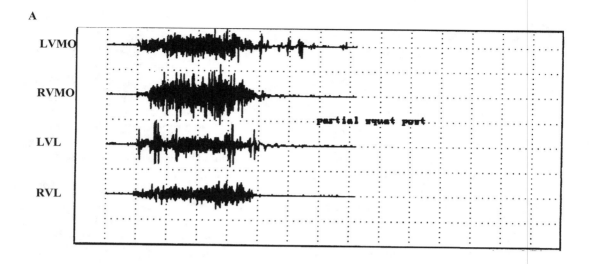

B

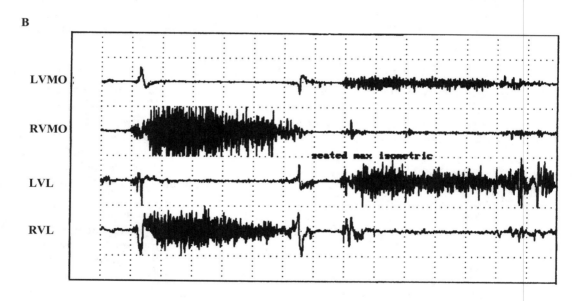

continues

Figure 14–B–2 Effects of SEMG-triggered NMES on SEMG activity of the (**L**) left and (**R**) right (**VMO**) vastus medialis oblique and (**VL**) vastus lateralis. (**A**) Activity from the same patient shown in Figure 14–4, after a 20-minute application of SEMG-NMES. (**B and C**) Activity from a different patient during seated maximal effort isometric quadriceps setting before and after a 20-minute application of SEMG-NMES.

Figure 14–B–2 continued

C

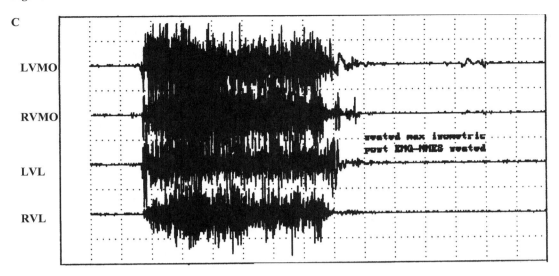

LVMO

RVMO

LVL

RVL

rested max isometric
post EMG-NMES rested

- Integrate SEMG feedback training with indicated physical agents, manual therapies, orthoses, taping techniques, and home exercise programs.

- Consider also the potential utility and costs effectiveness of home SEMG trainer.

SUGGESTED READINGS

Boucher JP, King MA, Lefebvre R, Pepin A. Quadriceps femoris muscle activity in patellofemoral pain syndrome. *Am J Sports Med*. 1992;20:527–532.

Cerny K. Vastus medialis oblique/vastus lateralis muscle activity ratios for selected exercises in persons with and without patellofemoral pain syndrome. *Phys Ther*. 1995;75:672–683.

Cuddeford T, Williams AK, Medeiros JM. Electromyographic activity of the vastus medialis oblique and vastus lateralis muscles during selected exercises. *J Orthop Sports Phys Ther*. 1996;4:10–15.

Fitzgerald GK, Karst G, Malone T, Wilk K, Rothstein J. Conference. *Phys Ther*. 1997;76:956–966.

Hodges P, Richardson C. The influence of isometric hip adduction on quadriceps femoris activity. *Scand J Rehabil Med*. 1993;25:57–62.

Ingersoll C, Knight K. Patellar location changes following EMG biofeedback or progressive resistance exercises. *Med Sci Sports Med*. 1991;23:1122–1127.

Karst GM, Jewett PD. Electromyographic analysis of exercises proposed for differential activation of medial and lateral quadriceps femoris muscle components. *Phys Ther*. 1993;73:286–295.

LeVeau BF, Rogers C. Selective training of the vastus medialis muscle using EMG biofeedback. *Phys Ther*. 1980;60:1410–1415.

Powers CM, Landel R, Perry J. Timing and intensity of vastus muscle activity during functional activities in subjects with and without patellofemoral pain. *Phys Ther*. 1996;76:946–955.

Soderberg GL, Duesterhaus Minor S, Arnold K, et al. Electromyographic analysis of knee exercise in healthy subjects and in patients with knee pathologies. *Phys Ther*. 1987;67:1691–1696.

Souza DR, Gross MT. Comparison of vastus medialis oblique: vastus lateralis muscle integrated electromyographic ratios between healthy subjects and patients with patellofemoral pain. *Phys Ther*. 1991;71:310–320.

Wise HH, Fiebert IM, Kates J. EMG biofeedback as treatment for patellofemoral pain syndrome. *J Orthop Sports Phys Ther*. 1984;6:95–103.

Index